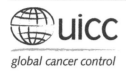

uicc

global cancer control

PROGNOSTIC FACTORS
IN CANCER

THIRD EDITION

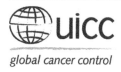

global cancer control

PROGNOSTIC FACTORS IN CANCER

THIRD EDITION

Edited by

Mary K. Gospodarowicz
Brian O'Sullivan
Leslie H. Sobin

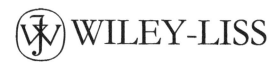

A JOHN WILEY & SONS, INC., PUBLICATION

DISCLAIMER

While the authors, editors, and publisher believe that drug selection and dosage and the specification and usage of equipment and devices, as set forth in this book, are in accord with current recommendations and practice at the time of publication, they accept no legal responsibility for any errors or omissions, and make no warranty, express or implied, with respect to material contained herein. In view of ongoing research, equipment modifications, changes in governmental regulations and the constant flow of information relating to drug therapy, drug reactions, and the use of equipment and devices, the reader is urged to review and evaluate the information provided in the package insert or instructions for each drug, piece of equipment, or device for, among other things, any changes in the instructions or indication of dosage or usage and for added warnings and precautions.

For general information on our other products and services or for technical support, please contact our Customer Care Department within the United States at (800) 762-2974, outside the United States at (317) 572-3993 or fax (317) 572-4002.

Wiley also publishes its books in a variety of electronic formats. Some content that appears in print may not be available in electronic formats. For more information about Wiley products, visit our web site at www.wiley.com.

Library of Congress Cataloging-in-Publication Data

Prognostic factors in cancer / edited by M.K. Gospodarowicz, B.
   O'Sullivan, L.H. Sobin. — 3rd ed.
     p. ; cm.
   Includes bibliographical references and index.
   ISBN-13 978–0–470–03801–7 (pbk.)
   ISBN-10 0–470–03801–2 (pbk.)
   1. Cancer—Prognosis. I. Gospodarowicz, M. K. (Mary K.)
II. O'Sullivan, B. (Brian) III. Sobin, L. H.
   [DNLM: 1. Neoplasms—diagnosis. 2. Prognosis. QZ 241 P964
2006]
   RC262.P688 2006
   616.99'4075—dc22
2005035951

◼◼◼ CONTENTS

v

PREFACE

Medicine is a science of uncertainty and an art of probability,
—*Sir William Osler, 1904*

This monograph is the result of an effort by the International Union Against Cancer (UICC) to study prognostic factors related to cancer. It is an extension of the long-term work on the TNM classification, and the follow-up to the first and second editions of *Prognostic Factors in Cancer* published in 1995 and 2001, respectively. As in previous editions, the anatomic extent of disease and histologic type are the most important indicators of prognosis for cancer patients and provide the main criteria for selection of therapy. However, it is recognized that they may not be sufficient in themselves to provide a powerful prognostic assessment. Many other factors also have a profound impact on the prognosis of cancer patients.

The purpose of the third edition is to consolidate the previously developed framework for the consideration of prognosis and prognostic factors and for the application of prognostic factors to clinical practice for most tumor sites. As in the second edition, the book has two parts. Part A, Principles of Prognostic Factors, deals with the importance of prognosis, principles of documentation of prognosis, and the methodology of studying prognostic factors. New chapters dealing with the role of prognostic factors in population-based cancer control and in terminal care are included. Furthermore, with the explosion of new knowledge of molecular medicine, the impact of new molecular factors is discussed.

Part B, Prognostic Factors in Specific Cancers, includes site or tumor-specific chapters that provide a general overview of the relevant literature on prognostic factors. There are new chapters on gastrointestinal stromal tumors, multiple myeloma, and retinoblastoma, which have been included. The authors were asked to follow the template suggested in Chapter 1.2. Each site-specific chapter has a summary table that classifies the prognostic factors according to subject or topic and relevance. Each chapter was streamlined to include a concise summary of disease presentation and staging, management, prognostic factors, and any relevant treatment controversies.

As in the second edition, within clinical relevance-based classification, we emphasize "essential" prognostic factors that are mandatory to select treatment as prescribed by published evidence- or consensus-based clinical practice guidelines under conditions where access to best standard of care is available. Examples of such guidelines are referenced beneath the prognostic factor grids in each chapter. To facilitate reading, we have also provided a glossary of selected terms used in this book.

We hope that this third edition of *Prognostic Factors in Cancer* will be of value in (1) demonstrating the breadth of this field; (2) stimulating the study of prognostic factors; (3) bringing perspective to those working in this arena; and (4) summarizing the currently accepted prognostic factors for individual tumor sites and types.

ACKNOWLEDGMENTS

The Editors thank the International Union Against Cancer (UICC) for its support and express appreciation to its secretariat for arranging meetings and facilitating communications.

This publication was made possible by grant number U58/CCU923976-02 from the United States Centers for Disease Control and Prevention (CDC). Its contents are the responsibility of the authors and do not necessarily represent the official views of the CDC.

MARY K. GOSPODAROWICZ, *Toronto, Canada*
BRIAN O'SULLIVAN, *Toronto, Canada*
LESLIE H. SOBIN, *Washington, DC*

■ CONTRIBUTORS

EDITORS

Mary K. Gospodarowicz, Professor and Chair, Department of Radiation Oncology, University of Toronto, Princess Margaret Hospital/University Health Network, 610 University Avenue, Toronto, Ontario M5G 2M9 Canada

Brian O'Sullivan, Professor, Department of Radiation Oncology, University of Toronto, Princess Margaret Hospital/University Health Network, 610 University Avenue, Toronto, Ontario M5G 2M9 Canada

Leslie H. Sobin, Professor of Pathology, Uniformed Services University of the Health Sciences, Co-Chair, Department of Hepatic and Gastrointestinal Pathology, Armed Forces Institute of Pathology, 6825 16th Street NW, Washington, DC 20306-6000 USA

ASSOCIATE EDITORS

Douglas G. Altman, Professor of Statistics in Medicine, Centre for Statistics in Medicine, Wolfson College Annexe, Oxford University, Linton Road, Oxford OX2 6UD UK

Frederick L. Greene, Clinical Professor of Surgery, University of North Carolina School of Medicine, Chairman, Department of General Surgery, Carolinas Medical Center, Charlotte, NC 1000 Blythe Blvd., Charlotte, North Carolina 28232 USA

Patti A. Groome, Associate Professor, Department of Community Health and Epidemiology, Queen's Cancer Research Institute, Queen's University, 10 Stuart Street, Kingston, Ontario K7L 3N6 Canada

Christian Wittekind, Professor and Director of the Institute of Pathology, University Clinic of Leipzig, Liebigstrasse 26, D-04103 Leipzig, Germany

Eng-Siew Koh, Clinical Fellow, Department of Radiation Oncology, University of Toronto, Princess Margaret Hospital/University Health Network, 610 University Avenue, Toronto, Ontario M5G 2M9 Canada

ALL AUTHORS

Douglas G. Altman, Professor of Statistics in Medicine, Centre for Statistics in Medicine, Wolfson College Annexe, Oxford University, Linton Road, Oxford OX2 6UD UK

Sylvia L. Asa, Professor, Department of Laboratory Medicine and Pathobiology, University of Toronto, Pathologist-in-Chief, University Health Network and Toronto Medical Laboratories, 610 University Avenue, Suite 4-302, Toronto, Ontario M5G 2M9 Canada

Richard J. Battafarano, Assistant Professor, Division of Cardiothoracic Surgery, Department of Surgery, Washington University School of Medicine, One Barnes-Jewish Plaza, 3108 Queeny Tower, St. Louis, MO 63110 USA

Henrik C. Bauer, Professor of Orthopedic Oncology, Department of Orthopaedics, Karolinska Hospital, SC-17176 Stockholm, Sweden

Trevor W. Beer, Consultant Dermatopathologist, Cutaneous Pathology, 26 Leura St, Nedlands, Western Australia 60109 Australia

Andrea Bezjak, Associate Professor, Department of Radiation Oncology, University of Toronto, Princess Margaret Hospital/University Health Network, 610 University Avenue, Toronto, Ontario M5G 2M9 Canada

Eric Bouffet, Professor of Pediatrics, Division of Haematology/Oncology, University of Toronto, Director of the Pediatric Brain Tumor Program, Hospital for Sick Kids, 555 University Avenue, Toronto, Ontario M5G 1X8 Canada

Jean Bourhis, Professor and Chair, Department of Radiotherapy, Institut Gustave Roussy, 39 rue Camille Desmoulins, Villejuif 94805 France

Michael Brada, Professor of Clinical Oncology, The Institute of Cancer Research and The Royal Marsden NHS Trust, Downs Road, Sutton, Surrey SM2 5PT UK

James D. Brierley, Associate Professor, Department of Radiation Oncology, University of Toronto, Princess Margaret Hospital/University Health Network, 610 University Avenue, Toronto, Ontario M5G 2M9 Canada

Michael D. Brundage, Associate Professor, Department of Oncology, Queen's University, Kingston Regional Cancer Centre, 25 King Street West, Kingston, Ontario, K7L 5P9 Canada

Charles N. Catton, Associate Professor, Department of Radiation Oncology, University of Toronto, Princess Margaret Hospital/University Health Network, 610 University Avenue, Toronto, Ontario M5G 2M9 Canada

Helen S. L. Chan, Professor of Pediatrics, Division of Hematology/Oncology, University of Toronto, Senior Scientist, Division of Cancer Research, Research Institute, Hospital for Sick Kids, 555 University Ave, Toronto, Ontario, M5G 1X8 Canada

Karen K. L. Chan, Assistant Professor, Department of Obstetrics and Gynecology, Queen Mary Hospital, The University of Hong Kong, Queen Mary Hospital Hong Kong, 102 Pokfulam Road, Hong Kong, China

Peter W. Chung, Assistant Professor, Department of Radiation Oncology, University of Toronto, Princess Margaret Hospital/University Health Network, 610 University Avenue, Toronto, Ontario M5G 2M9 Canada

Carolyn C. Compton, Adjunct Professor of Pathology, Johns Hopkins Medical Institute, Director of Biorepositories and Biospecimen Research, National Cancer Institute, Building 31, Suite 10A/31, 31 Center Drive, Bethesda, MD 20892 USA

Juanita M. Crook, Professor, Department of Radiation Oncology, University of Toronto, Princess Margaret Hospital/University Health Network, 610 University Avenue, Toronto, Ontario M5G 2M9 Canada

Michael Crump, Associate Professor, Department of Medical Oncology and Hematology, University of Toronto, Princess Margaret Hospital/University Health Network, 610 University Avenue, Toronto, Ontario M5G 2M9 Canada

Bernard J. Cummings, Professor, Department of Radiation Oncology, University of Toronto, Princess Margaret Hospital/University Health Network, 610 University Avenue, Toronto, Ontario M5G 2M9 Canada

Louis Jean Denis, Professor em. Urology, Vrije Universiteit Brussel, Director of Oncologic Centre Antwerp, Lange Gasthuisstraat 35–37, 2000 Antwerp, Belgium

Patricia Disperati, Translational Research Fellow, Leukemia Program, Princess Margaret Hospital/University Health Network, 610 University Avenue, Toronto, M5G 2M9 Canada

Anthony W. Fyles, Professor, Department of Radiation Oncology, University of Toronto, Princess Margaret Hospital/University Health Network, 610 University Avenue, Toronto, Ontario M5G 2M9 Canada

Brenda L. Gallie, Professor, Departments of Molecular Medical Genetics, Medical Biophysics and Ophthalmology, University of Toronto, Head Retinoblastoma Program/ Hospital for Sick Kids, Ontario Cancer Institute, Princess Margaret Hospital/University Health Network, 610 University Avenue, Toronto M5G 2M9 Canada

Adam S. Garden, Associate Professor, Radiation Oncology, Professor and Section Chief, Head and Neck Radiation Oncology, University of Texas, M.D. Anderson Cancer Center, 1515 Holcombe Blvd., Houston, TX 77030 USA

Paula Ghaneh, Senior Lecturer in Surgery, Division of Surgery and Oncology, University of Liverpool, 5th Floor UCD Building, Daulby Street, Liverpool L69 3GA UK

Christophe Ghysel, Senior Resident, Department of Urology, University Hospital of KU Leuven, UZ Gasthuisberg, Herestraat 49, B-3000 Leuven, Belgium

Paul Glare, Associate Professor, Director of Central Sydney Palliative Care Service, Royal Prince Alfred Hospital, Missenden Road, Camperdown, NSW 2050 Australia

Mary K. Gospodarowicz, Professor and Chair, Department of Radiation Oncology, University of Toronto, Princess Margaret Hospital/University Health Network, 610 University Avenue, Toronto, Ontario M5G 2M9 Canada

Frederick L. Greene, Clinical Professor of Surgery, University of North Carolina School of Medicine, Chairman, Department of General Surgery, Carolinas Medical Center, Charlotte, NC 1000 Blythe Blvd., Charlotte, North Carolina 28232 USA

Patti A. Groome, Associate Professor, Department of Community Health and Epidemiology, Queen's Cancer Research Institute, Queen's University, 10 Stuart Street, Kingston, Ontario K7L 3N6 Canada

Norma C. Gutiérrez, Consultant Physician in Hematology, Servicio de Hematología, Hospital Universitario de Salamanca, Paseo de San Vicente, 58, 37007 Salamanca, Spain

Neville F. Hacker, Professor of Gynaecological Oncology, University of New South Wales, Director, Gynaecological Cancer Centre, Royal Hospital for Women, Barker Street, Randwick 2031 Australia

Ian Harley, Clinical Fellow, Division of Gynecologic Oncology, Department of Obstetrics and Gynecology, University of Toronto, Princess Margaret Hospital/ University Health Network, 610 University Avenue, Toronto, Ontario M5G 2M9 Canada

Jan Hauspy, Clinical Fellow, Division of Gynecologic Oncology, Department of Obstetrics and Gynecology, University of Toronto, Princess Margaret Hospital/ University Health Network, 610 University Avenue, Toronto, Ontario M5G 2M9 Canada

Daniel F. Hayes, Professor, Clinical Director, Breast Oncology Program, University of Michigan Comprehensive Cancer Center, 6312 Cancer Center, 1500 E. Medical Center Drive, Ann Arbor MI 48109-0942 USA

Peter J. Heenan, Clinical Associate Professor, Visiting Research Fellow, Department of Pathology, University of Western Australia, Consultant Dermatopathologist, Queen Elizabeth II Medical Centre, 26 Leura St., Nedlands, Western Australia 6009 Australia

Fernanda G. Herrera, Clinical Fellow, Department of Radiation Oncology, University of Toronto, Princess Margaret Hospital/University Health Network, 610 University Avenue, Toronto, Ontario M5G 2M9 Canada

David C. Hodgson, Assistant Professor, Department of Radiation Oncology, University of Toronto, Princess Margaret Hospital/University Health Network, 610 University Avenue, Toronto, Ontario M5G 2M9 Canada

Simon Horenblas, Professor of Urologic Oncology, Head, Department of Urology, Netherlands Cancer Institute-Antoni van Leeuwenhoek Hospital, Plesmanlaan 121, 1066 CX Amsterdam, The Netherlands

Philip J. Johnson, Professor of Oncology and Translational Research, Cancer Research UK Institute for Cancer Studies, University of Birmingham, Vincent Drive, Edgbaston, Birmingham B15 2TT UK

Steven Joniau, Associate Professor, Department of Urology, University Hospital of the Katholieke Universiteit Leuven, Consultant Urologist, Department of Urology, University Hospital Leuven, Herestraat 49, 3000 Leuven, Belgium

Vikas Khetan, Retinoblastoma Fellow, Hospital for Sick Kids, 555 University Avenue, Toronto, Ontario M5G 1X8 Canada

Haytham Khoury, Clinical Fellow, Ontario Cancer Institute, Princess Margaret Hospital, 610 University Ave, Toronto, Ontario, M5G 2M9 Canada

Paul Kleihues, Professor, Department of Pathology, University Hospital Zurich, 8091 Zurich, Switzerland

Eng-Siew Koh, Clinical Fellow, Department of Radiation Oncology, University of Toronto, Princess Margaret Hospital/University Health Network, 610 University Avenue, Toronto, Ontario M5G 2M9 Canada

Geoffrey G. Liu, Department of Environmental Health, Harvard School of Public Health, Department of Medicine, Harvard Medical School, 665 Huntington Ave., FXB 115, Boston, MA, 02114 USA.

William J. Mackillop, Professor and Chair, Department of Community Health and Epidemiology, Abramsky Hall, 21 Arch Street, Queen's University, Kingston, Ontario K7L 3N6 Canada

Donald E. Marsden, Associate Professor of Obstetrics and Gynaecology, University of New South Wales, Deputy Director, Gynaecological Cancer Centre, Royal Hospital for Women, Barker Street, Randwick 2031 Australia

Howard L. McLeod, Professor, Department of Medicine, Division of Oncology, Washington University School of Medicine, Director, Alvin J. Siteman Cancer Center Pharmacology Core, Campus Box 8069, 660 South Euclid Avenue, St. Louis, MO 63110 USA

Michael F. Milosevic, Associate Professor, Department of Radiation Oncology, University of Toronto, Princess Margaret Hospital/University Health Network, 610 University Avenue, Toronto, Ontario M5G 2M9 Canada

Mark D. Minden, Professor, Department of Medical Oncology, University of Toronto, Princess Margaret Hospital/University Health Network, 610 University Avenue, Toronto, Ontario M5G 2M9 Canada

Guiseppe Minniti, Research Fellow, Specialist in Clinical Oncology, Department of Radiotherapy, Neurooncology Unit, The Royal Marsden NHS Trust, Fulham Road, London, SW3 6JJ UK

John P. Neoptolemos, Professor of Surgery, Head of Division of Surgery and Oncology, Royal Liverpool University Hospital, Daulby Street, Liverpool, L69 3GA UK

Hextan Y. S. Ngan, Professor, University of Hong Kong, Head, Division of Gynaecology Oncology, University of Hong Kong, Queen Mary Hospital, Room 605 6/F, Prof. Block, Pokfulham Rd., Hong Kong, SAR, China

Franco E. Odicino, Department of Obstetrics & Gynecology, Division of Gynecologic Oncology, University of Brescia, Spedali Civili, P.le Spedali Civili 1, 25123 Brescia Italy

Hiroko Ohgaki, Head, Pathology Group, International Agency for Research on Cancer (IARC), World Health Organization, 150 cours Albert Thomas, 69372 Lyon Cedex 08 France

Brian O'Sullivan, Professor, Department of Radiation Oncology, University of Toronto, Princess Margaret Hospital/University Health Network, 610 University Avenue, Toronto, Ontario M5G 2M9 Canada

Daniel H. Palmer, Senior Lecturer, University of Birmingham, Honorary Consultant in Medical Oncology, University Hospital Birmingham NHS Foundation Trust, Vincent Drive, Edgbaston, Birmingham B15 2TT UK

Brunella Pasinetti, Department of Obstetrics & Gynecology, Division of Gynecologic Oncology, University of Brescia, Spedali Civili, P.le Spedali Civili 1, 25123 Brescia, Italy

David G. Payne, Associate Professor, Department of Radiation Oncology, University of Toronto, Princess Margaret Hospital/University Health Network, 610 University Avenue, Toronto, Ontario M5G 2M9 Canada

Sergio Pecorelli, Professor, University of Brescia, Chief, Department of Obstetrics & Gynecology, Head, Division of Gynecologic Oncology, University of Brescia, Spedali Civili, P.le Spedali Civili 1, 25123 Brescia, Italy

Michael Poulsen, Associate Professor, University of Queensland, Southern Zone Radiation Oncology, Mater Centre, 31 Raymond Tce, South Brisbane, Queensland, 4101 Australia

Jesús San Miguel Professor, University of Salamanca, Head, Servicio de Hematología, Hospital Universitario de Salamanca, Paseo de San Vicente, 58, 37007 Salamanca, Spain

Hans-Joachim Schmoll, Professor, Universitätsklinik für Innere Medizin IV, Hämatologie/Onkologie, Martin-Luther-Universität Halle, Ernst-Grube-Straße 40, 06120 Halle, Germany

Carol L. Shields, Professor of Ophthalmology, Thomas Jefferson University, Co-Director, Ocular Oncology Service, Wills Eye Hospital, 840 Walnut Street-Suite 1440, Philadelphia, PA 19107 USA

Jerry A. Shields, Professor of Ophthalmology, Thomas Jefferson University, Director, Ocular Oncology Service, Wills Eye Hospital,, 840 Walnut Street-Suite 1440, Philadelphia, PA 19107 USA

Stefan Sleijfer, Department of Medical Oncology, Erasmus MC – Daniel den Hoed, University Medical Centre, Groene Hilledijk 301, 3075 EA Rotterdam, The Netherlands

Lena Specht, Associate Professor of Oncology, Chief Oncologist, Department. of Oncology, Section 3994, The Finsen Centre, Rigshospitalet, Copenhagen University Hospital, 9 Blegdamsvej DK-2100 Copenhagen, Denmark

Hubert J. Stein, Professor, Paracelsus Private Medical University, Chairman, Department of Surgery, University Hospital Salzburg, Müllner Hauptstr. 48, A-5020 Salzburg, Austria

Fernando J. Suarez-Saiz, Clinical Fellow, Medical Oncology, Ontario Cancer Institute, Princess Margaret Hospital/University Health Network, 610 University Avenue, Toronto, Ontario M5G 2M9 Canada

Richard Sylvester, Assistant Director, Biostatistics, European Organisation for Research and Treatment of Cancer, AISBL-IVZW, Avenue E. Mounierlaan, 83/11, Bruxelles 1200 Brussels, Belgium

Kevin Fai Tam, Division of Gynaecology Oncology, Department of Obstetrics & Gynaecology, University of Hong Kong, Queen Mary Hospital, 102 Pokfulam Road, Hong Kong, SAR, China

Eng Huat Tan, Senior Consultant, Department of Medical Oncology, National Cancer Centre Singapore, 11 Hospital Drive, Republic of Singapore 169610

Giancarlo Tisi, Department of Obstetrics & Gynecology, Division of Gynecologic Oncology, University of Brescia, Spedali Civili, P.le Spedali Civili 1, 25123 Brescia, Italy

Cornelis J.H. van de Velde, Professor of Surgery, Leiden University Medical Center, Department of Surgery, P.O. Box 9600, 2300 RC Leiden, The Netherlands

Adrian P.M. van der Meijden, Professor, Bosch Medi Centrum, Department of Urology, Jeroen Bosch Hospital, Groot Ziekengasthuis, P. O. Box 90153, 5211 NL 's Hertogenbosch, The Netherlands

J.H.J.M. van Krieken, Professor, Radboud University Nijmegen Medical Centre, Department of Pathology, P.O. Box 9101, Nijmegen, The Netherlands

Hendrik van Poppel, Professor and Chairman Department of Urology, University Hospital of the Katholieke Universiteit Leuven, Herestraat 49, B – 3000 Leuven, Belgium

Nirmal K. Veeramachaneni, Resident, Department of Surgery, Division of Cardiothoracic Surgery, Washington University School of Medicine, 660 South Euclid Avenue, St. Louis, MO 63110 USA

Jaap Verweij, Professor, Experimental Chemotherapy and Pharmacology, Department of Medical Oncology, Erasmus University Medical Centre, Groene Hilledijk 301, 3075 EA Rotterdam, The Netherlands

Burkhard H. von Rahden, Surgical Fellow, Department of Surgery, University Hospital Salzburg, Paracelsus Medical University (PMU) Salzburg, Müllner Hauptstrasse 48, A-5020 Salzburg, Austria

John N. Waldron, Assistant Professor, Department of Radiation Oncology, University of Toronto, Princess Margaret Hospital/University Health Network, 610 University Avenue, Toronto, Ontario M5G 2M9 Canada

Lisa Wang, Biostatistician, Clinical Study Coordination and Biostatistics, Ontario Cancer Institute/Princess Margaret Hospital, 610 University Avenue, Toronto, M5G 2M9 Canada

Zhaoxi Michael Wang, Research Fellow, Occupational Health Program, Harvard School of Public Health, I-1404B, 677 Huntington Avenue, Boston, MA 02115 USA

Padraig R. Warde, Professor, Department of Radiation Oncology, University of Toronto, Princess Margaret Hospital/University Health Network, 610 University Avenue, Toronto, Ontario M5G 2M9 Canada

Joseph Wee, Head, Division of Clinical Trials & Epidemiological Sciences, National Cancer Centre Singapore, 11 Hospital Drive, Republic of Singapore 169610

Christian Wittekind, Professor and Director of the Institute of Pathology, University Clinic of Leipzig, Liebigstrasse 26, D-04103 Leipzig, Germany

Wei Zhou, Research Scientist, Department of Environmental Health, Harvard School of Public Health, 665 Huntington Ave. FXB 109, Boston, MA, 02114 USA

Lucia Zigliani, FIGO Annual Report Editorial Office, European Institute of Oncology, via Ripamonti 435, 20141 Milan, Italy

Emanuele Zucca, Professor, Oncology Institute of Southern Switzerland, Ospedale San Giovanni, 6500 Bellinzona, Switzerland

PRINCIPLES OF PROGNOSTIC FACTORS

CHAPTER 1

The Importance of Prognosis in Cancer Medicine

WILLIAM J. MACKILLOP

THE ROLE OF PROGNOSIS IN THE PRACTICE OF MEDICINE

It is the best thing, in my opinion, for the physician to apply himself diligently to the art of foreknowing.

—Hippocrates

Prognosis: The Oldest of the Clinical Skills

Diagnosis, prognosis, and therapeutics are the three core elements of the art of medicine.[1,2] Today, diagnosis and treatment may seem to be of transcending importance, but prognosis has been part of the practice of medicine much longer than diagnosis. Sick people have always been preoccupied by their prospects for recovery, and physicians acquired genuine skill in prognosis long before therapeutics had anything real to offer.[3,4] *Mantic prognosis*, the foretelling of the outcome of an illness based on omens and magic, has been widely practiced since the beginning of recorded history,[5] but scientific approaches to prognosis also began long ago. *Semiotic prognosis*, the foretelling of the outcome of an illness based on clinical findings, can be traced as far back as the Sumerian civilization of 2000 B.C.[3] and reached a high level of sophistication in Greece in the era of Hippocrates ~400 B.C.[6] The Hippocratic school recognized complexes of symptoms and signs that predicted a good or bad outcome, and was also aware that environmental factors and characteristics of the patient could influence the prognosis. Hippocratic knowledge resembles modern medical knowledge in that it was based on clinical observation and applied by pattern recognition.[6] However, Hippocratic prognostication differed significantly from modern prognostication in that the prognosis was inferred directly from the symptoms without passing through

Prognostic Factors in Cancer, Third Edition, edited by Mary K. Gospodarowicz, Brian O'Sullivan, and Leslie H. Sobin.
Copyright © 2006 John Wiley & Sons, Inc.

the process of diagnosis.[1,6] Although many of the symptom complexes described by Hippocrates are readily recognizable today as corresponding to specific diseases, Edelstein points out that "there is, in ancient medicine, no theory of disease *per se*".[6]

The Rise of Diagnosis

After Hippocrates, there were few real advances in the science of medicine for almost 2000 years. Therapeutics flourished, but remedies were almost always directed by theories that had no empirical basis.[3,4] Modern medicine began ~300 years ago when it was first clearly recognized that the right way to treat a patient could not be *deduced* from scientific theory, and that the effectiveness of treatment had to be *induced* by clinical observation.[7,8] Induction is the general process of inference that allows us to predict what will happen in a specific set of circumstances in the future, based on observations made in similar circumstances in the past.[7] To apply inductive reasoning in medicine, it is essential to have a means of classifying clinical problems into groups of "similar" cases. In the seventeenth century, Sydenham provided the first "nosology", or classification of human diseases into diagnostic groups, based on the symptoms reported by the patient and the signs elicited by the clinicians.[3,4,8] Diagnosis from then on provided the link to past experience that permitted a rational choice of therapy. In the eighteenth century, postmortem studies began to reveal the pathological changes that were responsible for specific clinical syndromes, and this led to a more objective clinicopathological classification of diseases.[4,8] Successive advances in science and technology have since permitted many further refinements to this system of diagnostic classification, although our system today remains imperfect. The classification of neoplastic disease presents particular problems, and even modern diagnostic criteria do not create truly uniform groups of cases.[9]

The Ellipsis of Prognosis

In the modern era, the perceived importance of prognosis appears to have declined. In the late nineteenth century the standard textbooks of medicine all included extensive introductory sections dealing with this aspect of medical practice alongside diagnosis.[10–13] Modern textbooks of medicine, on the other hand, do not accord it any special status. Christakis traced the decline in the emphasis on prognosis in the context of acute pneumonia through successive editions of Osler's textbook of medicine.[14] From being a dominant concern 100 years ago, it almost disappeared altogether by the middle of the twentieth century. Christakis described this phenomenon as the "ellipsis" of prognosis, and attributed it to increasingly successful therapies that made the details of the natural history of the illness seem less relevant to the clinician. The theoretical basis of prognosis also receives scant attention in modern textbooks of clinical epidemiology, while diagnosis is discussed extensively and quantitative methods for measuring its accuracy are provided.[15,16] As we shall see, however, it is naive to believe that advances in diagnosis have made prognosis irrelevant; diagnosis and prognosis are complementary rather than competing aspects of medical practice.

The Relationship between Diagnosis and Prognosis

Diagnosis means generalizing, transcending the particular; prognosis, however, means individualizing, allowing for the particular.

—Weissman, Theoretical Medicine and Bioethics

Prognosis differs from diagnosis in several ways. First, the goal of diagnosis is to discover a present fact, while the goal of prognosis is to predict the future. Second, the diagnosis may be static, but prognosis changes over time and may be modified by therapy. Third, the diagnosis is primarily a means to an end, providing a guide for therapy and prognosis; the prognosis, too, may guide therapy, but it is also an end in itself in that it directly meets the patient's need for information about the future. Finally, and perhaps most importantly, the diagnosis is an abstract notion of the disease that is independent of the individual case, while the prognosis describes the probable course of the illness in a particular patient.[17–20]

THE BASIS OF PROGNOSIS

An expert prediction of outcome is based upon an accurate diagnosis, knowledge of the natural history of the disease, the disease's response to treatment, and the progression of the disease in the patient in question.

—Bailey, Concise Dictionary of Medical-Legal Terms

This definition, provided by a contemporary medical dictionary, makes it clear that two different frames of reference are used in predicting the outcome(s) of an illness. The first is an external frame of reference, provided by past experience in similar cases. The second is an internal frame of reference, provided by the previous course of the illness in the individual case. Both are important in oncology; the former is the dominant source of information at the time of diagnosis, and the latter assumes increasing importance during the course of the illness.

The External Frame of Reference: Past Experience in Similar Cases

There is a natural division of the subject into two parts. The first embraces prognosis as considered in its relation to diagnosis, and comprehends those general conclusions as to the future that are drawn from the known tendency of any given disease. The second comprehends those particular circumstances, which belong to the individual case.

—Ash, The Cyclopedia of Practical Medicine

Figure 1.1 illustrates how past experience in similar cases serves as the basis for prognosis in the individual case. Two different pathways lead to the prognosis. The first (α), starts with the assignment of a diagnosis based on clinical and pathological findings (α_1). The general prognosis associated with this diagnosis, which is sometimes referred to as the *ontologic prognosis*,[21] is then induced from past experience in patients with the same diagnosis (α_2). The prognosis is then attributed to the individual

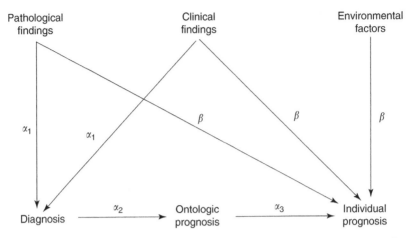

FIGURE 1.1   The basis of prognosis. The diagram illustrates the flow of information in establishing the prognosis in an individual case. The α pathway shows how diagnosis precedes and forms the basis for prognosis in modern medical practice. The β pathway shows how clinical findings were used to predict outcomes directly in the Hippocratic era. Today the β pathway serves to modify the ontologic prognosis established by the diagnosis.

case (α_3). The second pathway, labeled β in Figure 1.1, involves the application of past experience relating to aspects of the case that are *not* included in the abstract notion of the diagnosis. These attributes were formerly referred to as "prognostics,"[10] but today they are usually known as "prognostic factors". In ancient Greek medicine, before diagnosis became established, the β pathway was obviously the only route to the prognosis. In modern medicine, the β pathway usually operates in conjunction with the α pathway and serves to modify the ontologic prognosis to provide the *individual prognosis*. In modern oncology the β pathway also functions alone in some circumstances, for example, in terminal illness, when the primary diagnosis ceases to be relevant and the classical Hippocratic signs become the best indicators of impending death.[22] Note that the distinction between "diagnosis" and "prognostic factor" is sometimes blurred. Measures of the severity of the disease, such as the grade or stage of a cancer, may be considered as prognostic factors by some, while others see them as inherent aspects of the diagnosis.

The Internal Frame of Reference: The Previous Course of the Illness

The prognosis may also be inferred from the trajectory of the illness observed in the individual case.[1,21] Tumor growth rates in individual cases have been observed to remain relatively constant over time.[23,24] If a cancer has been observed to grow slowly in the past, it is therefore reasonable to infer that it will continue to grow slowly in the future. If the patient's functional status has declined rapidly, it will probably continue to decline rapidly. If the cancer has failed to respond to several forms of systemic treatment in the past, it is unlikely to respond to similar agents in the future. There is usually insufficient information available to use this form of reasoning at the time of diagnosis, but it becomes more and more important as the passage of time reveals the behavior of the disease. Although the primary frame of reference here is internal, it does rely on the external frame to some extent; we would not be able to infer the future behavior of an individual tumor from its previous behavior, if we did not know from past experience that the rate of tumor progression is generally fairly constant.

State- and Trait-Related Prognostic Factors

It has become conventional to classify prognostic factors in cancer medicine as tumor-, patient-, treatment-related, and environmental, depending on the source of the information. However, it is also conceptually useful to classify prognostic factors based on the way in which they relate to the prognosis. Cancer is a unidirectional, time-dependent process that causes morbidity and mortality by disruption of normal cellular function and organ function through the processes of invasion, metastasis, and the secretion of toxic products. At any point in time, the prognosis depends on how far the disease has already progressed and on its rate of progression. Prognostic factors can be broadly grouped into those that reflect the present extent of the cancer, and those that reflect its rate of progression. The former may be referred to as *state-related* and the latter as *trait-related prognostic factors*. Tumor volume, for example, is a state-related factor, while tumor doubling time is a trait-related factor. These two types of prognostic factor are complementary and both types of information are required to provide the best estimate of the prognosis. The effects of different types of treatment on prognosis may also be incorporated into this model. Surgery, for example, is a *state-modifying* therapy, while a hormonal agent that retards tumor cell proliferation is a *trait-modifying* therapy.

Formulating the Prognosis in Clinical Practice

As will become apparent in Part B of this book, there is a mass of information available about factors that are associated with the prognosis in most of the common malignancies. The practical challenge for the clinician is to recognize which factors are pertinent to the individual case, and to assign each an appropriate weight in formulating the prognosis. Little is known about the way in which doctors actually reach prognostic judgments in their day-to-day practice. It seems likely that doctors usually proceed by assigning the patient to a subgroup of cases that is sufficiently well defined to permit choice of therapy, and then attribute to the individual case, the average prognosis observed in this subgroup. Additional prognostic information may give the clinician a sense as to whether the prognosis of this case is likely to be better or worse than that of the average patient, but it is unusual for the clinician to actually calculate the prognosis based on all the information that is available. Many prognostic scoring systems have been designed with the intention of assisting clinicians in this task, but very few of them have been widely adopted. With the advent of microarray technology, which can generate huge volumes of information about the individual case that may complement the prognostic information provided by classical clinical pathological systems, it will be necessary for clinicians to become more adept and comfortable in using algorithms that will permit more of this information to be used in clinic.

THE DIMENSIONS OF THE PROGNOSIS

The prognosis is multidimensional. Bailey defines it as "a reasoned forecast concerning the course, pattern, progression, duration, and end of the disease."[20] The prognosis is a dynamic quantity that changes as events unfold. The *natural prognosis* may be modifiable by therapeutic intervention(s), in which case, several *conditional prognoses* may be applicable to a given case at one point, depending on the choice of treatment. Furthermore, the patient's future may be affected by more than one illness, and a comprehensive prognosis must reflect the probable outcomes of all competing causes of morbidity.

The Prognosis Is Multidimensional

The prognosis includes, but is not limited to, the issue of life and death. It may include any aspect of the future health or functional status of the patient. By the nineteenth century, the standard American and European medical textbooks all described the dimensions of prognosis. In that era, they were often referred to as the "objects of prognosis".[10–13,25,26] Today we would simply call them outcomes. In 1859, the following classic description of the types of questions that may have to be addressed in formulating the prognosis appeared in one of the standard textbooks of medicine:[12]

1. Will the disease end in death or recovery or will it continue indefinitely?
2. If it proves fatal, will death come quickly or slowly, and how will the patient die?
3. If the patient recovers, will some morbid condition remain either in the form of general ill health or some local problem?
4. How long will the illness last?
5. What events are likely to take place in its course, such as changes in symptoms, critical phenomena, the occurrence of complications?
6. Does having had the illness make the patient more or less susceptible to other illnesses?

This broad list of topics makes it clear that prognosis traditionally involved predicting not only survival, but many other outcomes as well. For a time in the 1960s and 1970s, when advances in chemotherapy made it seem that every cancer might soon be cured, the focus of prognosis in oncology seems to have narrowed to survival alone. Since the 1980s there has been a reawakening of interest in outcomes other

TABLE 1.1   Questions Ranked Most Important by Cancer Patients Who Are Faced with a Decision about Treatment[a]

Questions	Rank	Median Score
Will the treatment cause the disease to go into complete remission?	1	9.29
Will the treatment cure me of the disease so that I may live a normal life span?	2	9.26
Will the disease lead to my death if left untreated?	3	9.21
How fast will the disease spread if left untreated?	4	9.16
How long will I live if the disease is left untreated?	5	9.10
What organs of my body will be affected by the disease if left untreated?	5	9.10
Will I have to be admitted to the hospital for treatment?	7	8.70
Will the disease be painful if left untreated?	8	9.07
Is the equipment at this hospital up-to-date for treating this disease?	9	9.06
How quickly does the treatment affect the disease?	10	9.04
Will the disease (if left untreated) affect my ability to care for myself?	10	9.04
Will the untreated disease cause me to be dependent on others?	12	9.02
If I refuse treatment, will my physician continue to care for me?	13	8.99
Will the disease spread to my brain if left untreated?	14	8.97
How many patients with this disease are ever cured by this treatment?	15	8.96

Source: Reference 28.

[a]*Note*: Patients with ovarian cancer used a linear analog scale to indicate the relative importance of 57 questions about the illness and its treatment. This table shows their top 15 responses.

than survival, and the broader classical definition of prognosis fits well with contemporary concerns about quality of life.

Before formulating the prognosis, Roberts recommended that the doctor should decide what outcomes are most important in the individual case.[24] This sensible approach remains valid today, except that the patient, rather than the doctor, now seems to us the right person to judge what is important. Empirical studies have demonstrated that many different aspects of the prognosis are important to cancer patients and to their doctors.[27–30] Table 1.1 shows some information provided by a survey of patients with ovarian cancer who were asked to score the importance of a number of questions about the illness that had been identified as possibly relevant in preliminary surveys of patients, doctors, and nurses.[27,28] It is interesting that each type of prognostic issue identified by Roberts more than 100 years ago is represented on this empirically derived list of contemporary concerns. This study revealed that questions concerning the prognosis were generally ranked much higher by patients than questions about the diagnosis or the treatment. The aspects of the illness that were most important varied widely from one patient to the next, and the concerns of the individual could not easily be predicted based on the characteristics of the patient. Thus, the only way to find out what prognostic information patients want is to ask them.

The Prognosis is a Dynamic Quantity

> Perhaps the most important distinction between diagnosis and prognosis is to be made in terms of time. Diagnosis detemporalizes the disease process, and prognosis unrolls even a momentary state into a significant time sequence.
> —Buchanan, The Doctrine of Signatures: A Defense of Theory in Medicine

The prognosis changes as events unfold over time, and new information becomes available. When a patient who was treated initially for an early cancer with a good prognosis, develops evidence of distant metastases, the probability of long-term survival often drops to zero. On the other hand, when a patient with a locally advanced cancer with a relatively poor initial prognosis survives without recurrence for several years, the probability of subsequent long-term survival is often much higher than it was at the time of diagnosis. Consider the case of the patient treated radically for Stage IVA cervical cancer. At the outset there is a very high probability that she will die of the cancer, although there is a sufficient chance of cure to justify radical treatment. If she has a complete response to radiotherapy and there is no recurrence during the first few months, the outcome is much less certain. If she survives without recurrence for 5 years, there remains only a low probability that she will ever die of this cancer. Thus, we go from near certainty about a bad outcome, through complete uncertainty, to near certainty about a good outcome, over a period of a few years.

Conditional Prognosis

> The predictive inference depends on a dilemma between a prediction of the course of the trouble if left alone, and a prediction of the effect of the remedy if it is administered.
> —Buchanan, The Doctrine of Signatures: A Defense of Theory in Medicine

In a short story entitled, *El jardin de los senderos que se bifurcan* (The Garden of Branching Pathways), Jorge Luis Borges used his title theme as a metaphor for life.[31] Whenever a person faced a decision that would affect the future, one part of them took each of the two paths available, and each went on through life in a parallel universe. In reality, for any individual there will only be one future, but there may be several possible futures from which to choose. The course of an illness may be dependent on external factors over which the patient or doctor has control, and present actions may modify the future. Whenever a choice of paths is available to the patient, each comes with its own prognosis. The prognosis, *if* the patient chooses the primary radiotherapy, may be quite different from the prognosis *if* the patient chooses surgery, or the prognosis *if* the patient chooses no active treatment, and each of these *conditional prognoses* requires to be considered before a rational decision about treatment can be made. Whether or not formal decision analysis is employed at the bedside, the comparison of conditional prognoses is at the heart of all rational therapeutic decisions.

The Comprehensive Prognosis

Most contemporary and historical definitions of the prognosis insist that it is a prediction of the outcome of a particular case *of a disease*.[17-20] However, the patient's future may be determined by the outcomes of several different diseases. The term, comprehensive prognosis, is used here to describe predictions of what will happen *to the patient*. A comprehensive prognosis must reflect the expected outcomes of all potential competing causes of death and morbidity, and not merely those associated with the dominant illness. Consider, for example, how the probability of death from competing causes sometimes dominates treatment decisions in early prostate cancer, where no active treatment may be indicated if it appears that other illnesses pose a greater risk to the patient's life and health than the cancer. It is always useful to consider causes of morbidity other than the cancer, even if this only leads to the conclusion that the chance of another illness becoming the dominant issue is so unlikely as to be irrelevant. Doctors may do this unconsciously, but it is better dealt with explicitly. Errors in decision making may result if comorbidity is ignored, or if its importance is overestimated. The comprehensive prognosis, which incorporates all competing risks, is the correct basis for medical decision making, and it is the quantity that has most meaning for the patient.

THE IMPORTANCE OF PROGNOSIS IN ONCOLOGY

The prognosis plays a central role in medical decision making, and is also valuable to patients in making decisions about aspects of their lives unrelated to their medical care. Providing prognostic information is a medico–legal responsibility. Good prognostication also contributes to the efficiency of medical care, and an understanding of prognostic factors facilitates our ability to learn from clinical experience.

Medical Decision Making

> Whereas scientific knowledge is generalized and impersonal, medical practice takes place under conditions, which are singular, individual, and irreversible.
> —Weissman, Theoretical Medicine and Bioethics

Decision making in oncology is particularly difficult because the game is played for high stakes, and it is played for keeps. The potential benefits of cancer treatment are exceptional; unlike the situation in most other domains of medicine, cancer treatment can often eradicate the disease entirely. However, the morbidity associated with many forms of cancer treatment is also exceptional, and usually irreversible. Oncologists, therefore, rarely have the luxury of using a trial therapy to establish the correct course of action. The first treatment decision compromises all subsequent treatment decisions, and every effort has to be made to make the right choice the first time around.

The decision to treat is always based on the comparison of at least two conditional prognoses, the prognosis without treatment and the prognosis with treatment. The choice between two or more active treatment options is made by comparing the conditional prognoses associated with each course of action. This comparison may be made by formal decision analysis or more commonly, by some form of informal holistic judgment. In the past, doctors often made these decisions on behalf of the patient.

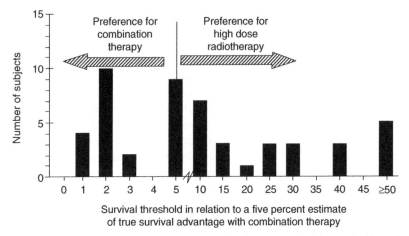

FIGURE 1.2   The effect of the prognosis on individual treatment decisions. The figure illustrates how much improvement in survival patients with Stage III nonsmall-cell lung cancer believe would be necessary for them to choose combined modality treatment as opposed to radiotherapy. The diagram shows a frequency distribution of the survival advantage at 3 years that made the combined approach seem superior to RT alone in a trade-off exercise. (From Brundage et al.[33])

Today, modern medical ethics emphasizes the patient's right to self-determination, and patients are increasingly involved with what were formerly medical decisions.[32] It is clear that, under apparently identical circumstances, different patients reach different decisions based on their personal values.[33,34] This is illustrated in Figure 1.2, which shows how different patients weigh gains in survival against increased toxicity, in choosing between more and less aggressive therapies for nonsmall-cell lung cancer. It illustrates how sensitive treatment decisions may be to prognostic information, and indicates that a fairly textured description of the probable outcomes of each alternative course of action may be required to permit the patients to make the best possible decision for themselves.

Personal Decision Making

Patients also need prognostic information to make decisions about other aspects of their lives. There are four distinct ways in which prognostic information can be useful in making personal decisions. First of all, knowing what the future may hold can provide an opportunity to take preemptive action to avoid a bad outcome. To use the weather as an analogy, the forecast may allow you to alter course to avoid a storm. In some instances, it may be possible for patients to modify their behaviors to decrease the risk of bad outcomes. Smoking cessation can decrease the risk of second primary cancers, and compliance with close follow-up, in some situations, can reduce the risk of death. Second, it may be useful to know what is coming in order to prepare for it; the forecast provides a chance to batten down the hatches and get ready for bad weather. Patients need to know their prognosis in order to make decisions about their finances, their employment, and sometimes their accommodation in order to prepare to meet their future needs. Relatives may also need to make important personal decisions in order to prepare for a care-giving role, or for life without the support of the patient. The prognosis may also provide the opportunity for the patient to make spiritual preparations for the end of their lives. Third, knowing what is to come in the longer term is useful in planning one's short-term agenda; if it is going to rain tomorrow, you will want to do the outdoor things today. With the threat of deteriorating health down the road, patients may want to take the opportunity to do things that they always promised themselves that they would do, but have previously postponed. Finally, and sometimes most importantly, there is knowing for the sake of knowing. The argument here is not a consequentialist one; the knowledge itself simply meets the psychological need to know.

Medico–Legal Perspective

He who is master of the art of prognosis, and shows himself such, will demonstrate such a superior knowledge, that the generality of men will commit themselves to the physician wholeheartedly.

—Hippocrates

In ancient Greek medicine, accurate prognosis was seen as a means of building patients' trust, of avoiding blame for bad outcomes, and of building a good reputation in the community.[6] These issues are still relevant in medical practice today, but potential liability for failure to provide prognostic information is an additional consideration. The physician is now expected to inform patients about the expected outcomes of any procedure or treatment before they are asked to give consent to it. Although practice varies around the world, this is an established principle under Anglo-American common law, and is also encoded as statute in some jurisdictions.[35] Failure to inform patients about the prognosis with respect to the potential benefits and material risks of treatment, and also about the risks associated with *not* undergoing treatment, may be deemed negligence.[35]

Health Policy Perspective

On a societal level, skill in prognosis is useful as a means of optimizing the use of resources. Accurate prognosis is a precondition for good medical decisions, and good decisions lead to efficient care, whereas bad decisions waste money. The use of aggressive forms of active treatment in situations where the prognosis is hopeless can obviously be very expensive, but undertreatment can also have adverse financial consequences. Overlooking the chance for cure in a potentially curable patient is not only a lethal error, it is also an expensive one, because the cost of dying of cancer can greatly exceed the cost of effective treatment. Prognostic information may also be useful in making allocational decisions. Some publicly funded healthcare systems have now begun to make decisions about which types of care they are willing to pay for, based on an economic appraisal of the benefits they achieve in the relationship to their cost. This type of decision making may be unfair unless the individual characteristics of the case can be factored into the equation. Consistently applying decisions at the level of the diagnostic group may seem sensible enough, but in circumstances in which individual characteristics of the case have a very large impact on outcome, it may prove too simplistic to be truly equitable. The principle of justice demands not only that like situations be treated alike, but also that situations that are unalike should not be treated as if they were the same.[32] Prognostic information is therefore essential for fair allocational decisions.

The Research Perspective

In cancer research, an understanding of prognostic factors is important in the design and analysis of clinical trials and retrospective reviews of clinical experience. Valid comparison of treatment and control groups requires that the expected outcome without treatment should be similar in both. Prognostic factors are used as eligibility criteria to ensure a relatively uniform study population, and they may also be used in the process of stratification that is undertaken to balance the case mix in each arm as far as possible. The more the variance in outcome due to prognostic factors other than the treatment can be controlled in the experiment, the more readily the effect of treatment itself can be determined. Identification of prognostic factors also allows identification of subgroups of cases that experience poor outcomes with standard treatment, in which experimental therapy should be tested. An understanding of prognostic factors is also important in cancer research because in some instances, prognostic factors may have a causal relationship to the outcome of the disease.

THE ACCURACY OF PROGNOSTIC JUDGMENTS

> The practical test of a true science is the power it confers of prevision, or of knowing now what will follow hereafter. When we can prognosticate with certainty, medicine will have become a science.
>
> —H. Hartshorne A system of medicine

Given that prognostic judgments are used as a basis for important decisions, we need to know how accurate they are. We may not yet be able to achieve the "certainty" in prognosis that Hartshorne envisaged as a characteristic of the scientific medicine, but we should at least be able to measure the predictive value of our prognostic judgments, and take this into account in our decision making. Although there is a very extensive literature about prognostic factors in cancer, there have been very few reports relating to the accuracy of prognostic judgments in practice in individual cases. This is much more of a challenge than predicting the outcome of groups of cases. Once the average outcome of a specific medical problem has been established in a large group of cases, the average outcome in another large group of similar cases may be predicted with great precision. However, a precise knowledge of the average outcome of an illness may have little predictive value in the individual case.

Measurements of Accuracy

The quality of prognostic judgments in medicine can be described using the terminology that is generally used to describe the quality of judgments and measurements in other fields. The terms *accuracy* or *accurate* are commonly employed to describe the closeness of a measurement or judgment to the true value of the quantity of interest,[36] and the same terms can also be used to describe how close a prognostic judgment comes to the outcome that is subsequently observed.[22,37] The term accurate can also be used to describe an instrument for making measurements.[36] The degree of accuracy of the instrument is measured by how closely, on average, its measurements approximate the corresponding true values in a series of observations.[36] Similarly, the term accuracy can be applied to the performance of a clinician in predicting the outcome of an illness.[22,37] The accuracy of the prognosticator is measured by how closely the predictions approximate the observed outcomes in a series of cases.[22,37] Accuracy may be affected by *random* and/or *systematic error*. The term *precision* describes the extent to which a measuring instrument, or prognosticator, is free of random error,[36,38] and the term *calibration* describes the extent to which it is free of systematic error.[37,39]

A prediction about the life expectancy of an incurable patient can be stated in months or years, and the outcome can be measured in the same units. Here, both the prediction and the outcome take the form of a continuous variable, and the accuracy of a prediction in an individual case is measured by how close it comes to the observed outcome. The accuracy of a series of such judgments is described by the average closeness of the predictions to the observed outcomes.[36] In contrast, predictions about the outcome of treatment in potentially curable patients are usually stated in terms of the chance of surviving, or of remaining disease-free, at some future time.[23,37] Here, the prediction takes the form of a probability expressed on a scale from 0 to 1, or from 0 to 100%. The outcome, however, is dichotomous; the patient either dies or does not die. The accuracy of such predictions is also measured by how close the prediction comes to the observed outcome, but somewhat different approaches are required to describe the accuracy of a series of such predictions.[22] One approach is to treat the prognostic judgments like the results of a diagnostic test, and calculate how well they *discriminate* between patients who will experience good or bad outcomes. The term *discrimination* is used to describe the extent to which a test or judgment distinguishes between two states. It is a concept borrowed from the signal-detection theory that has been widely used to evaluate diagnostic tests.[40,41] In the field of prognosis, it has been used to measure the ability of prognostic judgment to distinguish between those patients who will be alive, and those patients who will be dead at a specified time in the future.[42,43]

How Accurate are Prognostic Judgments in Oncology?

There have been several studies of the accuracy of clinical predictions about the duration of survival in cancer patients in the terminal and preterminal phases of the illness. All show these judgments to be imprecise. Several studies have also found evidence of poor calibration with a systematic tendency to overestimation of the duration

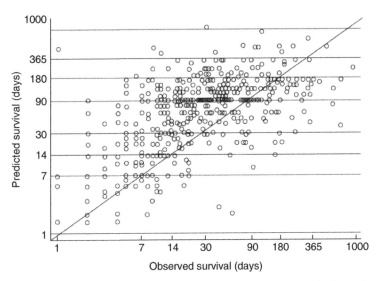

FIGURE 1.3   The Accuracy of Predictions of Survival in Terminally ill Patients. Predicted versus observed survival in 468 terminally ill hospice patients. The diagonal line represents perfect prediction. Patients above the diagonal line are those in whom survival was overestimated; Patients below the line are those in whom survival was underestimated. (From Christakis and Lamont.[44])

of survival (e.g., see Fig. 1.3),[44] but others have found no evidence of bias.[43] Most of these studies have been too small to provide sufficient power to identify characteristics of the doctor or the patient that are associated with the accuracy of the judgments. One larger scale study, the results of which are shown in Figure 1.3, found that doctors with more clinical experience were more accurate in their judgments, and also that prognostic judgments were more accurate when the doctor had known the patient for a longer of time.[44] One other interesting observation is that, toward the end of the patient's life, the accuracy of prognostic judgments increases. This phenomenon may be regarded as an example of what meteorologists call the "horizon effect", meaning that short-term forecasts are usually more accurate than long-term forecasts.[22]

There have been several studies of the accuracy of doctor's judgments about the probability of survival in acute-care medicine,[42,45,46–48] but there has been little comparable work in cancer or any of the other chronic diseases. Figure 1.4 shows the results of a prospective cohort study in which physicians' initial estimates of the probability of cure in a miscellaneous group of cases were compared to the outcomes observed after 5 years.[22] The calibration curves shown in the panels of Figure 1.4 illustrate how well doctors predict the outcomes of different subgroups of cases. Their predictions were generally well calibrated, with some evidence of systematic overestimation of the probability of survival among poorer prognosis patients, a finding that has been continued in two similar studies in lung cancer,[49] and in head and neck cancer.[50]

The doctor's ability to discriminate at the individual level between patients who would be cured and those who would not be cured is better described by the receiver

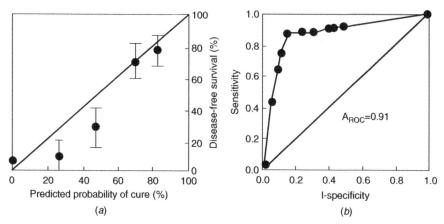

FIGURE 1.4   The accuracy of oncologists' judgments about the probability of cure in routine practice. Panel *a* shows calibration of doctors' estimates of probability of cure. The mean estimated probability of cure of subgroups of patients is plotted against the observed disease-free survival rate at 5 years ($\pm$S.E.). The solid diagonal represents the theoretical line of perfect calibration. Panel *b* shows the ROC curve that illustrates the relationship between the sensitivity and specificity of the doctors' estimates of probability of cure. The area under the ROC curve indicates the discrimination of those judgments. The diagonal line here shows the relationship that would be observed if there were no discrimination ($A_{ROC} = 0.5$). (From Mackillop and Quirt.[22])

operating characteristics curve (ROC curve) shown in Figure 1.4b. The area under the ROC curve (A_{ROC}) is a measure of the discrimination of the prognostic judgments.[21,22] An area of 1.0 indicates perfect discrimination, whereas an area of 0.5 indicates no discrimination.[21,22] For these data, $A_{ROC} = 0.91 \pm 0.09$, which indicates that there is a probability of 0.91 that the doctor, in assessing any randomly selected pair of cancer patients, one of whom is curable and the other not, will assign a higher probability of cure to the curable patient. Table 1.2 shows that the discrimination of doctors' predictions concerning the probability of cure of patients with cancer in this study was as good as short-term forecasts in acute-care medicine,[42,46-48] and better than cardiologists' 3-year infarct-free survival forecasts.[51,52] Furthermore, while prognosis is generally thought to be more of an art and less of a science than diagnosis, the level of discrimination of long-term forecasts in oncology compares very favorably with that of some diagnostic judgments.[53] Table 1.2 also shows that the accuracy of prognostic judgments in cancer medicine compares very favorably with the accuracy of forecasts in other spheres. The discrimination of predictions of 5-year disease-free survival were, for example, better than the discrimination of short-term weather forecasts.[54]

INHERENT LIMITATIONS TO THE ACCURACY OF PROGNOSIS

In interpreting the results of studies of the accuracy of prognosis in oncology, it is important that we consider how accurately we can ever expect to predict the outcome of cancer.

TABLE 1.2 The Discrimination of Human Judgments

Forecasters	Context	Prediction	Sources of Information	Area Under ROC Curve $A_{ROC} + SE$	Reference
Attending oncologists	Cancer patients in an ambulatory care setting	Probability of 5-year survival	The patient results of pretreatment investigations	0.91 ± 0.09	22
Senior cardiologists	Patients with $\geq$ obstruction of ≥ 1 major coronary artery	Probability of 3-year survival	Written case descriptions	0.74	51
Cardiology fellows	Patients with $\geq 75\%$ obstruction of ≥ 1 major coronary artery	Probability of 3-year survival	Written case descriptions	0.80	52
Board-certified critical-care fellows	Medical intensive-care-unit patients 24 h after admission	Probability of surviving until discharge	The patient The patient's chart Results of tests	0.899 ± 0.36	47
Critical-care fellows	Patients in a medical/surgical intensive care unit within 24 h of admission	Probability of surviving until discharge	The patient The patient's chart Results of tests	0.856 ± 0.028	46
Doctors who order blood cultures	Hospitalized patients who had a blood culture	Probability of a positive culture	The Patient The patient's chart	0.687 ± 0.073	53
Meteorologists	Weather	Probability of rain within next 12 h	Current meteorological data	0.871	54
Meteorologists	Weather	Probability of rain in 5–6 days	Current meteorological data	0.728	54

The outcome of an illness can only be predicted to the extent that it is predetermined. The maximum achievable accuracy of prognosis will fall short of 100% to the extent that the outcome of interest is determined by random events that have yet to occur. From what we know about the biology of cancer, it is unlikely that the course of the illness is completely determined at the time of diagnosis. Genetic plasticity is a characteristic of neoplasia, and tumors evolve stepwise by random mutation and natural selection.[55] There is no theoretical reason to believe that it is possible to predict when a metastatic, or drug-resistant, clone will develop, and these are the events that often determine the outcome of the illness. Furthermore, there are sound theoretical reasons to believe that it is impossible to predict whether a given dose of chemotherapy or radiotherapy will cure a particular case. Cell killing by cytotoxic agents involves random processes, and most exhibit first-order kinetics of cell killing.[56] It is therefore partly a matter of chance whether or not the last clonogenic cell is eliminated by a given dose of radiation or chemotherapy.[56] In studies using identical tumors transplanted into genetically identical laboratory animals, it has repeatedly been shown that it is possible to define a dose of radiation or chemotherapy that eradicates the cancer in 50% of the animals, and yet fails to cure it in the other 50%. This dose is referred to as the 50% tumor control dose (TCD_{50}), and it is often used to measure the sensitivity of tumors to cytotoxic agents. It is taken for granted in this context that the outcome in the individual animal is determined by random processes after the treatment is administered, and not by preexisting differences among the animals.

How, then, do we interpret a 50% cure rate following radiotherapy in a specific group of patients with squamous cancer of the oropharynx? The outcomes may have been entirely predetermined. One-half of the patients may have started treatment with a 100% probability of cure, while the other one-half started with a 0% probability of cure. If the molecular basis of these differences in radiocurability could have been identified, then the outcome could have been accurately predicted in every case. However, the outcome may not have been predetermined at all. All the patients may have started out with a 50% chance of cure, and the different outcomes that they experienced might have been decided by chance during treatment. In this case, the outcomes were entirely unpredictable. In fact, any combination of predetermination and chance could have produced the same results, and the predictability of the outcomes could therefore have ranged from 0 to 100%.

The difference between cancer outcomes that are predetermined, but as yet unknown, and those that that have yet to be decided, is analogous to the difference between the "scratch and win" feature on a lottery ticket that determines if it's a winner or a loser at the time you buy it, and the random draw that determines winners and losers after the fact. The extent to which cancer outcomes are established by the random draw sets the outer limits of the predictability of the prognosis in oncology.

CONCLUSION

Prognostic judgment remains an essential element of modern, medical practice. It meets patients' needs for information about the future that they can use to plan their lives, and it provides a basis for rational medical decisions. In the future, the potential to prognosticate accurately will be enhanced by the discovery of new molecular prognostic factors. Over the last 30 years, advances in clinical epidemiology have greatly improved the practice of oncology. Today, we understand much better how to establish the *generalizability* of clinical observations. In future, however, the challenge will be to increase the *particularizability* of medical knowledge in such a way that the individual characteristics of the patient and the tumor are appropriately factored into the prognosis and the treatment decision. This will require characterizing patients, not only in terms of the diagnostic group to which they belong, but also in terms of all those individual characteristics that may influence the outcome of treatment. We need better information and better ways of integrating the available information. Nonetheless, there are good reasons to believe that it will never be possible to prognosticate with certainty. The goal of prognostic factors research can only be to minimize uncertainty about cancer outcomes; there is little possibility of eliminating it.

REFERENCES

1. Buchanan S: In Edmund D. Pellegrino, Maycock PP Jr (eds.), *The doctrine of signatures: a defense of theory in medicine*, 2nd ed. Urbana and Chicago; University of Illinois Press, 1991.

2. Gibson AG: *The physician's art: an attempt to expand John Locke's fragment de arte medica*, Oxford; Clarendon Press, 1933.

3. Magner LN: *A history of medicine*, New York; Marcel Dekker, 1992.

4. McManus JFA: *The fundamentals of medicine: a brief history of medicine*. Springfield (IL), Charles C. Thomas, 1963.

5. Sigerist HE: *History of medicine*, New York; Oxford University Press, 1951–1961.

6. Temkin O, Temkin CL (eds.): *Ancient medicine: selected papers of Ludwig Edelstein*. Baltimore and London; Johns Hopkins University Press, 1967.

7. Howson C, Urbach P: *Scientific reasoning*. LaSalle, IL, Open Court Publishing Company, 1989.

8. Shryock RH: *The development of modern medicine: an interpretation of the social and scientific factors involved*. Madison; University of Wisconsin Press, 1979.

9. Mackillop WJ, O'Sullivan B, Gospodarowicz M: The role of cancer staging in evidence-based medicine, *Cancer Prev Control* 2:269–277, 1998.

10. Ash E: Prognosis, in Forbes J, Tweedie A, Conolly J (eds.): *The cyclopaedia of practical medicine*, vol. III. Philadelphia; Blanchard and Lea, 1859, pp. 699–706.

11. Hartshorne H: *A system of medicine*, vol. 1, Reynolds JR (ed.). Philadelphia; Henry C. Lea's Son, 1880, pp. 21–32.

12. Roberts FT: *A handbook of the theory and practice of medicine*, London; Lewis, 1885, pp. 10–21.

13. Flint A. *A treatise of the principles and practice of medicine*, 5th ed. Philadelphia; Henry C. Lea's Son, 1881, 98–109.

14. Christakis NA: The ellipsis of prognosis in modern medical thought. *Soc Sci Med* 44: 301–315, 1997.

15. Sacket DI, Haynes RB, Guyatt GH, Tugwell P: *Clinical epidemiology. A basic science for clinical medicine*, 2nd ed. Boston; Little, Brown, 1985.

16. Feinstein A: *Clinical epidemiology. The architecture of clinical research*. Philadelphia; W.B. Saunders, 1985.

17. *Encyclopaedia Britannica*. Chicago, 1998.

18. *The Oxford English Dictionary*, 2nd ed., Simpson JA, Weiner ESC (eds.). Oxford; Clarendon Press, 1989.

19. *Dorland's illustrated medical dictionary*. Philadelphia; Saunders, 1988.

20. Bailey JA: *Concise dictionary of medical-legal terms*. New York; The Parthanon Publishing Group, 1998.

21. Wiesemann C: The significance of prognosis for a theory of medical practice. *Theor Med Bioethics* 19:253–261, 1998.

22. Mackillop WJ, Quirt CF: Measuring the accuracy of prognostic judgments in oncology. *J Clin Epidemiol* 50:21–29, 1997.

23. Charbit A, Malaise EP, Tubiana M: Relation between pathological nature and growth rate of human tumours. *Eur J Cancer* 7:307–325, 1971.

24. Mackillop WJ: The growth kinetics of human tumours. *Clin Phys Physiol Meas* 11: 121–123, 1990.

25. Trousseau A, Cormack JR: Lectures on clinical medicine, vol. 2, London; The New Sydenham Society, 1868, pp. 32–39 (translated from 2nd ed.).

26. Holland H: *Medical notes and reflections*, 3rd ed. London; Longman, Brown, Green and Longmans, 1855.

27. Chammas S: MSc Thesis, Department of Community Health and Epidemiology, Queen's University, Kingston, Ontario, Canada 1991.

28. Feldman-Stewart D, Chammas S, Hayter C, et al.: An empirical approach to informed consent in ovarian cancer. *J Clin Epidemiol* 49:1259–1269, 1996.

29. Feldman-Stewart D, Brundage MD, Hayter C, et al.: What the prostate patient should know: variation in urologists' opinions. *Can J Urol* 4:438–444, 1997.

30. Feldman-Stewart D, Brundage MD, Hayter C, et al.: What prostate cancer patients should know: variations in professionals' opinions. *Radiother Oncol* 49:111–123, 1998.

31. Borges JL: *Ficciones*, Buenos Aires; Nuevo Mundo, 1946.

32. Applebaum PS, Lidz CW, Meisel A: *Informed consent. Legal theory and clinical practice*. New York; Oxford University Press, 1987.

33. Brundage MD, Davidson J, Mackillop WJ: Trading treatment toxicity for survival in locally advanced non-small cell lung cancer. *J Clin Oncol* 15:330–340, 1997.

34. Brundage MD, Davidson J, Mackillop WJ, et al.: Using a treatment trade-off method to elicit preferences for the treatment of locally advanced non-small cell lung cancer. *Med Decis Making* 18:256–267, 1998.

35. Sneiderman B, Irvine JC, Osborne PH: *Canadian medical law*. Agincourt; Ontario Carswell, 1989.

36. Sokal RR, Rohlf FJ: *Biometry*. San Francisco; Freeman, 1969.

37. Poses RM, Cebul RD, Centor RM: Evaluating of physicians' probabilistic judgments. *Med Decis Making* 8:223–240, 1988.

38. Rothman KJ: *Modern epidemiology*. Boston; Little, Brown, 1986.

39. Liechtenstein S, Fischoff B, Phillips LD: Calibration of probabilities: the state of the art in 1980, in Kahneuman D, Slovick P, Tversky A (eds.): *Judgment under uncertainty: heuristics and biases*. Cambridge; Cambridge University Press, 1982; pp. 306–334.

40. Swets JA: ROC analysis applied to the evaluation of medical imaging techniques. *Invest Radiol* 14:109–121, 1979.

41. Griner PF, Mayewski RJ, Mushlin AI: Selection and interpretation of diagnostic tests and procedures: principles and applications. *Ann Intern Med* 94:553, 1981.

42. McClish DK, Powell SH: How well can physicians estimate mortality in a medical intensive care unit? *Med Decis Making* 9:125–132, 1989.

43. Glare P, Virik K, Jones M, et al.: A systematic review of physicians' survival predictions in terminally ill cancer patients. *BMJ* 327:195–198, 2003.

44. Christakis NA, Lamont EB: Extent and determinants of error in doctors' prognoses in terminally ill patients: prospective cohort study. *BMJ* 320:469–479, 2000.

45. Knaus WA, Wagner DP, Lynn J: Short-term mortality predictions for critically ill hospitalized adults: science and ethics. *Science* 254:389–394, 1991.

46. Poses RM, Bekes C, Copare FJ, et al.: The answer to "What are my chances, doctor?" depends on whom is asked: prognostic disagreement and inaccuracy for critically ill patients. *Crit Care Med* 17:827–833, 1989.

47. Brannen AL, Godfrey LJ, Goetter WE: Prediction of outcome from critical illness: a comparison of clinical judgment with a prediction rule. *Arch Intern Med* 149:1083–1086, 1989.

48. Dolan JG, Bordley DR, Mushlin AI: An evaluation of clinicians' subjective prior probability estimates. *Med Decis Making* 6:216–213, 1986.

49. Quirt CF, Mackillop WJ: The accuracy of predictions of life expectancy in lung cancer. *Clin Invest Med* 19:1996.

50. Quirt CF, Hall S, Dixon P, et al.: Measuring the accuracy of prognostic judgments in head and neck cancer. *Clin Invest Med* 20:1997.

51. Kong DF, Lee KL, Harrell FE, et al.: Clinical experience and predicting survival in coronary disease. *Arch Intern Med* 149:1177–1181, 1989.

52. Lee KL, Pryor DB, Harrell FE, et al.: Predicting outcome in coronary disease: statistical models versus expert clinicians. *Am J Med* 80:553–560, 1986.

53. Poses RM, Anthony M: Availability, wishful thinking, and physicians' diagnostic judgments for patients with suspected bacteremia. *Med Decis Making* 11:159–168, 1991.

54. Stanski HR, Wilson LJ, Burrows WR: *Survey of common verification methods in meteorology. Environment Canada Atmospheric Environment Service Research Report*, No. (MSRB):89–85, 1989.

55. Nowell P: Mechanisms of tumour progression. *Cancer Res* 46:2203–2207, 1986.

56. Skipper HE, Schabel FM, Wilcox WS: Experimental evaluation of potential anticancer agents XIII: on the criteria and kinetics associated with "curability" of experimental leukemia. *Cancer Chemother Rep* 35:1–15, 1964.

CHAPTER 2

Prognostic Factors: Principles and Applications

MARY K. GOSPODAROWICZ, BRIAN O'SULLIVAN, and ENG-SIEW KOH

Since the beginning of time, humans have wanted to prognosticate, or "know before". In studies of cancer and other diseases, identification of prognostic factors is the present-day equivalent of predicting the future. Nonetheless, it would be implausible to believe that we can predict precisely for the individual patient. In reality, all we can provide are statements of probability, and even these are more accurate for groups of patients, the study of whom provides us with our knowledge about prognosis. The practical management of cancer patients requires us to make predictions and decisions for individuals, and the challenge of prognostication is to link the individual patient to the collective population of patients with the same disease. The rationale for prognostic factors and classifications of these factors with attention to those used in this book are outlined below. The potential endpoints relevant to oncology, the taxonomy of prognostic factors, and their applications in practice and, most importantly, a concept of a management scenario that forms the basis for defining prognosis at a given point in the course of disease, are presented. The "management scenario" is defined within a specific setting, since prognosis differs for different situations, taking account of the therapeutic milieu, the features of the host and disease, and the particular outcome under study. Prognostic factor research, like clinical trials, must observe essential principles of study assembly and analysis if meaningful conclusions are to be drawn.

RATIONALE FOR PROGNOSTIC FACTORS

The management of patients, or clinical practice, has four main components. Three comprise actions: namely, diagnosis, treatment, and prevention, and one is advisory, that of prognosis. Appraisal of a patient's prognosis is part of everyday practice, and studies

Prognostic Factors in Cancer, Third Edition, edited by Mary K. Gospodarowicz,
Brian O'Sullivan, and Leslie H. Sobin.

TABLE 2.1 **Application of Prognostic Factors**

Learning about the natural history of disease

Patient care
  Select appropriate diagnostic tests
  Select an appropriate treatment plan
  Predict the outcome for individual patient
  Establish informed consent
  Assess the outcome of therapeutic intervention
  Select appropriate follow-up monitoring
  Provide patient and caregiver education

Research
  Improve the efficiency of research design and data analysis
  Enhance the confidence of prediction
  Demarcate phenomena for scientific explanation
  Design future studies
  Identify subgroups with poor outcomes for experimental therapy
  Identify groups with excellent outcomes for simplified therapy
  Identify candidates for organ preservation trials

Cancer control programs
  Plan resource requirements
  Assess the impact of screening programs
  Introduce and monitor clinical-practice guidelines
  Monitor results
  Provide public education
  Explain variation in the observed outcomes

of prognostic factors are integral to cancer research. To consider management of an individual cancer case, the fundamental pieces of information required include the site of origin (e.g., lung or breast), and morphologic type or histology (e.g., adenocarcinoma or squamous cell carcinoma).[1-4] In addition, the outcome in a cancer patient depends on a variety of variables referred to as *prognostic factors*. These factors are defined as *variables that can account for some of the heterogeneity associated with the expected course and outcome of a disease*. Knowledge of prognostic factors helps us to understand the natural history of cancer. The range of applications for prognostic factors is outlined in Table 2.1.

CLASSIFICATIONS OF PROGNOSTIC FACTORS

There are well-defined and accepted classifications of diseases that include cancer. The best known is ICDO, widely used by cancer registries and administrative bodies. The World Health Organization (WHO) Classification of Tumors forms the basis for the histologic classification in cancer. The TNM (see Glossary) classifications published by the International Union Against Cancer (UICC) and the American Joint Committee on Cancer (AJCC) are the standard system for recording anatomic disease extent. In contrast to these evidence- and consensus-based agreements, these is no consensus on the optimal classification of prognostic factors. Although no formal system for classifying prognostic factors exists, numerous prognostic indexes and nomograms have been successfully implemented in clinical practice. Previously, we proposed an extremely simple framework for describing prognostic factors in cancer,[2,5] which included the subject-based classification developed to highlight the importance of nontumor related prognostic factors, and clinical relevance classification to highlight the factors indispensable for good clinical practice.

Subject-Based Classification

Most cancer literature equates prognosis with tumor characteristics. Examples include histologic type, grade, depth of invasion, or the presence of lymph-node metastasis. Cancer pathology and anatomic disease extent account for most variations in cancer outcome. However, factors not directly related to the tumor also affect the course of disease and the outcomes of interest. To consider all prognostic factors, we proposed three broad groupings that will be developed further in this edition: those factors that relate to disease or *tumor*, those that relate to the *host* or patient, and those that relate to the *environment* in which we find the patient. In this edition, we focus on prognostic factors that are relevant at the time of diagnosis and initial treatment, although in the management of cancer patients, determination of prognosis is required repeatedly at multiple situations along the course of the disease. These situations often reflect decision-making points, for example, about adjuvant therapy, management of recurrent cancer, and palliative or terminal care (see Chapter 5). A more comprehensive review of prognostic factors demonstrating the diversity of prognostic factors in each category in distinct cancers will follow in Part B of this book.

Tumor-Related Prognostic Factors   These include those directly related to the presence of the tumor or its effect on the host, and most commonly comprise those that reflect tumor pathology, anatomic disease extent, or tumor biology (Table 2.2). The fundamental factor to consider is definition of a particular cancer as a distinct disease entity. While histology forms the basis of tumor classification today, the recent revolution in molecular medicine has challenged today's classification and has led to redefinition of many cancers according to molecular and genetic tumor characteristics. These newer criteria have been now accepted in acute leukemia and subtypes of lymphoma. Most new tumor-related molecular factors, such as gene expression patterns, deal with disease characterization.

The second fundamental group of prognostic factors relate to the anatomic extent of disease, so-called "stage," classified according to the UICC TNM classification.[6] In addition to the TNM categories and stage groupings, factors describing disease extent, including tumor bulk, number of involved sites, or involvement of specific organs, and tumor histology, also have an impact on prognosis.[7–10]

Tumor pathology is crucial to the determination of prognosis in cancer. The histologic type has traditionally defined the disease under consideration, but additional factors, such as grade, pattern of growth, immunophenotype, and more recently gene

TABLE 2.2 **Examples of Tumor-Related Prognostic Factors**

1. Pathology
   Molecular tumor characteristics; gene expression patterns
   Morphologic classification (e.g., adenocarcinoma, squamous)
   Histologic grade
   Growth pattern (e.g., papillary vs. solid, cribriform vs. tubular vs. solid)
   Pattern of invasion (e.g., perineural, small vessel invasion)

2. Anatomic tumor extent
   TNM categories
   Tumor bulk
   Single versus multifocal tumor
   Number of sites of involvement
   Tumor markers (e.g., PSA, AFP, CEA)

3. Tumor biology
   Tumor markers (e.g., HER2-neu, CD20)
   Proliferation indices (e.g., S-phase fraction, MiB-1)
   Molecular markers (p53, rb, Bcl2)

4. Symptoms (related to the presence of tumor)
   Weight loss
   Pain
   Edema
   Fever

5. Performance status

expression patterns, also reflect the fundamental type of disease under consideration. In contrast, multifocality, presence of lymphatic or vascular invasion, infiltration patterns that also affect the outcome may relate both to type of disease and the extent.[11,12] Tumor markers like prostatic-specific antigen (PSA), alpha-feto protein (AFP), and beta human chorionic gonadotropin (βHCG) are used in everyday practice and strongly correlate with tumor bulk.[13–15] Hormone receptors, biochemical markers, expression of proliferation-related factors and, increasingly, molecular tumor characteristics that have been shown to affect outcomes for a variety of cancers relate to the type of cancer.[16–18] The presence of symptoms has generally been considered a host factor but it may also be a tumor related factor. A classic example is the presence of B-symptoms (night sweats, fever, and weight loss) in Hodgkin lymphoma.

Host-Related Prognostic Factors   These are factors present in the body of the host (patient) that are not directly related to malignancy, but through interference with the behavior of the tumor or their effect on treatment have the potential to significantly impact the outcome. These factors may generally be divided in demographic patient characteristics, such as age,[19] gender,[20] and racial origin,[21] comorbidity and coexistent illness,[22,23] especially those affecting the immune status,[24] performance status related to comorbid illness, and factors that relate to the host mental state, attitude, and compliance[25,26] with therapy. A history of prior cancer and treatment of that cancer also places survivors at risk for future events (Table 2.3).

TABLE 2.3   **Examples of Host-Related Prognostic Factors**

1. Demographics
   Age
   Race
   Gender
   Level of education
   Socioeconomic status
   Religion

2. Comorbidity
   Constant
      Inherited immune deficiency
      von Recklinghausen disease, etc.
   Changeable
      Coexistent illness (e.g., inflammatory bowel disease, collagen vascular disease)
      Weight
      Cardiac status
      Acquired immune deficiency
      Infection
      Mental health

2. Performance status

3. Compliance
   Social reaction to illness
   Influence of habits, drugs, alcohol, smoking, etc.
   Belief in alternative therapies

Environment-Related Prognostic Factors   The factors that operate external to the patient and could be specific either to an individual patient or, more frequently, to groups of patients residing in the same geographic area. Here, we can consider three categories of environmental factors: first, those that have a physician expertise focus, such as the choice of a specific treatment plan and caregiver skill; second a healthcare system focus including access[27,28] to cancer care, caliber of medical record keeping, internet access,[29] degree of clinical trial participation, and also the presence of ageism, which can all influence treatment selection and outcome. Finally, there are factors related to a society focus, such as a patient's socioeconomic,[30] and nutritional status, and the overall quality of care, including the presence of quality control programs,[31] which may impact the outcome (Table 2.4).

While a classification within the three subject-based categories may be a useful working model, the distinction between these groupings of prognostic factors is not always clear and many prognostic factors overlap these categories. For example, performance status may be related to the tumor, or, when compromised due to coexistent illness, could be a host-related prognostic factor. Similarly, the quality of treatment is a host-related factor if it relates to patient compliance, but is usually an environment-related factor relating to access to optimal medical care. An example of a prognostic factor that fits into all the subject-based categories is anemia[32] and all three could apply to the same patient. Anemia may be a direct result of the presence of tumor mass,

TABLE 2.4 Examples of Environment Related Prognostic Factors

	Related to		
	Treatment	Education	Quality
Physician	Choice of physician or specialty • Quality of diagnosis • Accuracy of staging Choice of treatment Expertise of physician, "narrow experts" Timeliness of treatment Ageism	Ignorance of medical profession Access to internet Knowledge, education of the patient Participation in clinical trials Participation in continuing education	Quality of treatment Skill of the physician Treatment verification
Healthcare system	Access to appropriate diagnostic methods Access to care • Distance • Waiting Lists • Monopoly control of access to care Availability of publicly funded screening programs	Continuing medical education Lack of audit of local results Access to internet Development of practice guidelines Dissemination of new knowledge	Quality of equipment Quality management in treatment facility Maintenance of health records Availability of universal health insurance Quality of diagnostic services Implementation of screening programs Promotion of error free environment
Society	Preference for unconventional therapies Socioeconomic status Distance from cancer center Insurance status Access to transportation, car, etc. Ageism	Literacy Access to information	Access to affordable health insurance Nutritional status of the population

as in superficial bladder cancer or cervix uteri cancer, because of persistent heavy bleeding. It may also be a host factor, as in a patient with thalassemia or anemia of chronic disease from an unrelated condition. However, in some parts of the world, as an *environmental* prognostic factor, anemia also may be a result of malnutrition.

Several prognostic factors, each individually giving predictions with relatively low accuracy, can be combined to provide a single variable of high accuracy. Such a variable is called a *prognostic index*. Other examples include the International Lymphoma Prognostic Index (IPI)[33] or the Eastern Cooperative Oncology Group (ECOG) performance status scale.

Clinical-Relevance-Based Classification

To consider the relevance of prognostic factors in clinical practice, prognostic factors in this book are placed in three distinct categories: *essential, additional*, and *new and promising factors*. *Essential* factors are those that are fundamental to decisions about the goals and choice of treatment, and include details regarding the selection of treatment modality and specific interventions. In this edition, we have asked the authors to classify as *essential* exclusively those factors that are required to meet a published clinical practice guideline. This was not possible in all the cases, and as for the other parameters, some variation in the interpretation of the proposed *additional* factors allow finer prognostication, but are not an absolute requirement for treatment related decision-making processes. Their role is to communicate prognosis, but they do not in themselves influence treatment choice. Finally, our *new and promising factors* are those that shed new light about the biology of disease, or the prognosis for patients, but for which currently there is, at best, incomplete evidence of an independent effect on outcome or prognosis.

Essential Prognostic Factors   The fundamental factors required to make treatment decision is the type of cancer defined by histology or molecular tumor characteristics. The second most important group of essential factors reflects the anatomic disease extent. The latter has been recognized for over 75 years, when the first attempts at staging classifications were made. Currently, the UICC TNM[6] and the AJCC[34] serve to facilitate worldwide communication about cancer. Many other essential factors have been identified including pathology, tumor biology, tumor-related symptoms, patient age, performance status, newer imaging methods,[35–37] and tumor markers[38] are also integral to the decision-making process in the choice of a treatment modality.

Additional Prognostic Factors   In addition to the essential factors, there are numerous variables that help to define the outcome more precisely, but are not required for general decisions about treatment. These include more detailed histologic features, host-related factors, including comorbid conditions and vital organ function, which influence the suitability for surgery, chemotherapy, or radiotherapy. Environment-related factors, such as the choice of an inferior treatment plan, poor quality diagnostic tests, or treatments themselves have the potential to compromise the outcome. Management in a specialized unit,[39] for example, in breast and colorectal cancer, has resulted in improved survival in population-based studies.

New and Promising Prognostic Factors The immense and rapid expansion of molecular biology has provided an abundance of opportunities to study new biologic prognostic factors,[40,41] which hold promise for future applications. Molecular factors, such as epidermal growth factor receptor (EGFR) status,[42,43] may be used to predict response to a treatment modality, or may present a target for therapy, such as imatinib in gastrointestinal stromal tumors.[44] Alternatively, they may assist in treatment stratification, such as MGMT status, which predicts for chemotherapy and radiotherapy responsiveness in glioblastoma multiforme.[45] Another category includes factors that predict for the presence of occult distant metastases. A more detailed discussion on prognosis in molecular oncology can be found in Chapter 6.

A combination of the subject-based and clinical-relevance-based classifications can be used to summarize in simple terms the prognostic factors for individual cancers for a selected management scenario, as depicted in the Summary Table.

MANAGEMENT SCENARIOS: FREEZING THE PROGNOSIS

Since prognosis is a dynamic process affected not only by time, but also other factors, such as the disease and intervention, it is thus useful to apply the concept of a *management scenario*, which freezes the prognostic attributes that exist at a given time point, enabling one to then consider how prognosis is influenced by the choice of the planned intervention and the outcome of interest (Fig. 2.1).

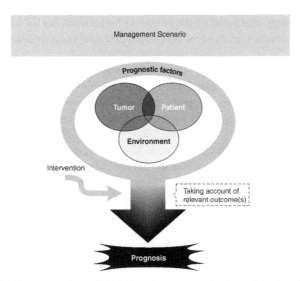

FIGURE 2.1 Representation of the interaction among the three domains of prognostic factors (tumor, host, and environment). The prognostic factors are expressed in the context of the proposed therapeutic intervention and for a given endpoint of interest (e.g., survival, response, local tumor control, organ preservation). In addition, the prognosis itself must be interpreted in the context of both the treatment (because it may change the prognosis) and the endpoint (which must be relevant to the prognosis).

For example, in *scenario 1* during a normal physical examination prior to lumpectomy, a patient is found to have a 2-cm breast cancer. Considering the overall survival as the outcome of interest, her prognosis equates to that of reported survival for clinical stage I breast cancer in her peer group (age, race, socioeconomic status) and in her geographic region. After the initial treatment is completed, the patient is in *scenario 2*. She has a pT1 pN0 tumor. Her prognosis is better than in scenario 1. She elects to be managed with partial mastectomy alone, her prognosis in scenario 2 is thus less favorable for local control than if she chose to have adjuvant radiation therapy. However, her prognosis for overall survival may not be affected by this decision. After some time, we can construct *scenario 3*. Thus, some years later she develops local recurrence and distant metastasis (scenario 3). Her prognosis for survival is now much worse than in previous scenarios. The progress of time may also affect positively the probability of survival.

Since the prognosis differs with a given scenario, prognostic factors should be considered within a given context or scenario, most commonly before a definitive treatment plan is formulated. Since treatment interventions also have a major impact on the outcome, it is important to discuss prognostic factors in the context of a specific treatment plan or therapeutic intervention.

ENDPOINTS RELEVANT TO CONSIDER IN CANCER PATIENTS

The relevant endpoints to consider in cancer include probability of cure, duration of survival, likelihood of response to treatment, probability of relapse, time to relapse, likelihood of local tumor control, likelihood of organ preservation, and possibility for symptom relief in a palliative context.[46] Therefore, the outcomes may be very heterogeneous. Moreover, some prognostic factors facilitate prediction of more than one outcome, while others predict selected outcomes only.

For example, the presence of bladder muscle wall invasion by a transitional cell carcinoma predicts for distant failure, while its absence virtually eliminates this probability. This knowledge permits clinicians to ignore the possibility of distant failure in patients with superficial bladder cancer both in diagnostic tests and therapeutic interventions. Another example is the number of involved nodal regions in stages I and II Hodgkin's disease that predict for risk of treatment failure, but not for survival. The number of tumors in superficial bladder cancer is predictive for recurrence, but has no impact on the overall survival.

Response to Treatment and Prognosis   Response to treatment is an outcome and as such it always reflects the prognosis. If a response to treatment had no impact on the outcome, such treatment by definition would be ineffective. However, since the knowledge of response is not available until after treatment is initiated, response should not be considered a prognostic factor for the scenario that preceded it.

Tumor response is an early endpoint in the assessment of treatment effectiveness. The four categories of response (complete response, partial response, stable disease, and progressive disease) were originally proposed by the World Health Organization

(WHO).[47] Although initially developed to assess the effects of drug therapy, these same criteria may easily be applied to the outcomes of surgical or radiotherapy interventions. For example, complete tumor resection with negative margins could be considered as a complete response to surgical intervention, while positive resection margins could be considered as a partial response to surgical intervention. Thus the extent of response is a surrogate for the anatomic extent of disease after the completion of therapy, and as such is a prognostic factor for further outcome. Since the knowledge of response is not available until after treatment is completed, it should not be considered a prognostic factor for the scenario that preceded it.

TAXONOMY: PROGNOSTIC FACTORS

In the English language, prediction, forecasting, and prognosis all indicate the probability of future events. In medical literature, however, the use of the terms, such as predictive, prognostic, and risk are being freely substituted for each other without much thought about consistent and accurate definitions.

In 1994, Burke[50] proposed that the general heading of *predictive factors* describe three subtypes: *a risk, a diagnostic*, and *a prognostic factor*. In his definition, a risk factor was a factor where the main outcome of interest was incidence and the predictive accuracy was <100%; the diagnostic factor was where the outcome of interest was the incidence and the predictive accuracy was almost 100% of disease. A prognostic factor was where the outcome of interest was death and the predictive accuracy was variable. This classification did not consider the temporal attributes of prediction and is associated with too narrow a view of relevant endpoint for patients with cancer. In epidemiological literature, a *risk factor* is defined as "a clearly defined occurrence or characteristic that has been associated with the increased rate of a subsequently occurring disease"; thus it is limited to patients who currently do not have a disease. In contrast, a *prognostic factor* refers to a probability of future event in patients who do currently have a disease.

Henderson and Patek[51] and others defined the term "predictive" as "prognosis for a measurable response" of overt tumor reduction following a treatment intervention and uses the term "predictive factor" as distinct from "prognostic" factor. The authors then consider a prognostic factor in the narrow context of a probability of cure or prolongation of survival. An example of a prognostic factor that is not a predictive factor is the number of involved axillary lymph nodes in breast cancer.[8] A high number of lymph nodes is associated with inferior survival, but the number of involved lymph nodes has no impact on response to treatment. In contrast, a factor that is both predictive and prognostic is the estrogen receptor status in breast cancer that predicts for response to hormonal therapy, but also prognosticates for a better survival. It is debatable whether such a distinction in terminology, which focuses on a single intermediate outcome (a measurable response to cytotoxic treatment) instead of defined endpoint relating to overall prognosis (e.g., local tumor control, survival), should be embraced.

Examples of clinical situations where response is not an indication for the use of treatment include: chemotherapy in an asymptomatic patient with Stage III follicular small-cell lymphoma; androgen deprivation therapy in an asymptomatic patient with T1 prostate cancer; and radiation therapy in stage IV Hodgkin's lymphoma.

Surrogate Diagnostic Factors versus Prognostic Factors   With better understanding of the mechanisms by which prognostic factors predict the future, new endpoints other than long-term survival have emerged. For example, the forecasting of the probability of occult distant metastasis allows for a better understanding of the pattern of failure and targeting of treatment efforts. Where the probability of the presence of occult metastatic disease at the time of diagnosis is concerned, however, these factors predict for the current state and not for a future event. Two examples of such factors are the PSA level[13] and the Gleason score in localized prostate cancer, which are considered as *prognostic* when survival or treatment failure probabilities are the endpoints of interest, but seen as *surrogate diagnostic factors* when they help discriminate different states at the present time. The reason is that they may help determine the probability of the presence of subclinical disease (e.g., disease lymph-node involvement) as an endpoint of interest.

Time-Dependent Prognostic Factors   Time-dependent prognostic factors are variables that become available over the time course of the patient's disease. While they may be very predictive of outcome, they are also problematic because they risk disturbing the context of relevant disease outcome evaluation and decision making.[52] This is because it may be impossible to separate real "causality" in the relationship between a time-dependent factor and an outcome of interest from a mere "association" caused by another factor common to them both. Therefore, if not undertaken carefully, the clinical interpretation of time-dependent prognostic factors may be incorrect. In some cases, prognostic factors associated with a subsequent scenario have been considered together with prognostic factors at diagnosis. For example, the postradiotherapy PSA nadir level has been included in Cox models of prognostic factors in localized prostate cancer. In truth, the PSA nadir is a surrogate for response to radiotherapy,[13] and as such belongs to a different management scenario occurring subsequently.

APPLICATION OF PROGNOSTIC FACTORS

Prognostic factors are used in daily clinical practice, in research, and in cancer control. In everyday clinical practice, the influence of prognostic factors dominates all the steps in decision making and the comprehensive management of patients with cancer, including selection of the primary goal of management, the most appropriate treatment modality, and the adjustment of treatment according to disease severity. Knowledge of prognostic factors allows clinicians to select treatment options that allow preservation of organs or function without compromising cure and survival.

The implementation of evidence-based clinical practice guidelines[53] will also serve to improve the quality of decision making and in turn the outcomes in cancer patients. It is thus necessary to know the prognostic factors in a relevant context in order to evaluate compliance with such guidelines to then examine their impact.

Prognostic Factors and Milieu

The prognostic factors that are defined as essential for decision making depend on their relevance to the issues in cancer care in a particular milieu, that is, the practice of cancer care in the first world or conversely in developing countries,[54] where the main issues are related to cancer prevention and early detection. Factors that predict for organ preservation and those that contribute to finesse in defining the prognosis may not be important in places with limited diagnostic equipment, and where funding for evaluation of assessment of response to treatment is not available. The milieu where the patient and healthcare professional are located thus impacts on the interplay of *essential, additional*, and *new and promising factors*. Moreover, progress in such situations does not require new discovery, but rather economic development, education, and a continued process to ensure improved access.

FUTURE RESEARCH INTO PROGNOSTIC FACTORS

To be relevant to the clinical practice, prognostic factors must either have a significant impact on cancer outcome, or be used to select treatment methods. It is likely that with progress in treatment, and improved outcomes, prognostic factors will be more relevant for selection of treatment. However, knowledge of prognostic factors is also required to minimize the impact of treatment. Improved staging methods, and especially more accurate characterization of microscopic disease extent will allow a more homogeneous grouping of patients with similar disease characteristics, and the tumor-related prognostic factors for an individual disease may change. Knowledge of genetic factors will further add to the improved prediction of outcome and greater individualization of therapeutic interventions. However, grouping of patients into similar categories will continue to be required to assess the impact of new technology of patient assessment and new therapies on the outcome.

■■■■■■ **SUMMARY TABLE**

Examples of Prognostic Factors in Cancer

Prognostic Factors	Tumor Related	Host Related	Environment Related
Essential	Anatomic disease extent Histologic type	Age	Availability of access to a radiotherapy facility
Additional	Tumor bulk Tumor marker level	Race Gender Cardiac function	Expertise of a surgeon
New and promising	EGFR (lung, head and neck) Gene expression patterns	Germline p53 mutation	Access to information

REFERENCES

1. Byar D: Identification of prognostic factors, in Buyse ME SM, Sylvester RJ (eds.): *Cancer clinical trials*. New York: Oxford University Press, 1984, pp. 423–443.

2. Gospodarowicz M, O'Sullivan B: Prognostic Factors: Principles and Application, in Gospodarowicz M, Henson DE, Hutter RVP, et al. (eds.): *Prognostic Factors in Cancer*. 2nd ed. New York; Wiley-Liss, 2001, pp. 17–36.

3. Stockler M, Tannock I: Guide to studies of diagnostic tests, prognostic factors, and treatments, in Tannock I, Hill, R. (eds.): *The basic science of oncology*, 3rd ed. Toronto; McGraw-Hill, 1998, pp. 466–492.

4. Riley RD, Abrams KR, Sutton AJ, et al.: Reporting of prognostic markers: current problems and development of guidelines for evidence-based practice in the future. *Br J Cancer* 88:1191–1198, 2003.

5. Gospodarowicz M, O'Sullivan, B, Bristow, et al.: Host, and Environment-related Prognostic Factors, in Gospodarowicz M, Henson DE, Hutter RVP et al. (eds.): *Prognostic Factors in Cancer*, 2nd ed. New York; Wiley-Liss, 2001, pp. 71–94.

6. Sobin LH WC: *TNM classification of malignant tumors*. 6th ed. New York; Wiley-Liss, 2002.

7. Schmoll HJ, Souchon R, Krege S, et al.: European consensus on diagnosis and treatment of germ cell cancer: a report of the European Germ Cell Cancer Consensus Group (EGC-CCG), *Ann Oncol* 15:1377–1399, 2004.

8. Truong PT, Berthelet E, Lee J, et al.: The prognostic significance of the percentage of positive/dissected axillary lymph nodes in breast cancer recurrence and survival in patients with one to three positive axillary lymph nodes. *Cancer* 103:2006–2014, 2005.

9. Compton CC: Colorectal carcinoma: diagnostic, prognostic, and molecular features. *Mod Pathol* 16:376–388, 2003.

10. Berglund M, Thunberg U, Amini RM, et al.: Evaluation of immunophenotype in diffuse large B-cell lymphoma and its impact on prognosis. *Mod Pathol* 18:1113–1120, 2005.

11. Baak JP, van Diest PJ, Voorhorst FJ, et al.: Prospective multicenter validation of the independent prognostic value of the mitotic activity index in lymph node-negative breast cancer patients younger than 55 years. *J Clin Oncol* 23:5993–6001, 2005.

12. Truong PT, Yong CM, Abnousi F, et al.: Lymphovascular invasion is associated with reduced locoregional control and survival in women with node-negative breast cancer treated with mastectomy and systemic therapy. *J Am Coll Surg* 200:912–921, 2005.

13. D'Amico AV, Renshaw AA, Sussman B, et al.: Pretreatment PSA velocity and risk of death from prostate cancer following external beam radiation therapy. *JAMA* 294:440–447, 2005.

14. Gorog D, Regoly-Merei J, Paku S, et al.: Alpha-fetoprotein expression is a potential prognostic marker in hepatocellular carcinoma. *World J Gastroenterol* 11:5015–5018, 2005.

15. Paramasivam S, Tripcony L, Crandon A, et al.: Prognostic importance of preoperative CA-125 in International Federation of Gynecology and Obstetrics stage I epithelial ovarian cancer: an Australian multicenter study. *J Clin Oncol* 23:5938–5942, 2005.

16. DiGiovanna MP, Stern DF, Edgerton SM, et al.: Relationship of epidermal growth factor receptor expression to ErbB-2 signaling activity and prognosis in breast cancer patients. *J Clin Oncol* 23:1152–1160, 2005.

17. Wang Y, Klijn JG, Zhang Y, et al.: Gene-expression profiles to predict distant metastasis of lymph-node-negative primary breast cancer. *Lancet* 365:671–679, 2005.

18. Buscarini M, Quek ML, Gill P, et al.: Molecular prognostic factors in bladder cancer. *BJU Int* 95:739–742, 2005.

19. Hurria A, Leung D, Trainor K, et al.: Factors influencing treatment patterns of breast cancer patients age 75 and older. *Crit Rev Oncol Hematol* 46:121–126, 2003.

20. Batevik R, Grong K, Segadal L, et al.: The female gender has a positive effect on survival independent of background life expectancy following surgical resection of primary non-small cell lung cancer: a study of absolute and relative survival over 15 years. *Lung Cancer* 47:173–181, 2005.

21. Chlebowski RT, Chen Z, Anderson GL, et al.: Ethnicity and breast cancer: factors influencing differences in incidence and outcome. *J Natl Cancer Inst* 97:439–448, 2005.

22. Maas HA, Kruitwagen RF, Lemmens VE, et al.: The influence of age and co-morbidity on treatment and prognosis of ovarian cancer: a population-based study. *Gynecol Oncol* 97:104–109, 2005.

23. Janssen-Heijnen ML, van Spronsen DJ, Lemmens VE, et al.: A population-based study of severity of comorbidity among patients with non-Hodgkin's lymphoma: prognostic impact independent of International Prognostic Index. *Br J Haematol* 129:597–606, 2005.

24. Straus DJ: Prognostic factors in the treatment of human immunodeficiency virus-associated non-Hodgkin's lymphoma. *Recent Results Cancer Res* 159:143–148, 2002.

25. Verkooijen HM, Fioretta GM, Rapiti E, et al.: Patients' refusal of surgery strongly impairs breast cancer survival. *Ann Surg* 242:276–280, 2005.

26. Cathcart CS, Dunican A, Halpern JN: Patterns of delivery of radiation therapy in an inner-city population of head and neck cancer patients: an analysis of compliance and end results. *J Med* 28:275–284, 1997.

27. Mackillop WJ, Zhang-Salomons J, Groome PA, et al.: Socioeconomic status and cancer survival in Ontario. *J Clin Oncol* 15:1680–1689, 1997.

28. Jemal A, Ward E, Wu X, et al.: Geographic patterns of prostate cancer mortality and variations in access to medical care in the United States. *Cancer Epidemiol Biomarkers Prev* 14:590–595, 2005.

29. Till JE, Phillips RA, Jadad AR: Finding Canadian cancer clinical trials on the Internet: an exploratory evaluation of online resources. *CMAJ* 168:1127–1129, 2003.

30. Freeman HP: Poverty, culture, and social injustice: determinants of cancer disparities. *CA Cancer J Clin* 54:72–77, 2004.

31. Sauven P, Bishop H, Patnick J, et al.: The National Health Service Breast Screening Programme and British Association of Surgical Oncology audit of quality assurance in breast screening 1996–2001. *Br J Surg* 90:82–87, 2003.

32. Munstedt K, Johnson P, Bohlmann MK, et al.: Adjuvant radiotherapy in carcinomas of the uterine cervix: the prognostic value of hemoglobin levels. *Int J Gynecol Cancer* 15:285–291, 2005.

33. Hermans J, Krol AD, van Groningen K, et al.: International Prognostic Index for aggressive non-Hodgkin's lymphoma is valid for all malignancy grades. *Blood* 86:1460–1463, 1995.

34. *AJCC Cancer Staging Manual.* 6th ed.: Springer-Verlag, 2002.

35. Borst GR, Belderbos JS, Boellaard R, et al.: Standardised FDG uptake: a prognostic factor for inoperable non-small cell lung cancer. *Eur J Cancer* 41:1533–1541, 2005.

36. Hutchings M, Mikhaeel NG, Fields PA, et al.: Prognostic value of interim FDG-PET after two or three cycles of chemotherapy in Hodgkin lymphoma. *Ann Oncol* 16:1160–1168, 2005.

37. Jackson AS, Parker CC, Norman AR, et al.: Tumor staging using magnetic resonance imaging in clinically localised prostate cancer: relationship to biochemical outcome after neo-adjuvant androgen deprivation and radical radiotherapy. *Clin Oncol (R Coll Radiol)* 17:167–171, 2005.

38. Lam JS, Shvarts O, Leppert JT, et al.: Renal cell carcinoma 2005: new frontiers in staging, prognostication and targeted molecular therapy. *J Urol* 173:1853–1862, 2005.

39. Smith ER, Butler WE, Barker FG, 2nd: Craniotomy for resection of pediatric brain tumors in the United States, 1988 to 2000: effects of provider caseloads and progressive centralization and specialization of care. *Neurosurgery* 54:553–563; discussion 56 3–555, 2004.

40. Poon RT, Fan ST, Wong J: Clinical significance of angiogenesis in gastrointestinal cancers: a target for novel prognostic and therapeutic approaches. *Ann Surg* 238:9–28, 2003.

41. Russo A, Bazan V, Iacopetta B, et al.: The TP53 Colorectal Cancer International Collaborative Study on the Prognostic and Predictive Significance of p53 Mutation: Influence of Tumor Site, Type of Mutation, and Adjuvant Treatment. *J Clin Oncol* 23:7518–7528, 2005.

42. Shepherd FA, Rodrigues Pereira J, Ciuleanu T, et al.: Erlotinib in previously treated non-small-cell lung cancer. *N Engl J Med* 353:123–132, 2005.

43. Bentzen SM, Atasoy BM, Daley FM, et al.: Epidermal growth factor receptor expression in pretreatment biopsies from head and neck squamous cell carcinoma as a predictive factor for a benefit from accelerated radiation therapy in a randomized controlled trial. *J Clin Oncol* 23:5560–5567, 2005.

44. Van Glabbeke M, Verweij J, Casali PG, et al.: Initial and late resistance to imatinib in advanced gastrointestinal stromal tumors are predicted by different prognostic factors: a European Organisation for Research and Treatment of Cancer-Italian Sarcoma Group-Australasian Gastrointestinal Trials Group study. *J Clin Oncol* 23:5795–5804, 2005.

45. Hegi ME, Diserens AC, Gorlia T, et al.: MGMT gene silencing and benefit from temozolomide in glioblastoma. *N Engl J Med* 352:997–1003, 2005.

46. Toscani P, Brunelli C, Miccinesi G, et al.: Predicting survival in terminal cancer patients: clinical observation or quality-of-life evaluation? *Palliat Med* 19:220–227, 2005.

47. *WHO handbook for reporting results of cancer treatment*, Geneva: World Health Organization Offset Publication, 1979.

48. Zagars GK, Ballo MT, Pisters PW, et al.: Surgical margins and reresection in the management of patients with soft tissue sarcoma using conservative surgery and radiation therapy. *Cancer* 97:2544–2553, 2003.

49. Smitt MC, Nowels K, Carlson RW, et al.: Predictors of reexcision findings and recurrence after breast conservation. *Int J Radiat Oncol Biol Phys* 57:979–985, 2003.

50. Burke HB: Increasing the power of surrogate endpoint biomarkers: the aggregation of predictive factors. *J Cell Biochem Suppl* 19:278–282, 1994.

51. Henderson IC, Patek AJ: The relationship between prognostic and predictive factors in the management of breast cancer. *Breast Cancer Res Treat* 52:261–288, 1998.

52. McShane LM, Altman DG, Sauerbrei W, et al.: Reporting recommendations for tumor marker prognostic studies (REMARK). *J Natl Cancer Inst* 97:1180–1184, 2005.

53. Woolf SH: Evidence-based medicine and practice guidelines: an overview. *Cancer Control* 7:362–367, 2000.

54. Magrath I, Shanta V, Advani S, et al.: Treatment of acute lymphoblastic leukaemia in countries with limited resources; lessons from use of a single protocol in India over a twenty year period. *Eur J Cancer* 41:1570–1583, 2005.

CHAPTER 3

Studies Investigating Prognostic Factors: Conduct and Evaluation

DOUGLAS G. ALTMAN

Prognostic markers can help to identify patients with different risks of specific outcomes, facilitate treatment choice, and aid patient counseling. They may be simple measures, such as stage of disease or tumor size, but are often more complex, such as abnormal levels of proteins or genetic mutations. Most prognostic marker studies include assessments of the association of one or more markers with overall survival or disease-free survival. While these studies often explore several factors simultaneously, many examine the prognostic importance of a single specified tumor marker. Some studies examine in particular the ability of markers to predict outcome of patients receiving a particular treatment, so-called predictive markers.

This chapter considers studies of single prognostic and predictive markers both from the perspective of how best to carry out such studies and how to appraise published research articles. Many of the issues discussed do, however, also apply to prognostic studies more broadly, such as exploratory studies of many possible factors and studies that aim to develop a prognostic model (risk score).

THE PROGNOSTIC LITERATURE

Prognostic markers are widely studied in cancer. Each year many thousands of studies are published assessing the association of one or more markers with patient prognosis, usually overall survival or disease-free survival. How useful are all these studies?

For each cancer, many markers have been studied. For example, a review of the literature for neuroblastoma found that 130 different markers had been investigated in 211 studies, with a median of one publication per marker.[1] For more common cancers,

Prognostic Factors in Cancer, *Third Edition*, edited by Mary K. Gospodarowicz, Brian O'Sullivan, and Leslie H. Sobin.
Copyright © 2006 John Wiley & Sons, Inc.

such as in the breast or colon, there is a very large literature and even more markers have been investigated.[2] Yet large numbers of studies do not necessarily bring the hoped for resolution of uncertainty. The authors of a review of p53 overexpression as a possible prognostic marker in bladder cancer found 168 publications from 117 studies including >10,000 patients, yet were unable to reach a clear conclusion: "After 10 years of research, evidence is not sufficient to conclude whether changes in p53 act as markers of outcome in patients with bladder cancer."[3]

Although there are a few notable exceptions, including estrogen receptor status and c-erbB-2 for breast cancer[4] and prostate specific antigen (PSA) for prostate cancer, overall this major research effort has as yet yielded rather little across all cancers.[5–7] One important reason for this unfortunate situation is the poor methodological quality of many studies, as discussed later in this chapter. In addition, when there are several published studies for a single marker, their results are frequently conflicting. Inconsistent findings may be due to variation in some or all of patient characteristics, laboratory methods, and statistical methods. In addition, there is considerable chance variability because such studies tend to be much smaller than they need to be to provide reliable results. While small studies are not in principle problematic (i.e., biased), they are a major concern because evidence is accumulating that smaller studies are less likely to be published if they have nonsignificant results (i.e., the literature is distorted by "publication bias").[8]

Unfortunately, methodological issues are compounded by the generally poor standard of reporting in published articles, seriously impeding efforts to make sense of the literature.[9] Recent guidelines (REMARK) are intended to improve quality and completeness of reporting of prognostic studies in cancer.[10]

The following sections review aspects of some of the key elements of the REMARK guidelines relating to study design, data analysis, and interpretation of studies of single markers. There follows a discussion of reporting prognostic studies. This chapter draws on reviews of published prognostic studies[9,11–13] and previous discussion articles.[14–20]

STUDY DESIGN

For all types of research, it is strongly advisable to develop a detailed study protocol specifying objectives and key aspects of how the study will be done, covering in particular study design, laboratory methods, data to be collected, and methods for statistical analysis. Such considerations are just as appropriate for a retrospective as a prospective study and should not be linked only to the need to secure funding. The following sections consider some of the most important aspects in more detail.

Study Objectives

Studies of a particular possibly prognostic marker can be carried out for various reasons and with varying aims. The literature would be easier to assess if there was a standard way of classifying studies as there is for clinical trials, and a classification for prognostic studies proposed by Altman and Lyman[15] is shown in Table 3.1. A particularly

TABLE 3.1   Types of prognostic marker studies[15]

Phase I

Exploratory studies (hypothesis generating) that seek an association between a prognostic marker and characteristics of disease thought to have prognostic importance.

Phase II

Exploratory studies attempting to use values of a prognostic marker to:
(a) discriminate between patients at high and low risk of disease progression or death; or to
(b) indicate which subsets of patients are likely to benefit from therapy.

Phase III

Confirmatory studies of *a priori* hypotheses attempting to use values of a prognostic marker to
(a) discriminate between patients at high and low risk of disease progression or death; or to
(b) indicate which subsets of patients are likely to benefit from therapy.

critical distinction is between Phase II studies, which are exploratory studies seeking evidence of relation to patient outcome (possibly in relation to treatment), and Phase III studies, which are confirmatory studies testing hypotheses developed from Phase II studies. There is nothing wrong with exploratory research. Many of the problems in the literature arise, however, from researchers conducting Phase II studies and interpreting them as if they had been Phase III. It is not possible to get reliable answers that way. Investigators may then compound the problems by basing their interpretation on just their own data rather than putting their study into the context of the available literature. The best way to address uncertainty in the literature is to review all the evidence.[21]

Researchers should consider carefully what type of prognostic study they are planning. The primary objectives, as well as any secondary questions, should be stated precisely in advance of the study. Prespecification helps to focus the study and also helps to avoid the adverse effects of multiple testing associated with unspecified or untargeted searches of the data.

Prognostic studies are observational and so provide evidence that is inherently less reliable than randomized trials. Nonetheless, there is a strong case for making every effort to limit potential biases and to emulate the design standards of a randomized trial to the extent possible. Thus, for example, prognostic studies will be much stronger if they have attributes such as clearly defined inclusion criteria for patients, standardized laboratory methods for the whole sample, high quality data, complete follow up, and so on.

Sample Selection

A reliable prognostic study ideally requires a well-defined "inception" cohort of patients at the same stage of their disease, commonly at the time of first diagnosis of cancer. Apart from stage of cancer there may be additional selection criteria, such as age while exclusion criteria might include prior cancer or nonstandard treatment. Eligible patients should not be excluded because of missing data or loss to follow up. Rather, they should be included in the study cohort and if necessary excluded from analyses.

Patients should not be sampled in relation to their survival experience (e.g., taking only patients with either very short or very long survival) as this sampling strategy leads to bias.[22] Only unselected cases or random samples from a given population will produce unbiased survival estimates.

In prospective studies, eligible patients are enrolled, complete baseline measurements are made in a standardized way, and they are followed for an adequate length of time to allow a comparison of survival experience in relation to baseline tumor marker values. Some randomized trials sensibly incorporate the collection of tumor markers for prognostic studies; otherwise prospective studies are rare.

While prospective studies are the ideal, the large majority of prognostic studies in cancer are necessarily retrospective, using existing clinical data possibly combined with new assay results based on analysis of stored tissue samples. Such studies have the considerable advantage of the ready availability of a cohort with a long enough follow up for assessment of a substantial number of outcome events (e.g., deaths or recurrences). Their main disadvantage is the lower quality of the data: the cohort may not be complete, measurements may not be standardized, and baseline data may be incomplete. Also, treatments given to patients may vary, with the choice of treatment partly related to prognostic information under study.

Sample Size

Sample size specification and power calculations seem to have received little attention in many prognostic studies, perhaps because they are usually performed on preexisting data sets. Yet adequate sample size is as important here as for other types of research.

Several authors have addressed the issue of sample size for prognostic studies.[23-27] The calculations for survival time outcomes can be complex, with the need to consider, among other things, the length of follow up, the number of expected events, and the likely loss to follow up, as well as the size of effect being sought. Use of specialist statistical software is recommended (preferably by means of seeking expert advice from a statistician), but simple approaches to sample size estimation have been described.[25,28] In particular, sample size calculations can be simplified by considering the power to detect a specified outcome difference at a fixed point in time, such as the 2 year survival rate.

An important consideration is that the power of a study with time-to-event data depends on the number of observed events not the number of patients. Thus a small sample with long follow up may well yield better information than a large study with short follow up. It follows that a study will have less power to investigate rarer endpoints; in the present context, this means that there is more power to investigate recurrence than death.

Published prognostic studies are often rather small.[1,3] For example, a systematic review of studies of p53 and bladder cancer found that the studies were generally far too small even to have adequate statistical power to detect a (quite large) hazard ratio of 2.[3]

When several variables are investigated, as in many exploratory (Phase II) studies, there are additional considerations. The sample size needs to be large enough to override the problems of multiple comparisons in the selection of variables and the comparison of models, issues discussed below. A commonly applied rule of thumb is that the data set should include at least 10 outcome events per candidate variable.

For phase III studies, the aim should not be primarily to achieve statistical significance (i.e., $p < 0.05$), but rather to obtain a reasonably precise estimate of the magnitude of the effect. If a study is confirmatory of the prognostic importance of the variable, it needs to do so reliably. Likewise, if a study fails to confirm the prognostic importance in previous studies, it needs to do so unambiguously. Confirmatory studies should therefore be considerably larger than earlier exploratory studies. While a large sample size is desirable and will increase precision, it cannot help overcome deficiencies in the completeness of data or the relevance of the study.

Predictive factor studies seek evidence that a prognostic factor is predictive of the patient's outcome after a specified treatment. This question requires comparison of the prognostic impact of the marker in groups who did and did not receive the specified treatment. As such, the analysis is one of interaction and a standard statistical result is that the sample size needs to be about four times as large as a conventional prognostic study for the equivalent statistical power. It is perhaps not surprising that convincing evidence of predictive factors is rare.

Quality of Measurements

Clinical investigators should be aware of the properties of assays for the markers they are investigating. Accurate and precise measurement of the values of prognostic markers may not always be possible. Measurement error is very important because it will lead to underestimation of the value of a prognostic marker and so will reduce the power of a study to detect a real prognostic effect. In addition, different assays for measuring a marker may differ systematically from one another. Studies comparing different assay methods provide important background information to prognostic studies.[29]

Some assessments necessarily incorporate subjectivity and so there may also be variation between observers. An example is microvessel counts in studies of tumor angiogenesis.[30] In such cases, it could be useful to take the average of two or three readings, as reduction of measurement error will increase the power of the study, and hence the reliability of the findings. A similar difficulty applies to the assessment of the histologic and nuclear grade of breast malignancies, indicating the desirability of using single reviewers or reference laboratories to reduce between observer variability.

Selection of Variables

When examining the prognostic importance of one or more markers it will generally be necessary also to collect information about the patient (demographic and clinical characteristics), the tumor, and the treatment received. It is important to ascertain the extent to which tumor markers are associated with other characteristics (including known prognostic variables) and to take account of other factors when investigating the relation to outcome (patient prognosis).

For retrospective studies, the variables that are available will depend on what has been routinely collected over several years. Key information may thus be missing completely, available only after a certain date, or recorded incompletely. By contrast, in prospective studies, often randomized trials, the investigators can specify the important baseline variables, and it is likely that they will be available for almost all patients.

In general, the prognostic importance of a marker is considered in relation to other information available at baseline (i.e., at the start of the period of follow up) as described below. It is incorrect to include in conventional regression models variables (covariates) not known at that time, such as compliance with therapy, tumor response, or change in marker over time. Events observed after the start of the follow-up period should be considered as outcomes, not as explanatory variables.[31]

Patient Outcomes

The most common outcomes studied in prognostic evaluations of tumor markers are death from any cause (often called overall survival), cancer death, and some variant of the notion of disease recurrence. Of these, only all-cause mortality is completely objective. Cancer death may be preferred, as among older patients there could be a considerable number of deaths from other causes. Recurrence is frequently studied. It has the statistical advantage of being more common, and hence giving a study greater power, but suffers from variation in definition. Many studies consider the relation of tumor markers with the risk of both recurrence and death.

ANALYSIS

Basic Principles

The association of a marker with known prognostic variables, such as stage of cancer, is often considered first. While a correlation does imply that the marker is likely to be related to prognosis, a strong correlation may suggest that it is not likely to add anything new.

The main analysis will consider whether the new marker is prognostic and whether it adds meaningfully to the prognostic value of existing factors. These questions are addressed by univariate and multivariate analyses, respectively. Analysis of the association with patient outcome requires use of methods designed for time-to-event data. Because of censoring (the nonobservation of the event of interest after a period of follow up) a proportion of the survival times of interest will usually be unknown. The analysis assumes that those patients whose observation times are censored at a certain time have the same survival prospects as those who continue to be followed; that is, the censoring is unrelated to prognosis. Many books[32,33] and journal articles[34–37] describe the rationale for and illustrate various methods of analysis and give much more information than can be included here. Input from a statistician is advisable for all but the simplest analyses.

Univariate and multivariate analysis will now be considered in turn, followed by consideration of problems associated with continuous variables, missing data, and multiplicity.

Univariate Analysis

In a univariate analysis, the outcome of interest (e.g., time to death) is compared for groups with different values of the tumor marker. The most common methods for analyzing single variables are Kaplan–Meier survival curves and logrank tests.

It is customary in cancer studies to show the data graphically using Kaplan–Meier (cumulative) survival curves, but it may be more helpful to show cumulative incidence curves especially when events are rare.[37,38] The logrank test is the most widely used method of comparing two or more survival curves, which yields a p value for the null hypothesis of no relation between the marker and survival.

Kaplan–Meier curves and logrank tests require values of a variable to be grouped. As noted below, it is preferable to have more than two groups. It is also possible to avoid grouping and keep the variable continuous by using a univariate version of regression analysis, described in the next section. That analysis has the advantage of being directly comparable to the results from the multivariate analysis, both in how the variable was handled and also in providing a hazard ratio associated with different levels of the tumor marker. However, a hazard ratio can also be obtained using the values obtained when performing a logrank test, and it is certainly desirable to produce an estimate of prognostic strength in addition to the p value from the test.[37]

While univariate analysis is of interest, knowing that a marker is associated with patient prognosis is of limited use. Much more important is whether it adds usefully to what is already known—does it provide prognostic information beyond that from known prognostic variables? To answer that question we need a more complex analysis.

Multivariate Analysis

A multivariable analysis considers whether a tumor marker has an additional (independent) effect when other variables are taken into consideration. This analysis serves to identify a set of variables all of which may be considered to be prognostic for the cancer in question, and also forms the basis for a prognostic model and the creation of a risk score or risk groups.

The most common method for multivariate analysis is Cox (proportional hazards) regression. That method is called semiparametric as no assumption is made about the distribution of the survival times. As its name suggests, the method assumes that the relative risk of the event in two groups remains constant at all times of follow up. The quantity called "risk" here is the hazard, which is related to, but not the same as the survival probability: The hazard ratio is the ratio of the rates at which people have the event in the two groups.[39] Alternative, fully parametric methods exist for analysis survival data[35,36]; they should probably be used rather more often.

Regression models yield a set of variables all of which are statistically significant and thus, seemingly important. In fact, variables are usually incorporated into a regression model when they meet the criterion of $p < 0.05$. Variables that only just achieve this criterion are unlikely to be especially important.

In multivariate analysis, the marker of interest is included in a multiple regression model along with other variables. How should these variables be chosen? As noted above, prognostic studies are often exploratory and so the variables considered in such an analysis generally include both those known *a priori* to be prognostic in this disease and others where such evidence is lacking. A common approach to analysis is to use a variable selection algorithm, most often "stepwise selection", to reduce the set of candidate variables to a subset of "important" ones. This simple idea invokes several difficulties, however.

An important criticism of using stepwise selection methods to develop a model is that because of the play of chance important variables may fail to be detected, and conversely the chosen model may include variables that are not truly prognostic. Also, the results will tend to be overoptimistic because the best model is being selected from a large number of possibilities. Both of these problems are especially likely in small studies. An important additional analysis for a new marker is thus to consider its prognostic ability in a model together with all previously defined prognostic variables (e.g., age, stage, performance status) regardless of whether those variables happen to be statistically significant in the current data set. Such an analysis is not often seen, but it should be routinely presented.[10]

Predictive factors can be investigated in much the same way, but additionally a term needs to be added to the model indicating the interaction between the marker and treatment received. It is not sufficient to show that the marker is associated with outcome in a cohort of patients receiving a particular treatment. To distinguish a predictive marker from a prognostic marker it is necessary to show that the marker predicts response to that particular treatment by comparison with other treatments.

From a regression model, a risk score can be constructed, which is a weighted combination of the numerical values of the variables in the model (the regression coefficients are the weights). Those scores may be grouped to create, say, three or four risk groups that may help to inform clinical decision making. But before a prognostic model (or risk groups derived from it) is used to inform clinical decisions, it is important to assess how well it predicts. While the fit of the model to the original data can be explored,[24,35] the only reliable way to assess the performance of a regression model is to evaluate it on a completely new data set, in a so-called "validation" study.[40] Because of various aspects of selection from multiple possibilities in the modeling process, the apparent importance of a marker may be illusory and not all such findings survive evaluation in further studies.

In time, many studies may be published looking at the same marker, and so a meta-analysis of these should lead to a more reliable answer than could be derived from a single study.[21] However, meta-analysis may not provide a clear answer; those studies may be heterogeneous in study methods and may have methodological flaws. In addition, it is likely that not all conducted studies have been published. Such "publication bias" is discussed below.

Handling Continuous Variables

Although we usually expect risk to increase or decrease consistently as the level of a marker increases, many researchers prefer to divide patients into high- and low-risk groups. Patients are often divided into two equal groups by splitting at the median value, but there is no *a priori* reason to suppose that half of the patients are at higher risk.[41,42] While not incorrect, dichotomization discards a considerable amount of information and seems foolhardy when studies are generally too small in the first place.

Some investigators wish to determine the cut-point for a new marker that best distinguishes risk groups. They address the cut-point problem by computing a statistical significance level for all possible cut-points, and then selecting the cut-point with the smallest significance level. This "optimal cutpoint" approach is deeply problematic and the results may be completely misleading. The true type I error (false positive) rate for this procedure is close to 40% rather than the nominal 5%.[43] Further, because the binary variable based on the selected cut-point is used in subsequent multiple regression analyses involving that factor, the bias is transferred to that analysis and the marker will receive undue weight in the analysis. The regression coefficients and p values are all biased because the cut-point was preselected using the same data. No reliable information can come from a data-based choice of cutpoint, and such studies may also contaminate the results of subsequent meta-analyses. If it is really necessary to create two groups then a cut-point reported from other studies or the sample median (or some other centile) can be used without introducing bias.

While it may be convenient to group the patients into risk groups, categorizing a variable discards information, especially if only two groups are created. The use of several categories is preferable as it retains more information and allows some idea of how the risk varies across the range of values of the marker.[34,44] An alternative approach is to evaluate prognostic importance without introducing any cut-points at all.[42] Representing the marker as a continuous variable has the considerable advantage of retaining all the information, but many researchers are rightly unhappy to assume that the relation with outcome is linear (i.e., the risk, measured by the log hazard ratio, increases linearly as the variable increases). The assumption of linearity can be tested, but unfortunately the conventional use of an additional quadratic term in the model is not always satisfactory. Newer methods of regression splines[45,46] or fractional polynomial models[47] can be used effectively for this purpose. These approaches give a reliable assessment of the nature of the relation between values of the marker and risk, and so provide valuable information about how patient outcome varies with level of the marker. Cut-points, if needed, can then be defined.

Multiplicity

When multiple statistical assessments are made in a study, the chance of obtaining a "significant" result is increased, and the risk of a false-positive finding increases. For example, if 20 unimportant markers are assessed then, by chance, we would expect one marker to be wrongly deemed "significant" at the conventional 5% significance level. Developing a regression model by choosing the best predictors from a larger set of candidate variables, as is commonly done, may yield overoptimistic results. Small, underpowered studies are particularly at risk of overly optimistic reported effect sizes and significance levels due to the multiple testing inherent in stepwise variable selection. As already discussed, choosing cutpoints for one or more variables based on the data will increase the problem considerably, and the problems are further exacerbated by selective reporting, as discussed below.

One consequence of the optimism associated with selection from many analyses is that the promise of many apparently prognostic markers fails to be supported by further studies.[48]

Missing Data

Prognostic studies generally require data on many patient and tumor characteristics, including the markers being investigated. It is not usually possible to get complete data for all patients, especially with the retrospective design that is typical when investigating prognosis. The importance of missing data is not widely appreciated. Even when the amount of missing data is not great for any variable, the proportion of patients with full data can be quite low and multivariable analysis will be based on a considerably reduced sample. Further, observations are unlikely to be missing at random and so the results may be biased. As an example, prostate cancer patients without a p53 determination had a significantly worse survival than those who had one. Strategies for coping with missing data have been discussed.[49,50] An option of increasing interest is to impute (estimate) the missing data.[49]

Analysis of time to event data (survival analysis) allows inclusion of all patients up to the time when they are lost to follow up. Thus incompleteness of the data is hidden, unlike the case with a binary or continuous outcome. A simple measure is available that is useful to indicate the completeness of a data set.[51]

REPORTING A PROGNOSTIC STUDY

Unfortunately, in addition to the methodological problems just outlined, many published articles describing tumor marker studies have not been reported adequately: they often lack sufficient information to allow a full appreciation of the methods used, assessment of the methodological quality of the study, or the generalizability of the study results.[11,26] Indeed, the study results themselves may well also be reported inadequately.[3,9] Such reporting deficiencies are increasingly being highlighted by systematic reviews of the published literature.[1,3,9]

The considerations addressed in the preceding sections and the literature cited heavily influenced the content of recent REMARK guidelines for reporting studies of tumor markers shown in Table 3.2.[10] Other, more specialized guidance has been published. For example, guidelines have been presented for reporting prognostic studies with missing covariate data.[13] Adherence to these recommendations would greatly improve the literature on markers in the future.

TABLE 3.2   Reporting Recommendations for Tumor Marker Prognostic Studies (REMARK)

Introduction

1. State the marker examined, the study objectives, and any prespecified hypotheses.

Materials and Methods

PATIENTS

2. Describe the characteristics (e.g., disease stage, comorbidities) of the study patients, including their source and inclusion and exclusion criteria.
3. Describe treatments received and how chosen (e.g., randomized, rule based).

SPECIMEN CHARACTERISTICS

4. Describe type of biological material used (including control samples), and methods of preservation and storage.

ASSAY METHODS

5. Specify the assay method used and provide (or reference) a detailed protocol, including specific reagents or kits used, quality control procedures, reproducibility assessments, quantitation methods, and scoring and reporting protocols. Specify whether and how assays were performed blinded to the study endpoint.

STUDY DESIGN

6. State the method of case selection, including whether prospective or retrospective and whether stratification or matching (e.g., by stage of disease, age) was used. Specify the time period from which cases were taken, the end of the follow-up period, and the median follow-up time.
7. Precisely define all clinical endpoints examined.
8. List all candidate variables initially examined or considered for inclusion in models.
9. Give rationale for sample size; if the study was designed to detect a specified effect size, give the target power and effect size.

STATISTICAL ANALYSIS METHODS

10. Specify all statistical methods, including details of any variable selection procedures and other model-building issues, how model assumptions were verified, and how missing data were handled.
11. Clarify how marker values were handled in the analyses; if relevant, describe methods used for cutpoint determination.

(Continued)

TABLE 3.1 *(Continued)*

Results

DATA

12. Describe the flow of patients through the study, including the number of patients included in each stage of the analysis (a diagram may be helpful) and reasons for dropout. Specifically, both overall and for each subgroup extensively examined report the numbers of patients and the number of events.

13. Report distributions of basic demographic characteristics (at least age and sex), standard (disease-specific) prognostic variables, and tumor marker, including numbers of missing values.

ANALYSIS AND PRESENTATION

14. Show the relation of the marker to standard prognostic variables.

15. Present univariate analyses showing the relation between the marker and outcome, with the estimated effect (e.g., hazard ratio, survival probability). Preferably provide similar analyses for all other variables being analyzed. For the effect of a tumor marker on a time-to-event outcome, a Kaplan–Meier plot is recommended.

16. For key multivariate analyses, report estimated effects (e.g., hazard ratio) with confidence intervals for the marker and, at least for the final model, all other variables in the model.

17. Among reported results, provide estimated effects with confidence intervals from an analysis in which the marker and standard prognostic variables are included, regardless of their statistical significance.

18. If done, report results of further investigations, such as checking assumptions, sensitivity analyses, and internal validation.

Discussion

19. Interpret the results in the context of the pre-specified hypotheses and other relevant studies, include a discussion of limitations of the study.

20. Discuss implications for future research and clinical value.

Source: Reference 10.

Publication Bias

Small studies will yield unreliable results. Some will show small, nonsignificant effects and others will show larger, significant effects. Preferential publication of statistically significant findings, known as publication bias, is a well-recognized phenomenon for randomized trials. It seems certain that this bias affects prognostic studies too. Selective reporting of statistically significant tumor marker studies would lead to larger effects being seen in smaller studies, and the literature would be biased toward overestimating the prognostic importance of tumor markers. As Simon wrote: "… the literature is probably cluttered with false-positive studies that would not have been submitted or published if the results had come out differently".[17]

Evidence is accumulating of publication bias in prognostic studies. For example, in a systematic review of studies of Bcl2 in nonsmall cell lung cancer, almost all the smaller studies showed a statistically significant relationship between Bcl2 and risk of dying, with large hazard ratios, whereas the three large studies were all nonsignificant and showed a much smaller effect.[52] A recent review of the prognostic importance of TP53 status in head and neck cancer showed clearly that published studies had larger effects than unpublished studies.[8]

Publication bias distorts the medical literature leading to erroneous, inflated assessments of the prognostic importance of tumor markers. If the value of the literature is to improve there is a clear need for fewer, larger, better studies, preferably prospective, with results published regardless of the findings.

DISCUSSION

Loi et al.[53] suggested that the two most crucial questions for the oncologist today are "who to treat" and "how to treat each individual". Prognostic studies offer the potential to help answer both these important questions, but there are many difficulties in obtaining reliable information about tumor markers.[54] Those difficulties are well illustrated by the increasing numbers of systematic reviews of the published literature; these may fail to produce a clear message despite >100 published studies to consider.[1,3]

Prognostic research is becoming of increasing importance with a more direct impact on clinical practice and clinical trials than in the past. Getting reliable information about the prognostic strength of tumor markers is certainly not easy, however, as is illustrated by the preceding discussion. Unfortunately, many investigations are too small, poorly designed and analyzed, and incorrectly interpreted. Greater attention is needed especially in the planning and analysis of such studies.

In order to provide valid and clinically useful results, more prognostic factor studies should be planned and conducted as confirmatory investigations with prespecified hypotheses and consideration given to limiting and controlling problems of multiplicity. When studies are not conducted in that way, they should be clearly identified as exploratory (Phase I or II) investigations that require confirmation (Phase III studies). Stepwise regression analysis and cutpoints for continuous measures should be handled with care and preferably avoided. Interaction tests should be provided to support claims that the effect of treatment or a marker varies among subsets of patients or that a marker is predictive of response to a particular treatment. The p values should not be used as the sole statistical summary. Confidence intervals should be used when reporting results.

Studies of poor quality obscure rather than clarify the picture regarding the prognostic importance of tumor markers. As with randomized trials, reliable conclusions about a marker are more likely to arise from large, carefully designed, possibly collaborative, confirmatory phase III studies than from a series of undersized studies using a variety of laboratory and statistical methodology and clinical inclusion criteria. If sound scientific principles of careful study design, adequate study size, scrupulous data collection and documentation, and appropriate analysis strategies are not adhered to, the field will flounder. The necessity of large, definitive prospective studies or prospectively planned meta-analyses for tumor marker research must be recognized.[55]

In addition, the reporting of prognostic studies must be improved. The recent REMARK guidelines[10] present a framework for reporting studies and also for reviewers and editors to assess submitted manuscripts. Adherence to these guidelines should greatly assist readers to judge what was done and the reliability of the findings.

Finally, this chapter has focused on acquiring reliable information about specific tumor markers. As noted, even data on thousands of patients may not always lead to clear conclusions. In recent years, microarray technology has allowed researchers to investigate thousands of markers on <100 patients. While microarray studies hold much promise, it should be evident that a single study of that type cannot be expected to come up with a definitive answer about which markers are prognostic.

REFERENCES

1. Riley RD, Burchill SA, Abrams KR et al.: A systematic review and evaluation of the use of tumor markers in paediatric oncology: Ewing's sarcoma and neuroblastoma. *Health Technol Assess* 7: 1–162, 2003.

2. Esteva FJ, Hortobagyi GN: Prognostic molecular markers in early breast cancer. *Breast Cancer Res* 6: 109–118, 2004.

3. Malats N, Bustos A, Nascimento CM et al.: P53 as a prognostic marker for bladder cancer: a meta-analysis and review. *Lancet Oncol* 6: 678–686, 2005.

4. Hayes DF, Thor AD: c-erbB in breast cancer: development of a clinically useful marker. *Semin Oncol* 29: 231–245, 2002.

5. Hayes DF, Bast RC, Desch CE et al.: Tumor marker utility grading system: a framework to evaluate clinical utility of tumor markers. *J Natl Cancer Inst* 88: 1456–1466, 1996.

6. Bast RC, Jr., Ravdin P, Hayes DF et al.: 2000 update of recommendations for the use of tumor markers in breast and colorectal cancer: clinical practice guidelines of the American Society of Clinical Oncology. *J Clin Oncol* 19: 1865–1878, 2001.

7. Schilsky RL, Taube SE: Tumor markers as clinical cancer tests—are we there yet? *Semin Oncol* 29: 211–212, 2002.

8. Kyzas PA, Loizou KT, Ioannidis JP: Selective reporting biases in cancer prognostic factor studies. *J Natl Cancer Inst* 97: 1043–1055, 2005.

9. Riley RD, Abrams KR, Sutton AJ et al.: Reporting of prognostic markers: current problems and development of guidelines for evidence-based practice in the future. *Br J Cancer* 88: 1191–1198, 2003.

10. McShane LM, Altman DG, Sauerbrei W et al.: Reporting recommendations for tumor marker prognostic studies (REMARK). *J Natl Cancer Inst* 97: 1180–1184, 2005.

11. Altman DG, De Stavola BL, Love SB et al.: Review of survival analyses published in cancer journals. *Br J Cancer* 72: 511–518, 1995.

12. Sauerbrei W, Royston P, Bojar H et al.: Modelling the effects of standard prognostic factors in node-positive breast cancer. German Breast Cancer Study Group (GBSG). *Br J Cancer* 79: 1752–1760, 1999.

13. Burton A, Altman DG: Missing covariate data within cancer prognostic studies: a review of current reporting and proposed guidelines. *Br J Cancer* 91: 4–8, 2004.

14. Simon R, Altman DG: Statistical aspects of prognostic factor studies in oncology. *Br J Cancer* 69: 979–985, 1994.

15. Altman DG, Lyman GH: Methodological challenges in the evaluation of prognostic factors in breast cancer. *Breast Cancer Res Treat* 52: 289–303, 1998.

16. Gasparini G, Pozza F, Harris AL: Evaluating the potential usefulness of new prognostic and predictive indicators in node-negative breast cancer patients. *J Natl Cancer Inst* 85: 1206–1219, 1993.

17. Simon R: Evaluating prognostic factor studies, in Gospodarowicz MK, Henson DE, Hutter RVP et al. (eds.): *Prognostic factors in cancer*. 2nd ed. New York: Wiley-Liss, 2001, pp. 49–56.

18. Gion M, Boracchi P, Biganzoli E et al.: A guide for reviewing submitted manuscripts (and indications for the design of translational research studies on biomarkers). *Int J Biol Markers* 14: 123–133, 1999.

19. Pajak TF, Clark GM, Sargent DJ et al.: Statistical issues in tumor marker studies. *Arch Pathol Lab Med* 124: 1011–1015, 2000.

20. Hall PA, Going JJ: Predicting the future: a critical appraisal of cancer prognosis studies. *Histopathology* 35: 489–494, 1999.

21. Altman DG, Riley RD: Primer: an evidence-based approach to prognostic markers. *Nature Clin Practice Oncol* 2: 466–472, 2005.

22. Kivela T, Grambsch PM: Evaluation of sampling strategies for modeling survival of uveal malignant melanoma. *Invest Ophthalmol Vis Sci* 44: 3288–3293, 2003.

23. Schmoor C, Sauerbrei W, Schumacher M: Sample size considerations for the evaluation of prognostic factors in survival analysis. *Stat Med* 19: 441–452, 2000.

24. McShane LM, Simon R: Statistical methods for the analysis of prognostic factor studies, in Gospodarowicz MK, Henson DE, Hutter RVP, et al. (eds.): *Prognostic factors in cancer*. 2nd ed. New York: Wiley-Liss, 2001, pp. 37–48.

25. Fayers PM, Machin D: Sample size: how many patients are necessary? *Br J Cancer* 72: 1–9, 1995.

26. Skovlund E: A critical review of papers from clinical cancer research. *Acta Oncol* 37: 339–345, 1998.

27. Pajak TF, Clark GM, Sargent DJ et al.: Statistical issues in tumor marker studies. *Arch Pathol Lab Med* 124: 1011–1015, 2000.

28. Vaeth M, Skovlund E: A simple approach to power and sample size calculations in logistic regression and Cox regression models. *Stat Med* 23: 1781–1792, 2004.

29. Douglas-Jones AG, Morgan JM, Appleton MA et al.: Consistency in the observation of features used to classify duct carcinoma *in situ* (DCIS) of the breast. *J Clin Pathol* 53: 596–602, 2000.

30. Hansen S, Grabau DA, Sorensen FB et al.: Vascular grading of angiogenesis: prognostic significance in breast cancer. *Br J Cancer* 82: 339–347, 2000.

31. Rochon J: Issues in adjusting for covariates arising postrandomization in clinical trials. *Drug Inf J* 33: 1219–1228, 1999.

32. Schumacher M, Hollander N, Schwarzer G et al.: Prognostic factor studies, in Crowley J (ed.): *Handbook of Statistics in Clinical Oncology*. New York: Marcel Dekker, 1999, pp. 321–378.

33. Parmar M, Machin D: *Survival analysis*. Chichester, UK: John Wiley & Sons Ltd, 1995.

34. Clark TG, Bradburn MJ, Love SB et al.: Survival analysis part IV: further concepts and methods in survival analysis. *Br J Cancer* 89: 781–786, 2003.

35. Bradburn MJ, Clark TG, Love SB et al.: Survival analysis part III: multivariate data analysis—choosing a model and assessing its adequacy and fit. *Br J Cancer* 89: 605–611, 2003.

36. Bradburn MJ, Clark TG, Love SB et al.: Survival analysis part II: multivariate data analysis—an introduction to concepts and methods. *Br J Cancer* 89: 431–436, 2003.

37. Clark TG, Bradburn MJ, Love SB et al.: Survival analysis part I: basic concepts and first analyses. *Br J Cancer* 89: 232–238, 2003.

38. Pocock SJ, Clayton TC, Altman DG: Survival plots of time-to-event outcomes in clinical trials: good practice and pitfalls. *Lancet* 359: 1686–1689, 2002.

39. Kay R: An explanation of the hazard ratio. *Pharmaceut Stat* 3: 295–297, 2005.

40. Altman DG, Royston P: What do we mean by validating a prognostic model? *Stat Med* 19: 453–473, 2000.

41. Knorr KL, Hilsenbeck SG, Wenger CR et al.: Making the most of your prognostic factors: presenting a more accurate survival model for breast cancer patients. *Breast Cancer Res Treat* 22: 251–262, 1992.

42. Royston P, Altman DG, Sauerbrei W: Dichotomizing continuous predictors in multiple regression: a bad idea. *Statistics in Medicine* 25: 127–141, 2006.

43. Altman DG, Lausen B, Sauerbrei W et al.: Dangers of using "optimal" cutpoints in the evaluation of prognostic factors. *J Natl Cancer Inst* 86: 829–835, 1994.

44. Brown J, Machin D: Statistics and clinical oncology. *Clin Oncol (R Coll Radiol)* 12: 202–205, 2000.

45. Harrell FE, Jr., Lee KL, Matchar DB et al.: Regression models for prognostic prediction: advantages, problems, and suggested solutions. *Cancer Treat Rep* 69: 1071–1077, 1985.

46. Durrleman S, Simon R: Flexible regression models with cubic splines. *Stat Med* 8: 551–561, 1989.

47. Sauerbrei W, Royston P: Building multivariable prognostic and diagnostic models: transformation of the predictors by using fractional polynomials. *J R Stat Soc* 162: 71–94, 1999.

48. Hilsenbeck SG, Clark GM, McGuire WL: Why do so many prognostic factors fail to pan out? *Breast Cancer Res Treat* 22: 197–206, 1992.

49. Clark TG, Altman DG: Developing a prognostic model in the presence of missing data: an ovarian cancer case study. *J Clin Epidemiol* 56: 28–37, 2003.

50. Vach W: Some issues in estimating the effect of prognostic factors from incomplete covariate data. *Stat Med* 16: 57–72, 1997.

51. Clark TG, Altman DG, De Stavola BL: Quantification of the completeness of follow-up. *Lancet* 359: 1309–1310, 2002.

52. Martin B, Paesmans M, Berghmans T et al.: Role of Bcl-2 as a prognostic factor for survival in lung cancer: a systematic review of the literature with meta-analysis. *Br J Cancer* 89: 55–64, 2003.

53. Loi S, Buyse M, Sotiriou C, Cardoso F: Challenges in breast cancer clinical trial design in the postgenomic era. *Curr Opin Oncol* 16: 536–541, 2004.

54. Boracchi P, Biganzoli E: Markers of prognosis and response to treatment: ready for clinical use in oncology? A biostatistician's viewpoint. *Int J Biol Markers* 18: 65–69, 2003.

55. McShane LM, Altman DG, Sauerbrei W: Identification of clinically useful cancer prognostic factors: what are we missing? *J Natl Cancer Inst* 97: 1023–1025, 2005.

Prognostic Factors in Population-Based Cancer Control

PATTI A. GROOME

Cancer control is directed to the entire time course of the disease and is defined through its objectives:

> Cancer control aims to prevent cancer, cure cancer, and increase survival and quality of life for those who develop cancer, by converting the knowledge gained through research, surveillance and outcome evaluation into strategies and actions[1]

As shown in Figure 4.1, the cancer trajectory moves from host susceptibility to the development of presymptomatic disease, its diagnosis, treatment, and hopefully, its cure. The targets of cancer control, as listed in our definition, occur at different points along the trajectory and it is useful to think about the separate issues that arise when trying to control cancer at these various time points. Prognosis applies to the period posttreatment and is, therefore, distinct from the natural history of the disease, which

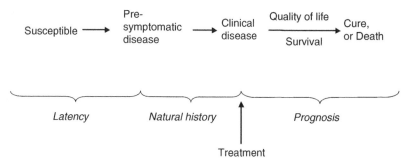

FIGURE 4.1 The cancer trajectory and its relationship to prognosis.

Prognostic Factors in Cancer, Third Edition, edited by Mary K. Gospodarowicz, Brian O'Sullivan, and Leslie H. Sobin.
Copyright © 2006 John Wiley & Sons, Inc.

describes the disease trajectory in the absence of human intervention. As implied in the definition, "those who develop cancer" are the group to whom improvements in the probability of cure, survival, and quality of life are targeted. These outcomes are the key ones in our study of the determination and impact of prognostic factors.

The last aim, to prevent cancer, is targeted to the prevention of the occurrence of the cancer. But as defined by J.M. Last in The Dictionary of Epidemiology,[2] prevention can be conceptualized more broadly as:

> Actions aimed at eradicating, eliminating, or minimizing the impact of disease and disability, or if none of these is feasible, retarding the progress of disease and disability.[2]

So, as with the definition of cancer control, prevention spans the disease trajectory and linking cancer control to prevention reminds us that cancer control is a public health activity. Last goes on to refine his definition:

> The concept of prevention is best defined in the context of levels, traditionally called primary, secondary, and tertiary prevention...primary prevention aims to reduce the incidence of disease, secondary prevention aims to reduce the prevalence of disease by shortening its duration, and tertiary prevention aims to reduce the number and/or impact of complications.[2]

These definitions are more applicable to the infectious or incurable chronic diseases. In the cancer setting, they are more aptly defined thus: secondary prevention as early detection and treatment, and tertiary prevention as targeting prolonged survival and increased quality of life. Figure 4.2 maps the prevention levels onto our disease trajectory. Since prognosis relates to the entire period postdiagnosis, secondary and tertiary prevention are the areas of cancer control that can be enhanced by the knowledge provided to us by studying prognosis.

The implementation of strategies, programs, interventions meant to reduce the impact of cancer are often delivered to populations of people rather than to individuals. Most

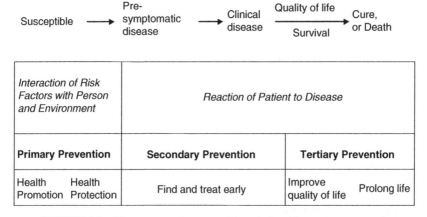

FIGURE 4.2   The cancer trajectory and its relationship to cancer control.

often, primary preventive strategies are targeted to an entire population, usually in a defined geographical region. For example, smoking control programs are often launched in communities and can involve such strategies as public education campaigns, enforcement of tobacco legislation, targeted youth smoking prevention strategies, and programs to support smokers in their quit attempts. Secondary and tertiary prevention are aimed at cancer patient populations. The unbiased selection of a cancer population is how we conceive of the term "population-level" used in this chapter's title. How prognosis facilitates cancer control in unbiased (entire) cancer populations is, therefore, the subject of this chapter.

THE IMPACT OF CANCER CONTROL ACTIVITIES

The success of preventive measures is largely determined by observing changes in the incidence and mortality of the cancer in the entire population of a particular geopolitical region and by observing changes in the outcomes experienced by that population's members who have had cancer.

Decreased Incidence through Prevention

Primary prevention is achieved when a cancer that would have previously occurred does not. But primary prevention of a cancer cannot be determined for an individual because we cannot know that such a cancer would have occurred in that person in the presence of the risk factor that is the target of the primary prevention campaign. Changes in population-level cancer incidence are therefore used to measure the impact of prevention strategies. Since these strategies are often targeted to whole populations, the population focus is appropriate. Most commonly, the focus of primary preventive efforts is lifestyle risk factors or environmental risk factors and associations between changes in the risk factor exposure burden and changes in incidence are the subject of the related cancer control studies. However, when a cancer can be detected through screening, its incidence may *increase* simply due to the detection of cases earlier in the disease course (lead time bias) and/or the detection of more slowly growing tumors that may not have been detected in the past (length bias). So the interpretation of changes in the incidence of those cancers that have effective screening tools (breast, prostate, colon, and cervical) need to consider developments in cancer screening programs in addition to public health campaigns waged against modifiable risk factors.

Decreased Mortality through Prevention, Screening and Effective Treatment

Mortality, which is measured in the entire population, is affected both by the underlying incidence of cancer and the survival and/or cure rates among those who develop the cancer. Here, prevention through screening (early detection) and effective treatment are key interventions (Fig. 4.2). Prognosis is relevant to the study of changes in cancer mortality as it is an expression of the probability of cure or the expected survival duration. Refinements of prognostic predictions are made through the study of the impact of relevant prognostic factors. At the population level, variations in the spectrum of prognostic factors present among persons with cancer will be associated with variations in the mortality rate of that cancer as it is measured in the entire population.

EXPANSION OF CANCER CONTROL BEYOND THE STUDY OF DISEASE ETIOLOGY

Traditionally, cancer control efforts at the population level have focused on reducing cancer incidence by identifying cancer risk factors and implementing population-level interventions targeted at those factors. Cancer registries, university departments of epidemiology, and public health schools and agencies have held the mandate for these activities. But as we have seen, cancer control also targets the period after a cancer has occurred. How does one extend the population-level mandate, which is crucial to reductions in cancer mortality, to this postdiagnostic setting?

Cancer Survival and the Role of Prognostic Factors

Many cancer registries now provide information about cancer survival across the cancer spectrum. For example, the Scottish Cancer Registry reports on trends in cancer survival by disease site so that they can track the effects of improvements in cancer screening and treatment: both crucial aspects of cancer control that relate to secondary prevention of the disease.[3] Since prognosis is defined as the expected course of the disease after diagnosis and treatment, survival information by disease site provides the most basic prognostic information for a given cancer. Reporting is usually in the form of survival curves, relative survival estimates, 5-year survival rates, and median survival duration. One realizes very quickly, however, that further definition of the case groups is needed beyond disease site to understand the survival trends observed. Sex, age, tumor stage, and type of treatment are some of the first that come to mind.[3] When one is reporting on cancer survival, these factors are prognostic; that is, they have the potential to refine ones ability to prognosticate. Other prognostic factors that have been incorporated into population-level cancer control activities are geographic location (both within and between countries) and socioeconomic status.[4,5]

The Spectrum of Disease in a Cancer Population

Prognostic factors are measured in individuals with cancer, but we can also conceptualize the prognostic profile of a population of patients. As before, "populations" of patients can be defined by region of residence within a country, across countries, over time, or by any other unbiased grouping of interest. Another term we can use to describe this profile is the "spectrum of disease" in a population.[6] The disease spectrum can vary across populations as a result of underlying differences in the nature of the disease, its hosts, or the environment in which the patients find themselves. The disease spectrum can also vary over time as screening programs are implemented, more effective treatments are found, or treatment becomes more (or less) widely available. So the disease spectrum, or prognostic profile, of a population of patients with a particular cancer can be influenced by the quality of the cancer care resources provided to those patients. Describing and comparing the spectrum of disease in a population to other times and settings provides a means to assess the quality of the cancer care system and, therefore, the quality of cancer control efforts in a given jurisdiction at a given point in time.

Prognostic Characterization of Subgroups

From a population point of view, a good prognostic factor is one that, through its study, can have an impact on the control of cancer. Table 4.1 provides a checklist of the qualities such variables should have. These qualities differ somewhat from what would be contained in such a list if the focus were on an individual patient, such as it is in the conduct of clinical medicine. In the population-level context, system issues become important and the perspective is a public health one. The sorts of issues that one may be concerned about are based on a public health perspective and need to be considered just as much as those issues that are clinically relevant. So what kinds of variables are prognostically relevant from a public health perspective? We have already mentioned a few: age, sex, race, socioeconomic status, tumor stage, treatment, era, geographic residence, are all studied now by some cancer surveillance systems. How do these achieve the criteria outlined in Table 4.1? Starting from the bottom of our list, variables that identify groups of patients who may be more or less susceptible to inadequate care are of interest from a population cancer control perspective. Age, sex, race, and socioeconomic status are all relevant to these concerns and differences in cancer survival between countries may be explained by differing abilities to provide care to these more susceptible subgroups. In the context of accessibility to a timely diagnosis, tumor stage can be conceived as a disease outcome (a marker of a diagnosis made later in the disease course) and studied in relation to these prognostic identifiers as well. Programs targeted at earlier diagnosis involve accessibility to screening when such a test is available, accessible high-quality healthcare, and

TABLE 4.1   A Checklist of the Qualities Prognostic Factors Should Have

---

A good population-level prognostic variable should:
Have an impact on the disease outcome in individual patients and in the whole population of
    such patients
Be measurable accurately
Differentiate populations in their experience of the disease
Differentiate populations on some underlying characteristic relevant to the disease prognosis
Help to control disease by
    helping to develop health policy, and/or
    helping to plan and deliver cancer care

Source:
• Adapted from: Bhopal RS: *Concepts of epidemiology: An integrated introduction to the ideas, theories, principles and methods of epidemiology.* New York, Oxford University Press, 2002, p. 7.

educational–awareness campaigns, especially for those cancers that only declare themselves symptomatically. Treatment is not normally considered a prognostic factor when ones perspective is on the individual patient, but when its accessibility and/or quality varies among different subgroups whose disease presentation is identical, treatment variations among groups become prognostic.

Importance of a Population-Based Perspective

It is self-evident that in order to study the impact of prognostic factors at the population level, we need to study representative populations of patients. Selection bias will be present when we use control group data from randomized trials for this purpose, as patients in trials are explicitly selected and often selectively approached for their involvement. Analogously, the problems of single institution information to understand prognosis at the population level is problematic since typically, institutions who collect and report on the outcomes of their cancer patients are quite different with regard to their case mix, treatment policies, and levels of experience than institutions who do not report. Again, cancer registries are the obvious choice to conduct prognostic surveillance at the population level.

THE IMPORTANCE OF CANCER REGISTRIES IN POST-DIAGNOSIS CANCER CONTROL

Good data collection and reporting at the population level are needed to properly conduct cancer control activities and the enhancement of cancer registries is one obvious way to accomplish this goal. There are examples of registries that contain variables that are prognostically important from a public health perspective; the most notable being the program of SEER registries in the United States, to which others are often compared.[5] It is difficult, time consuming, and expensive to create such registries, however, as they employ cancer registrars to collect data from patient charts. Alternatively, many registries are passive, that is, their data are compiled from other, existing sources. In this context, the registry is dependant on data collected for other purposes. Such data often do not contain information on important prognostic factors. In particular, stage and details of treatment may not be available. Their absence undermines a registry's ability to understand survival patterns and mortality rate variations.

Enhancement of the Prognostic Information in Registries

Most cancer registry activities continue to be focused on the reporting of age–sex standardized cancer incidence and mortality and many registries, particularly in developing countries, do not contain any other information about the cancer cases they identify.[7] Cancer control efforts, therefore, are hampered by an inability to interpret trends. Are changes in incidence a function of increased screening or are they due to a real increase in cancer risk? Are mortality trends a function of improved survival, lead-time and length biases, or changes in incidence? Other registries, primarily in developed countries, have been capturing cancer stage for varying lengths of time and have also enhanced their traditional data capture with information about treatment that allows monitoring and planning of cancer services provision, either through routine capture of these data or through periodic treatment surveys.[8-10]

Inclusion of Molecular Information for Cancer Control

As documented in the site-specific chapters that follow, molecular information on malignant tumors is becoming increasingly important for our understanding of cancer prognosis. Although population-based registries have yet to collect this information, there have been a number of large-scale tumor banking efforts launched in the last few years.[11-13] These tumor banks are designed to provide a resource for cancer research targeted at cancer control across the disease trajectory. Typically, these tumor banks are also collecting comprehensive clinical information about the patient, their treatment, and the disease outcome in order that the tissue characteristics are understood in context. Aspects of cancer control that can benefit from these tissue resources include the prediction of outcome and identifying new prognostic factors. Whether these tumor banks provide information that is generalizable outside the patients seen at the institutions from which the samples came has not yet been addressed; that is, none are explicitly population based.

CONCLUSIONS

In addition to explaining differences in the disease outcomes experienced among individual cancer patients, prognostic factors can also explain differences in the outcomes experienced among populations of cancer patients. Prognostic factors that are relevant for the assessment of an individual's prognosis may or may not be relevant when we try to understand outcome differences among populations of patients. In this context, factors that describe the care received and access to care in a population can be as or more relevant than those that describe the individual case. Cancer registries are increasingly aware of their role in understanding cancer control as it relates to secondary and tertiary prevention. Efforts to enhance registries with the relevant data for these purposes need to be encouraged and supported.

REFERENCES

1. Luciani S, Berman NJ: Canadian strategy for cancer control. *Chronic Dis Can* 21: 23–25, 2000.
2. Last JM (ed.) *A dictionary of epidemiology*. 3rd ed. New York, Oxford University Press, 2001.
3. Black RJ, Sharp L, Kendrick SW: Trends in cancer survival in Scotland. Edinburgh: Information & Statistics Division, Directorate of Information Services, National Health Service in Scotland, 1993.

4. Scottish Cancer Intelligence Unit. Trends in cancer survival in Scotland 1971–1995. Edinburgh: Information & Statistics Division, The National Health Service in Scotland, 2000.

5. SEER cancer statistics review, 1975–2002. Ries LAG, Eisner MP, Kosary CL, et al. (eds.). http://seer.cancer.gov/csr/1975_2002/, based on November 2004 SEER data submission, posted to the SEER website 2005. Accessed 2005. Bethesda, MD, National Cancer Institute.

6. Bhopal R: *Concepts of epidemiology: an integrated introduction to the ideas, theories, principles and methods of epidemiology.* Oxford, Oxford University Press, 2002.

7. International Association of Cancer Registries. http://www.iacr.com.fr. Accessed September 2005.

8. Thames Cancer Registry. http://www.thames-cancer-reg.org.uk. Accessed September 2005.

9. SEER Cancer Registries. http://www.seer.cancer.gov. Accessed September 2005.

10. Burton RC: Cancer control in Australia: Into the 21st century. *Jpn J Clin Oncol* 32(Suppl 1): S3–S9, 2002.

11. National Translational Cancer Research Network. http://www.ntrac.org/Initiatives/NCTR/NCTR.aspx. Accessed September 2005.

12. National Cancer Institute, Cooperative Human Tissue Network. http://www-chtn.ims.nci.nih.gov. Accessed September 2005.

13. BC Cancer Research Centre, Tumour Tissue Repository. http://www.bccrc.ca/ttr/index.html. Accessed September 2005.

CHAPTER 5

Prognostic Factors in Terminal Cancer

PAUL GLARE

The three great branches of clinical science are diagnosis, prognosis, and treatment.[1] While prognostication became increasingly undervalued in comparison to diagnostics and therapeutics by much of modern medicine during the twentieth century,[2] an accurate prognosis is a key skill the physician can bring to the management of patients with terminal cancer.

When considering the clinical science of prognosis, it is important to remember that prognosis refers to the relative probabilities of a patient developing the alternative outcomes of the natural history of their disease.[3] While life expectancy is the usual outcome under consideration in patients with terminal cancer, and the main focus of this chapter, it is important to remember that there are many other outcomes that the physician needs to be able to predict to ensure that the dying patient's care is optimized. Fries and Ehrlich referred to these as the Five D's of prognosis (Table 5.1).[4]

Accurate survival predictions in patients with terminal cancer are important for several reasons. First, prognosis may be used as a criterion for hospice admission. Second, it is necessary to respond to the awkward question "Doctor, how much time

TABLE 5.1   The "Five D's of Prognosis" and Their Relevance to Terminal Cancer

Prognostic Dimension	Examples of Clinical Questions in Terminal Cancer
Death	Doc, how long have I got?
Disability	Will this patient walk again after the cord compression is treated?
Discomfort	Will this pain respond to morphine?
Drug (therapeutic) toxicity	Will the sedation resolve if I rotate the opioids?
Dollar cost	Will palliative care be less expensive than oncologic treatment?

Source:
• Adapted from Ref. 4.

Prognostic Factors in Cancer, Third Edition, edited by Mary K. Gospodarowicz, Brian O'Sullivan, and Leslie H. Sobin.
Copyright © 2006 John Wiley & Sons, Inc.

do I have?".[5] Third, it may be required for research design and analysis, and for good clinical decision making in patients with advanced disease. Not only does the physician need prognostic information, but patients with advanced disease also base their treatment choices on their perceived prognosis.[6] Some of the trend to over-aggressively treat patients with advanced cancer being seen in recent years,[7] might be avoided if physicians were better prognosticators.

Despite the importance of accurate predictions of life expectancy to the terminally ill, modern physicians seem reluctant to prognosticate and there is evidence that they may prefer to avoid doing so wherever possible.[8] There are a number of reasons that may account for this, including the fact that they are not taught prognostication in medical school, their prognoses are usually inaccurate,[9] and there may be broader cultural or religious imperatives against it.

A hypothetical model for formulating the prognosis in oncology has been proposed by Mackillop, illustrating the flow of information as the prognosis is established for an individual case.[10] Diagnosis and characterization of the primary cancer precedes and forms the basis of the disease's generic prognosis (e.g., 6 months median survival for stage IV nonsmall cell lung cancer), which is then modified for the individual patient by taking other factors, such as their symptoms and comorbidities, into account (e.g., generic prognosis individualized to 1–2 months for a patient with stage IV nonsmall cell lung cancer who has severe COPD, has lost weight, and is depressed).

Formulating Prognosis in Terminal Cancer

Applying such a model to clinical practice requires, as for any other clinical assessment, the collection and interpretation of clinical data. They include the history, the physical examination, and the results of diagnostic tests. Two different types of interpretive function can be used for making clinical assessments. That which is used most commonly in prognostication in terminal cancer is *subjective* judgment, where the physician consciously combines and processes the data to render a judgment about the prognosis. This may also be called "clinical acumen". The other type of interpretive function involves *actuarial judgment*, with input of the data into a statistically derived index or tool, eliminating the need for the human judge.[11]

Prognostic Factors

There are many potential prognostic factors that can be statistically analyzed to improve predictions of survival. These can be conveniently categorized according to whether they are tumor, patient, or environment related. In patients with terminal disease (defined as a predicted survival <3 months), these factors appear to be different to those relevant in advanced cancer (with predicted survival <12 months). Factors that are important in patients with terminal cancer are summarized in Table 5.2. The Prognostic Factors Working Group of the European Association of Palliative Care (EAPC) has recently identified these as performance status, various symptoms (notably anorexia, dyspnea, delirium) and abnormalities on basic laboratory parameters (leukocytosis, lymphopenia, and elevated C-reactive protein). The EAPC have made evidence-based recommendations to assist clinicians in formulating a prognosis in terminal

TABLE 5.2   Clinical Prognostic Factors in Patients with Advanced Cancer, According to Consistency of Evidence

Definite correlation with survival in terminal cancer	Correlation has been indicated but not confirmed, or else correlated in less advanced disease but not terminal cancer, or else contradictory data	Factors with controversial correlation with survival in terminal cancer
Clinical prediction of survival	Characteristics primary site secondary sites	Multidimensional quality of life questionnaires
Performance status	Patient characteristics age gender marital status	
Signs and symptoms of cancer cachexia syndrome anorexia weight loss dysphagia xerostomia	Symptoms Pain Nausea	
Other symptoms Delirium dyspnoea	Signs Tachycardia Fever Proteinuria	
Some biological factors Leucocytosis Lymphocytopenia C-reactive protein	– Anemia – Hypoalbuminemia – Prehypoalbuminemia – Serum calcium level – Serum sodium level – LDH and other enzymes[a] Comorbidity	

[a]Lactate dehydrogenase = LDH.

cancer patients, and have graded the strength of the evidence as B (consistent level III studies or one level II study).[12]

Tumor-Related Factors

Tumor-related factors, such as the primary site, size, grade, and metastatic sites, are important determinants of survival in advanced cancer. In addition, the disease-free interval imparts additional information. For example, patients with metastatic breast cancer or prostate cancer typically follow a more indolent course than those with lung cancer or pancreas cancer. Several prognostic models for advanced cancer have been developed that take factors into account.[13–16] In patients with terminal cancer, however, tumor-related factors appear to become less important than other factors.[17–23]

Patient-related factors that might affect prognosis include demographics, comorbidities, performance status, symptoms, psychological status, quality of life, and laboratory parameters. Demographic factors, such as age and gender, can be important in earlier stage disease, but appear to become less important in advanced cancer. The impact of comorbidities on survival of cancer patients has been recognized for >30 years,[24] but few studies to date have investigated their importance in advanced disease[25,26] and it is not clear whether they are important in terminal cancer. The importance of clinical signs and symptoms in predicting survival was recognized nearly 40 years ago[27] and has been confirmed subsequently in terminal cancer.[18–23,28–38] Performance status (PS) has long been recognized as a predictor of outcomes in cancer,[39] and over the past half-century many studies have shown its importance as a survival predictor in advanced cancer[18,19,23,29,30,32,33,36]. Many different scales have been developed for measuring performance status. One of the first studies to demonstrate an association between PS and survival measured PS by the Karnofsky Performance Status (KPS) scale in >150 advanced cancer patients in the late 1970s.[40] In this study, a KPS score <50 on admission was uniformly associated with a survival of <6 months. The U.S. National Hospice Study, conducted in the 1980s, found that the KPS score accounted for only a small amount of the variability in observed survival, but its contribution was highly significant.[30] Furthermore, each increase in the KPS level (e.g., from 10 to 20) added ~2 weeks to the remaining life span of participants in the study. The KPS scores could be used to group the study participants into survival risk classes (KPS score 10–20: median survival 2 weeks; KPS score 30–40: 7 weeks; KPS score ≥50: 12 weeks).

Subsequently, many authors confirmed an association between PS and survival whether measured by KPS,[18,19,23,29,30,32,33,41,42] the ECOG scale,[32,43,44] or a measure of functional status.[31,45,46] While PS is considered a very reliable prognostic factor to predict a poor short-term survival in the presence of low scores, initially high scores are not necessarily predictive of a long survival. While patients with an initially good PS can demonstrate a rapid deterioration in PS, typically over the final 2 months of life, a much slower decline may be seen in some cases. In a patient with advanced cancer, unless the decline in PS is associated with some acute, reversible problem, such as anemia, sepsis, or a side effect of treatment, it usually indicates the commencement of the terminal phase. This pattern is the typical "death trajectory" of patients with terminal cancer.[47,48] A recent modification of the KPS, called the Palliative Performance Scale (PPS), has been developed as a new tool for measuring physical status in patients referred to hospice,[49] and is becoming increasingly popular as a prognostic aid. The authors who developed the PPS showed it could predict various outcomes in terminal cancer, including short-term survival. In their population, patients admitted to an in-patient hospice unit had an average survival of only 2 days if the PPS score on admission was 10 (defined as "unconscious with no oral intake" and "for mouth care only"), while ~60% of those with a PPS score of 40 on admission ("mostly in bed" or "sitting in a chair") had an average survival of 10 days. Similar types of results have been obtained with the PPS in other palliative care units, although the exact survival durations vary with the survival pattern of the population.[50–53] In an Australian study, the PPS was used to separate hospitalized patients with an overall median survival of ~1 month into three homogenous survival groups (PPS 10–20, median survival 6 days; PPS 30–50: 41 days; and PPS 60–70: 108 days).[51] A US study showed that the patient's PPS score at the time of hospice enrolment was a strong independent predictor of mortality (log rank test of Kaplan Meier survival curves $p < 0.001$) with 6-month mortality rates for 3 PPS categories were 96% (for PPS scores 10–20), 89% (for PPS scores 30–40), and 81% (for PPS scores > or = 50).[53]

Following on from the observation in the National Hospice Study that a good PS does not ensure long-term survival,[30] it was subsequently shown that the symptom profile can be used to supplement the prognostic information provided by the KPS score to accurately predict short-term survival.[23] The symptoms in that study that were predictive of survival were anorexia, weight loss, xerostomia, dysphagia, and dyspnoea. Perhaps not surprisingly, symptoms provided the most supplementary prognostic information in patients with higher KPS scores. For example, patients with a KPS score >50 and none of the five key symptoms had a median survival of ~6 months, which dropped to 2 months if all five symptoms were present. In patients with poor performance status (KPS 10–20), the addition of information on symptoms made little difference to the prognosis. The life expectancy was uniformly poor with or without symptoms (median survival 2 weeks vs. 6 weeks, respectively).

Many subsequent studies have shown an association between survival and a variety of these symptoms. They include anorexia,[18,23,31,35,48] weight loss,[25,35] dysphagia and difficulty in swallowing,[25,35] and xerostomia.[23] The cluster of poor performance and gastrointestinal symptoms, generally caused by the cancer cachexia syndrome, has been termed the Common Terminal Pathway of advanced cancer by some.[31,55–57] Consistent results are also found for dyspnea or breathlessness[18,20,21,23,35,48] and for cognitive failure or confusion,[23,28,34,35] which was not evaluated in the National Hospice Organization study. Results are less clear for other symptoms including nausea, constipation, dizziness, anxiety, depression, fever, pain, diarrhoea and for clinical signs like hemorrhage, pulse rate, respiratory rate, jaundice).[18,19,22,23,32,37,55] Perhaps surprisingly, pain is not usually considered to be predictive of poor survival in the late stages of cancer,[28,31,35,58] even though it is well known that pain increases in frequency and severity as cancer progresses.[59] However, episodes of severe, uncontrollable (unendurable) pain and breathlessness have been reported to be commoner in the last few weeks of life.[60] Treatment with opioids does not have any impact on survival rate according to several investigators.[32,61]

Quality of Life

The finding that certain symptoms adversely affect survival in advanced cancer naturally leads onto a consideration of quality of life (QOL) as a prognostic factor. While the impact of QOL on survival is clearer in the earlier stages of the disease (whether this is because patients with better quality of life have a survival advantage *per se*, or they just tolerate treatment better),[62] the EAPC Working Group concluded that the results are contradictory in far advanced disease.[12]

The role of psychological factors in cancer survival remains controversial and confusing. Over the past 20 years, well-known studies by Greer, Pettingale, and Speigel have identified psychosocial aspects considered to be important in cancer survivorship, such as the "fighting spirit".[63–65] In the palliative care setting, experienced healthcare professionals can all recount anecdotes of dying patients who seemed to hold on for an important event like the birth of a first grandchild and then let go or others who were "real fighters", remaining moribund for days until they eventually expired. A recent prospective study of psychosocial issues and breast cancer survival found a significantly increased risk of death from all causes by 5 years in women with a high scores for depression and helplessness/hopelessness, although there were no significant results found for "fighting spirit".[66] On the other hand, there has been the well-known study of newly diagnosed cancer patients by Cassileth, which found that "the inherent biology of the disease alone determines the prognosis."[67] Others have confirmed this finding more recently.[68]

In studies of QOL in patients with advanced cancer where an association with survival has been found, it is the physical symptom or physical well-being subscales of the QOL instruments that correlate best. For example, a significant association has been reported between patient-rated well being and survival time in women receiving treatment for advanced breast cancer.[62] Patient's perception of well being has been shown to be more important in predicting survival in advanced lung cancer than other predictors like KPS score or weight loss, using the Functional Living Index-Cancer (FLIC) instrument.[69] Patients with high FLIC scores lived twice as long (6 months) as those with low scores (3 months). The global health status item at the beginning of the SF-36 has been shown to be a predictor of survival in patients with advanced, but not terminal, cancer,[70] a finding that has also been seen in general populations.[71] Responses on the Symptom Distress Score, the Rotterdam Symptom Checklist, the Anderson Symptom Assessment Schedule, and the physical symptom subscale score of the Memorial Symptom Assessment Scale independently predicted a reduced survival.[58,72–74]

In patients with terminal cancer, QOL as a prognostic factor has not been fully investigated, although measuring multidimensional QOL in very ill patients is fraught with difficulties.[75] Nevertheless, a validated QOL instrument developed in Italy for use in hospice and palliative care settings, the Therapeutic Impact Questionnaire (TIQ), has been investigated. The TIQ consists of a global QOL question, as well as Likert scales that rate physical symptoms, function, psychological state, and family and social relationships. Only the patient-rated perception of cognitive function and global wellbeing has been shown to have independent prognostic value. Patients had median survivals of 137, 50, and 17 days for impairment of neither, one, or both scales, respectively.[34,76] These data again suggest that in patients with terminal cancer it is the physical–symptomatic component of QOL that correlates best with survival.

Biological Parameters

Biological parameters have not been as widely investigated as clinical ones in the terminally ill although a large number of laboratory abnormalities have been evaluated for their impact on survival. In patients with either advanced cancer or terminal cancer, leucocytosis[48,77,78] lymphocytopenia,[48,79] elevated C-reactive protein,[81–83] low pseudocholinesterase,[77] high-vitamin B12, and high bilirubin have shown significance in multivariate analysis, and the initial three parameters were confirmed in multiple studies. Other factors that are significant in advanced cancer, such as low serum albumin and prealbumin levels, lose their statistical significance in more terminal populations. This is probably because their association with survival is weaker than other features of cancer cachexia and malnutrition, such as poor performance, anorexia, and weight loss.[12] The cancer cachexia syndrome is the direct cause of death in approximately one-third of patients and contributes to mortality in up to 80%.[84] Recent preclinical work and some clinical studies indicate that proinflammatory cytokines play a role in its genesis.[85] Proinflammatory cytokines, such as IL-6, may prove to be useful prognostic markers.[86]

Environmental Factors

Various environmental factors can be considered as candidate prognostic factors for patients with advanced cancer. Some that have been identified include marital status, geography and socioeconomic status.[85] Marital status has been shown to modify the effect of QOL on survival in cancer patients.[68] Cancer treatment factors (type of treatment, response to treatment) and supportive care characteristics (interventions, opioid therapy,[32,61] place of care) are also candidate prognostic factors. Some multivariate analyses of prognostic factors in far advanced cancer have incorporated these types of variables,[20,30,21,24,25,34,39] but the data are inconsistent regarding their independent significance.

Accuracy of Clinical Prediction

The physician's clinical prediction of survival (CPS) can be classified as a type of environmental prognostic factor because it is external to the patient and may influence other aspects of care. The factors that physicians take into account when formulating a prognosis in terminal cancer are not well understood. However, an Italian survey of oncologists showed reliance on traditional prognostic factors, such as tumor characteristics.[88] The influence of the doctor's own psychology cannot be ignored when subjective judgment is being applied. Personal characteristics of the physician appear to influence the accuracy of a CPS. Older physicians and those with training in oncology or palliative care are more accurate, but a close physician–patient relationship blunts this accuracy.[89] It is possible that the greater accuracy of the survival estimates made by experienced physicians, compared to inexperienced ones, is because of the inclusion of PS and symptoms into prognostication. Other factors like response to treatment, disease-free interval, the impact of comorbidities, and the attitude of the patient may also be included. If this process can be better understood, it could be taught to young oncologists and inexperienced internists.

Nevertheless, the accuracy of such judgment has been studied for >30 years.[9,12,16–18,28,29,36,48,51,55,90–99] Most studies have looked at the difference between predicted survival and actual survival of patients after referral to palliative care services or admission to hospice. A recent systematic review of eight such studies,[9] involving >1500 predictions, showed that predictions were more than twice as likely to be overoptimistic (median predicted survival 6 weeks; median actual survival 4 weeks), correct to within a week in only 25% of cases and out by >1 month in another 25% of cases. However, despite the inaccuracy, there was a strong correlation between the predicted and actual survival, up to 6 months, with the correlation coefficient between CPS and actual survival ranging from 0.2 to 0.65 in the different studies. Physicians' subjective survival predictions are repeatedly found to retain statistical significance in multivariate models of prognostic factors in advanced cancer. Predictions of <4 weeks were the most precise and accurate, referred to by Mackillop as the "horizon effect" a term borrowed from meterology,[99] but predictions beyond 6 months had no relationship with observed survival (see Chapter 1).

Some authors have tried to compare the accuracy of CPS with PS, but the results are conflicting. One group found that KPS score was more strongly correlated with survival than CPS made at the initial visit,[100] while others reacted with the opposite conclusion.[28] The latter study showed that the CES and KPS score were closely correlated, with ~37% of the variation in the survival estimate being accounted for by changes in the performance status. Other investigators have confirmed this strong association between KPS score and CPS, to the point that performance status dropped out of their survival models. One problem with KPS score is that, like other clinical scales, it is scored with varying degrees of interrater reliability. This improves with training and care is need when scoring it.[30] Patient-rated KPS scores provide independent prognostic information in addition to physician rated KPS score.[44]

Until validated prognostic indices are available that provide precise prognostic information for a range of relevant time points in the trajectory of the cancer illness, subjective judgment will remain important and it is apparent that the CPS contains some useful prognostic information. There has been little research into what information physicians take into account when formulating a prognosis, but it may not be the most relevant information. CPS is best used in conjunction with other parameters and could be integrated into prognostic models and scores. Clinicians should consider using CPS in combination with other prognostic factors to improve the accuracy of their predictions. Training in prognostication could improve the accuracy of CPS.

Predictive Models

The identification of clinically relevant individual prognostic factors enables the construction of predictive models for short-term survival. A variety of prognostic models have been developed for patients with advanced cancer. Some are for specific cancers[13,14,101] while others are for heterogeneous populations.[15,102–104] Four studies have involved construction and development of such indices for patients with terminal cancer (Table 5.3).[28,48,54,105] Two of them have been validated: the Palliative Prognostic (PaP) Score[36,61,95,106] and the Palliative Prognostic Index (PPI).[96] Prognostic factors present in all the scores are symptoms related to nutritional status, cognitive function (cognitive failure, delirium, confusion), while dyspnoea and PS were reported in two

TABLE 5.3 **Prognostic Scores for Terminal Cancer**

Reference	Country	Name of Score	Factors Included	Prediction
28	Canada	Indicator of poor prognosis	Dysphagia, cognitive failure, weight loss	1-month survival
48	Italy	PaP	Clinicians prediction, symptoms, PS, white cell count	Probability of being alive in 30 days
96	Japan	PPI	PS, dyspnea, delirium, edema	3- and 6-week survival or not
105	Korea	Terminal Cancer Prognostic (TCP) score	Anorexia, confusion, diarrhea	None stated

of the scores. The PaP Score includes simple biological factors and judgment of survival, measured in weeks (up to 12 weeks), so that the score is used together with, rather than instead of, clinical judgment. The original version of the PaP Score did not include cognitive failure, which was subsequently demonstrated to subdivide each population categorized by the PaP Score into two further prognostic subgroups.[36] None of the scores constructed so far include psychological symptoms or quality of life scores.

The PaP Score was built and validated in two independent multicenter population studies and is the only one to include biological factors. It has been validated in several countries, in various settings, and in different disease phases. It was not constructed to include hematological malignancies. Points are awarded for the presence of symptoms (anorexia, dyspnoea), poor performance status, white cell abnormalities, and the CPS. These individual scores are summed to provide a total PaP score stratifying three groups with high, intermediate, and low chances of surviving for the next month. The PPI does not include CPS, and a study specifically addressed at comparing the prognostic accuracy of the PPI compared with CPS has been conducted.[96] This showed a significant improvement in accuracy with the tool. The process by which the PPI was developed was not as rigorous as the PaP Score. No studies have ever been conducted to compare the efficacy of different scores or the effect of prognostic scores on decision making.

An objective prognostic index that might obviate the need for assessing symptoms, performance status, or QOL has some advantages, and some progress is being made toward that end. The Prognostic Inflammatory Nutritional Index (PINI) is a validated prognostic index that has been associated with decreased short-term survival in both critically ill patients and advanced cancer patients.[107] One drawback with the PINI is that it requires measurement of laboratory parameters that are not performed routinely in most hospital biochemistry departments (i.e., alpha-acid glycoprotein and pre-albumin). More recently, the product of two acute-phase reactants, C-reactive protein and vitamin B12, termed BCI, has also been shown to be predictive of short-term survival in a sample of advanced cancer patients,[79] and has been validated in a palliative care population.[108]

More research is needed to validate the existing tools and demonstrate their usefulness in clinical practice. The type of prognostic information provided limits the utility of current indices. New developments in biostatistics and information technology are resulting in new web-based tools based on algorithms and nomograms derived from large patient databases that are currently being constructed by groups at Memorial Sloan Kettering Cancer Center (MSKCC) and Washington University at St Louis (WUSTL). The MSKCC group have web-based nomograms for breast, pancreas, lung, prostate, and renal cancers and sarcomas, although many of the predictions are for treatment decisions in early stage disease. Recently, prognostic nomograms have been developed by others to assist with decision making, such as patient selection for surgery in patients with more advanced disease.[104] The WUSTL group's Prognostigram uses SEER data to generate individualized survival curves based on age, gender, race, primary site, extent of disease, and comorbidities, but have not been widely validated.

Predicting life expectancy in terminally ill cancer patients is very important for patients, their families, clinicians, researchers, and policy makers. While clinicians will continue to depend on their subjective judgment when responding to difficult questions, such as Doc, how much time do I have?, objective prognostic factors, such as performance status, symptoms of the cancer cachexia syndrome, breathlessness, and cognitive impairment, and simple blood test results can be used to inform clinical acumen. Prognostic indices that combine these factors have been developed and validated, but have not yet been used to improve patient care. Accuracy of prognostication is a clinical skill that needs to be resurrected, as it is crucial to good end-of-life care in terminal cancer. It should be included in cancer medicine curricula.

REFERENCES

1. Hutchinson R: Prognosis: general principles. *Lancet* i:697–698, 1934.
2. Christakis NA: The ellipsis of prognosis in modern medical thought. *Soc Sci Med* 44:301–305, 1997.
3. Sackett DL, Haynes BR, Guyatt GH, et al.: *Clinical epidemiology: a basic science for clinical medicine*, 2nd ed. Boston:Little, Brown, 173, 1991.
4. Fries JF, Ehrlich GE, (eds): *Prognosis: contemporary outcomes of disease.* Bowie, MD: The Charles Press, 12, 1981.
5. Schapira L, Eisenberg PD, MacDonald N, et al.: A revisitation of "Doc, how much time do I have?" *J Clin Oncol* 21:8S–11S, 2003.
6. Weeks JC, Cook EF, O'Day SJ: Relationship between cancer patients' predictions of prognosis and their treatment preferences. *JAMA* 279:1709–1714, 1998.
7. Earle CC, Neville BA, Landrum MB, et al.: Trends in the aggressiveness of cancer care near the end of life. *J Clin Oncol* 22:315–321, 2004.
8. Christakis N: Professional norms regarding prognostication. In Christakis N. *Death foretold*. Prophecy and prognosis in medical care. Chicago:Chicago University Press, 1999: 84–106.
9. Glare P, Virik K, Jones M, et al.: A systematic review of physicians' survival predictions in terminally ill cancer patients. *BMJ* 327:195–200, 2003.

10. Mackillop WJ: The importance of prognostication in cancer medicine. In Gospodarowicz MJ (ed). *Prognostic factors in advanced cancer* (2nd ed.). New York, NY:Wiley-Liss, 2001:3–14.

11. Dawes RM, Faust D, Meehl PE: Clinical versus actuarial judgement. *Science* 243:1668–1674, 1989.

12. Maltoni M, Caraceni A, Brunelli C, et al.: Prognostic factors in advanced cancer patients: evidence based clinical recommendations — a study by the steering committee of the European Association of Palliative Care. *J Clin Oncol* 23:6240–6248, 2005.

13. Stanley KE: Prognostic factors for survival in patients with inoperable lung cancer. *JNCI* 65:25–32, 1980.

14. Yamamoto N, Watanabe N, Katsumata N, et al.: construction and validation of a practical prognostic index for patients with metastatic breast cancer. *J Clin Oncol* 16:2401–2408, 1998.

15. Chow E, Fung K, Panzarella T, et al.: A predictive model for survival in metastatic cancer patients attending an outpatient radiotherapy clinic. *Int J Radiat Oncol Biol Phys* 53:1291–1302, 2002.

16. Llobera J, Esteva M, Rifa J, et al.: Terminal cancer. Duration and prediction of survival time. *Eur J Cancer* 36:2036–2043, 2000.

17. Faris M: Clinical estimation of survival and impact of other prognostic factors on terminally ill cancer patients in Oman. *Support Care Cancer* 11:30–34, 2003.

18. Maltoni M, Pirovano M, Scarpi E, et al.: Prediction of survival of patients terminally ill with cancer. Results of an Italian prospective multicentric study. *Cancer* 75:2613–2622, 1995.

19. Forster LE, Lynn J: The use of physiologic measures and demographic variables to predict longevity among inpatient hospice applicants. *Am J Hospice Care* 6:31–34, 1989.

20. Heyse Moore LH, Ross V, Mullee MA: How much of a problem is dyspnoea in advanced cancer? *Palliat Med* 5:20–26, 1991.

21. Hardy JR, Turner R, Saunders M, et al.: Prediction of survival in a hospital-based continuing care unit. *Eur J Cancer* 30 (A):284–288, 1994.

22. Vitetta L, Kenner D, Kissane D, Sali A: Clinical outcomes in terminally ill patients admitted to hospice care: diagnostic and therapeutic interventions. *J Palliat Care* 17: 69–77, 2001.

23. Reuben DB, Mor V, Hiris J: Clinical symptoms and length of survival in patients with terminal cancer. *Arch Intern Med* 148:1586–1591, 1988.

24. Feinstein A: The pre-therapeutic classification of morbidity in chronic disease. *J Chron Dis* 23:455–469, 1970.

25. Patel U, Spitznagel E, Piccirillo J: Multivariate analysis to assess treatment effectiveness in advanced head and neck cancer. *Arch Otolaryungol Head Neck Surg* 128:497–503, 2002.

26. Tammemagi CM, Neslund-Dudas C, Simoff M, et al.: Lung cancer patients, age, race-ethnicity, gender and smoking predict adverse comorbidity, which in turn predicts treatment and survival. *J Clin Epidemiol* 57:597–609, 2004.

27. Feinstein AR: Symptoms as an index of biological behavior and prognosis in advanced cancer. *Nature* 209:241–245, 1966.

28. Bruera E, Miller MJ, Kuehn N, et al.: Estimate of survival of patients admitted to a Palliative Care unit: a prospective study. *J Pain Symptom Manage* 7:82–86, 1992.

29. Maltoni M, Nanni O, Derni S, et al.: Clinical prediction of survival is more accurate than the Karnofsky Performance Status in estimating life span of terminally-ill cancer patients. *Eur J Cancer* 30:764–766, 1994.

30. Mor V, Laliberte L, Morris JN, Wiemann M: The Karnofsky Performance Status Scale: an examination of its reliability and validity in a research setting. *Cancer* 53:2004–2007, 1984.

31. Schonwetter RS, Teasdale T, Storey P: The terminal cancer syndrome. *Arch Intern Med* 149:965–966, 1989.

32. Rosenthal MA, Gebski VJ, Kefford RF, Stuart-Harris RC: Prediction of life-expectancy in hospice patients: identification of novel prognostic factors. *Palliat Med* 7:199–204, 1993.

33. Allard P, Dionne A, Patvin D: Factors associated with length of survival among 1081 terminally ill cancer patients. *J Palliat Care* 11:20–24, 1995.

34. Tamburini M, Brunelli C, Rosso S, et al.: Prognostic value of quality of life scores in terminal cancer patients. *J Pain Symptom Manage* 11:32–41, 1996.

35. Morita T, Tsunoda J, Inoue S, et al.: Survival prediction of terminally ill cancer patients by clinical symptoms: development of a simple indicator. *Jpn J Clin Oncol* 29:156–159, 1999.

36. Caraceni A, Nanni O, Maltoni M, et al.: Impact of delirium on short term prognosis of advanced cancer patients. *Cancer* 89:1145–1149, 2000.

37. Pasanisi F, Orban A, Scalfi L, et al.: Predictors of survival in terminal cancer patients with irreversible bowel obstruction receiving home parenteral nutrition. *Nutrition* 17:581–584, 2001.

38. Rodrigus P, de Brouwer P, Raaymakers E: Brain metastases and non-small cell lung cancer. Prognostic factors and correlation with survival after irradiation. *Lung Cancer* 32:129–136, 2001.

39. Karnofsky DA, Burchenal JH: The clinical evaluation of chemotherapeutic agents in cancer. In MacLeod CM (ed): *Evaluation of chemotherapeutic agents*. Symposium Microbiology Section, NY Acad Med New York: Columbia University, 191–205, 1949.

40. Yates JW, Chalmer B, McKegney P: Evaluation of patients with advanced cancer using the Karnofsky Performance Status. *Cancer* 45:2220–2224, 1980.

41. Brown DJ, McMillan DC, Milroy R: The correlation between fatigue, physical function, the systemic inflammatory response, and psychological distress in patients with advanced lung cancer. *Cancer* 103:377–382, 2005.

42. Hwang SS, Scott CB, Chang VT, et al.: Prediction of survival for advanced cancer patients by recursive partitioning analysis: role of Karnofsky performance status, quality of life, and symptom distress. *Cancer Invest* 22:678–687, 2004.

43. Hoang T, Xu R, Schiller JH, et al.: Clinical model to predict survival in chemo-naive patients with advanced non-small-cell lung cancer treated with third-generation chemotherapy regimens based on eastern cooperative oncology group data. *J Clin Oncol* 23:175–183, 2005.

44. Loprinzi CL, Lauire JA, Wienand S, et al.: Prospective evaluation of prognostic variables from patient completed questionnaires. *J Clin Oncol* 12:601–607, 1994.

45. Bennett M, Ryall N: Using the modified Barthel index to estimate survival in cancer patients in hospice: observational study. *BMJ* 321:1381–1382, 2000.

46. Lunney JR, Lynn J, Foley DJ, et al.: Patterns of functional decline at the end of life. *JAMA* 289:2387–2392, 2003.

47. Mc Cusker J: The terminal period of cancer: definition and descriptive epidemiology. *J Chron Dis* 37:377–385, 1984.

48. Pirovano M, Maltoni M, Nanni O, et al.: A new Palliative Prognostic Score (PaP Score). A first step for the staging of terminally ill cancer patients. *J Pain Symptom Manage* 17:231–239, 1999.

49. Anderson F, Downing GM, Hill J, et al.: Palliative performance Scale (PPS): a new tool. *J Palliat Care* 12:5–11, 1996.

50. Virik K, Glare P: Validation of the Palliative performance Scale for inpatients admitted to a palliative care unit in Sydney, Australia (letter). *J Pain Symp Manage* 23: 455–457, 2002.

51. Morita T, Tsunoda J, Inoue S, et al.: Validity of the palliative performance scale from a survival perspective. *J Pain Symp Manage* 18:2–3, 1999.

52. Head B, Ritchie CS, Smoot TM: Prognostication in hospice care: can the palliative performance scale help? *J Palliat Med* 8:492–502, 2005.

53. Harrold J, Rickerson E, Carroll JT, et al.: Is the palliative performance scale a useful predictor of mortality in a heterogeneous hospice population? *J Palliat Med* 8:503–509, 2005.

54. Morita T, Tsunoda J, Inoue S, et al.: The Palliative Prognostic Index: a scoring system for survival prediction of terminally ill cancer patients. *Support Care Cancer* 7:128–133, 1999.

55. Viganò A, Bruera E, Jhangri GS, et al.: Clinical survival predictors in patients with advanced cancer. *Arch Intern Med* 160:861–868, 2000.

56. Wachtel T, Allen-Masterson SA, Reuben D, et al.: The end-stage cancer patient: terminal common pathway. *Hospice J* 4:43–80, 1988.

57. Viganò A, Bruera E, Suarez-Almazor ME: Terminal cancer syndrome: myth or reality? *J Palliat Care* 15:32–39, 1999.

58. Palmer JL, Fisch MJ: Association between symptom distress and survival in outpatients seen in a palliative care cancer center. *J Pain Symp Manage* 29:565–571, 2005.

59. Bonica JJ: Treatment of cancer pain: current status and future needs, in Fields HL, Dubner R, Cervero F (eds). *Advances in Pain Research and Therapy* Vol 9. New York: Raven Press, 589–616, 1985.

60. Ventafridda V, Ripamonti C, Tamburini M, et al.: Unendurable symptoms as prognostic indicators of impending death in terminal cancer patients. *Eur J Cancer* 26:1000–1001, 1990.

61. Maltoni M, Nanni O, Pirovano M, et al.: The Italian Mulitcenter Study Group on Palliative Care. Successful validation of the Palliative Prognostic Score in terminally ill cancer patients. *J Pain Symp Manage* 17:240–247, 1999.

62. Coates A, Gebski V, Signorini D, et al.: Prognostic value of quality of life scores during chemotherapy for advanced breast cancer. *J Clin Oncol* 10:1833–1838, 1992.

63. Greer HS, Morris T, Pettingale KW: Psychological response to breast cancer: effect on outcome. *Lancet* 2:785–787, 1979.

64. Pettingale KW, Morris T, Greer S, et al.: Mental attitudes to cancer: an individual prognostic factor. *Lancet* i:750, 1985.

65. Spiegel D, Bloom JR, Kraemer HC, et al.: Effect of psychosocial treatment on survival of patients with metastatic breast cancer. *Lancet* ii:888–891, 1989.

66. Watson M, Haviland JS, Greer S, et al.: Influence of psychological response on survival in breast cancer: a population-based cohort study. *Lancet* 354:1331–1336, 1999.

67. Cassileth BR, Lush EJ, Miller DS, et al.: Psychosocial correlates of survival in advanced malignant disease? *N Eng J Med* 312:1551–1555, 1985.

68. Ringdal GI, Götestam KG, Kaasa S, et al.: Prognostic factors and survival in a heterogeneous sample of cancer patients. *Brit J Cancer* 73:1594–1599, 1996.

69. Ganz PA, Lee JJ, Siau J: Quality of life assessment: an independent prognostic variable for survival in lung cancer. *Cancer* 67:3131–3135, 1991.

70. Shadbolt B, Barresi J, Craft P: Self-rated health as a predictor of survival among patients with advanced cancer. *J Clin Oncol* 20:2514–2519, 2002.

71. Soldo BJ, Hurd MD, Rodgers WL, et al.: Asset and Health Dynamics Among the Oldest Old: an overview of the AHEAD Study. [Journal Article] *J Gerontol Ser B-Psychol Sci Soc Sci* 52 Spec No:1–20, 1997.

72. Degner LF, Sloan A: Symptom distress in newly diagnosed ambulatory cancer patients and as a predictor of survival in lung cancer patients. *J Pain Symp Manage* 10:423–431, 1995.

73. Earlam S, Glover C, Fordy C, et al.: Relation between tumour size, quality of life, and survival in patients with colorectal liver metastases. *J Clin Oncol* 14:171–175, 1996.

74. Chang VT, Thaler HT, Ployak TA, et al.: Quality of life and survival. The role of multidimensional symptom assessment. *Cancer* 83:173–179, 1998.

75. Paci E, Miccinesi G, Toscani F, et al.: Quality of life assessment and outcome of palliative care. *J Pain Symp Manage* 21:179–188, 2001.

76. Toscani P, Brunelli C, Miccinesi G, et al.: Predicting survival in terminal cancer patients: clinical observation or quality-of-life evaluation? *Palliat Med* 19:220–227, 2005.

77. Maltoni M, Pirovano M, Nanni O, Marinari M, et al.: Biological indices predictive of survival in 519 terminally ill cancer patients. *J Pain Sympt Manage* 13:1–9, 1997.

78. Shoenfeld Y, Tal A, Berliner S, et al.: Leukocytoisis in non-hematological malignancies. A possible tumor-associated marker. *J Clin Res Clin Oncol* 111:54–58, 1986.

79. Geissbuhler P, Mermillod B, Rapin CH: Elevated serum vitamin B12 associated with CRP as a predictive factor of mortality in palliative care cancer patients: a prospective study over five years. *J Pain Sympt Manage* 20:93–103, 2000.

80. McMillan DC, Elahi MM, Sattar N, et al.: Measurement of the systemic inflammatory response predicts cancer-specific and non-cancer survival in patients with cancer. *Nutr Cancer* 41:64–69, 2001.

81. Falconer JS, Fearon KC, Ross JA, et al.: Acute-phase protein response and survival duration of patients with pancreatic cancer. *Cancer* 75:2077–2082, 1995.

82. O'Gorman P, McMillan DC, McArdle CS: Impact of weight loss, appetite, and the inflammatory response on quality of life in gastrointestinal cancer patients. *Nutr Cancer* 32:76–80, 1998.

83. Scott HR, McMillan DC, Forrest LM, et al.: The systemic inflammatory response, weight loss, performance status and survival in patients with inoperable non-small cell lung cancer. *Br J Cancer* 87:264–267, 2002.

84. Bruera E, Sweeney C: Cachexia and asthenia in cancer patients. *Lancet Oncol* 1:138–147, 2000.

85. Lee BN, Dantzer R, Langley KE, et al.: A cytokine-based neuroimmunologic mechanism of cancer-related symptoms. *Neuroimmunomodulation* 11:279–292, 2004.

86. Iwase S, Murakami T, Saito Y, et al.: Steep elevation of blood interleukin-6 (IL-6) is associated only with late stages of cachexia in cancer patients. *Eur Cytokin Netw* 15:312–316.

87. Iwashyna TJ, Zhang JX, Lauderdale DS, et al.: A methodology for identifying married couples in Medicare data: mortality, morbidity, and health care use among the married elderly. [see comments.]. [Journal Article] *Demography* 35:413–419, 1998.

88. Tanneberger S, Malavasi I, Mariano P, et al.: Planning palliative or terminal care: the dilemma of doctors' prognoses in terminally ill cancer patients. *Ann Oncol* 13:1320–1322, 2002.

89. Christakis NA, Lamont EB: Extent and determinants of error in doctors' prognoses in terminally ill patients: prospective cohort study. *Br Med J* 320:469–472, 2000.

90. Parkes CM: Accuracy of predictions of survival in later stages of cancer. *BMJ* 2:29–31, 1972.

91. Evans C, Mc Carthy M: Prognostic uncertainty in terminal care: can the Karnofsky Index help? *Lancet* 251:1204–1206, 1985.

92. Heyse-MooreLH, Johnson-Bell VE: Can doctors accurately predict the life-expectancy of patients with terminal cancer? *Palliat Med* 1:165–166, 1987.

93. Forster LE, Lynn J: Predicting life span for applicants to inpatient hospice. *Arch Intern Med* 148:2540–2543, 1988.

94. Oxenham D, Cornbleet MA: Accuracy of prediction of survival by different professional groups in a hospice. *Palliat Med* 12:117–118, 1998.

95. Glare P, Virik K: Independent prospective validation of the PaP Score in terminally ill patients referred to a hospital-based palliative medicine consultation service. *J Pain Symptom Manage* 22:891–898, 2001.

96. Morita T, Tsunoda J, Inoue S, et al.: Improved accuracy of physicians' survival prediction for terminally ill cancer patients using the Palliative Prognostic Index. *Palliat Med* 15:419–424, 2001.

97. Higginson IJ, Costantini M: Accuracy of prognosis estimates by four palliative care teams: a prospective cohort study. *BMC Palliat Care* 1:1–5, 2002.

98. Viganò A, Dorgan M, Bruera E, et al.: The relative accuracy of the Clinical Estimation of the duration of life for patients with end of life cancer. *Cancer* 86:170–176, 1999.

99. Mackillop WJ, Quirt CF: Measuring the accuracy of prognostic judgements in oncology. *J Clin Epidemiol* 50:21–29, 1997.

100. Viganò A, Dorgan M, Buckingham J, et al.: Survival prediction in terminal cancer patients : a systematic review of the literature. *Palliat Med* 14:363–374, 2000.

101. Tan CK, Law NM, Ng HS, et al.: Simple clinical prognostic model for hepatocellular carcinoma in developing countries and its validation. *J Clin Oncol* 21:2294–2298, 2003.

102. Knaus WA, Harrell FE, Lynn J, et al.: The SUPPORT prognostic model: onbjective estimates of survival for seriously ill hospitalised adults. *Ann Intern Med* 122:191–203, 1995.

103. Sloan JA, Loprinzi CL, Laurine JA, et al.: A simple stratification factor prognostic for survival in patients with advanced cancer: the good/bad/uncertain index. *J Clin Oncol* 19:3539–3546, 2001.

104. Nathan SS, Healey JH, Mellano D, et al.: J Survival in patients operated on for pathological fracture: implications for end of life orthopaedic care. *J Clin Oncol* 23:6072–6082, 2005.

105. Yun HY, Heo Ds, Heo BY, et al.: Development of terminal cancer prognostic score as an index in terminally ill cancer patients. *Oncol Rep* 8:795–800, 2001.

106. Glare PA, Eychmueller S, McMahon P: Diagnostic accuracy of the palliative prognostic score in hospitalized patients with advanced cancer. *J Clin Oncol* 22:4823–4828, 2004.

107. Nelson KA, Walsh D: The cancer anorexia-cachexia syndrome: a survey of the Prognostic Inflammatory and Nutritional Index (PINI) in advanced disease. *J Pain Symp Manage* 24:424–428, 2002.

108. Kelly L, Stone P: validation of the BCI prognostic index in palliative care patients: an interim analysis (abst). *Palliat Med* 19:155, 2005.

CHAPTER 6

Incorporating Molecular Oncology into Prognosis

GEOFFREY G. LIU, WEI ZHOU, ZHAOXI WANG, and HOWARD L. McLEOD

The past decade has seen an explosion of advances in molecular oncology, and their impact on clinical practice appears in various areas, particularly in the development of molecularly targeted drugs.[1,2] A major goal has been to incorporate some of these molecular advances into the prognostic systems. Despite progress, molecular prognostic factors have not been integrated well into clinical practice, particularly in the solid-tumor setting. In this chapter, we examine recent advances in major categories of molecular prognostic factors, address problems with integrating them into clinical practice, and describe possible remedies to the current situation.

Molecular prognostic factors can be categorized based on their involvement in specific biological pathways. However, common themes associated with the clinical implementation of molecular prognostic factors relate more to the type of biologic specimen being evaluated than to the biological pathway. Thus, we have divided molecular prognostic factors into DNA-, RNA-, and protein-based specimens, in addition to the molecular detection of occult tumor cells. A common (but false) assumption has been to consider molecular prognostic factor research to be synonymous with biomarker research. Biomarkers are an objectively measurable or evaluable characteristic that serves as an indication of biological or pharmacologic processes, or of therapeutic intervention. A good example of biomarker research that does not involve molecular oncology is the use of FDG–PET scanning to predict cancer outcomes. Molecular prognostic factors research comprises the triadic intersection of outcome research, biomarker research, and molecular biology (Fig. 6.1). Molecular prognostic factors may be causal in that they are directly associated with biological pathways that influence cancer biology. An example of a noncausal prognostic factor is PSA (prostrate specific antigen), which reflects general prostate cancer burden rather than a specific

Prognostic Factors in Cancer, *Third Edition*, edited by Mary K. Gospodarowicz, Brian O'Sullivan, and Leslie H. Sobin.

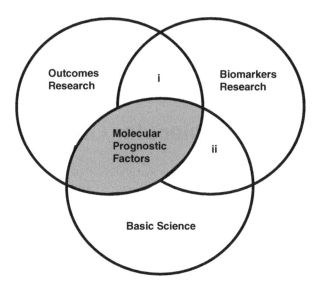

FIGURE 6.1   The relationship between biomarkers and molecular prognostic factors. An example for subset (i) is the use of FDG–PET scanning to predict overall survival. An example for subset (ii) is the use of circulating tumor cells to detect early cancer.

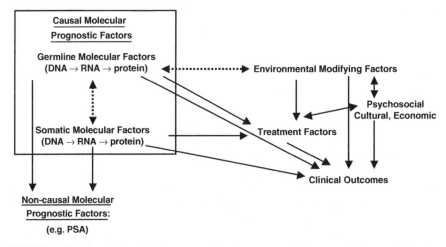

FIGURE 6.2   The relationship between molecular prognostic factors and other variables that affect clinical outcomes.

biological pathway. Difficulties in isolating true molecular prognostic factors rest with the intricate relationships between these molecularly based variables and environmental, treatment, psychosocial, cultural, and economic variables that also affect clinical outcome (Fig. 6.2). Another important differentiating factor is the concept of prognosis versus prediction. Both have value, but are used in distinct ways. For example, a prognostic marker helps choose whether a patient needs treatment, while a predictive marker aids in the selection of a specific treatment. Molecular cancer prognostic factors interface with clinical practice in a wide variety of ways, through the use of molecular variables to identify high-risk individuals, to detect disease in its early stages, to discover novel drugs (by identifying targets and pathways), to individualize therapy (pharmacogenomics), and to monitor patients. Since a multitude of molecular characteristics are being assessed as prognostic factors, we will also focus on how the technological advances in the postgenomics era can be integrated into clinical practice.

CURRENT STATE OF CLINICAL INTEGRATION OF MOLECULAR PROGNOSTIC FACTORS

DNA Tumor-Based Prognostic Factors

Tumor-based genetic factors have been associated with clinical prognosis across many cancer sites. Integration into classification systems for prognosis and treatment is well established in hematologic malignancies. For example, cytogenetic abnormalities are used to classify acute leukemias into risk categories that result in different prognostic categories that ultimately shape treatment options.[3] In solid tumors, greater heterogeneity and complexity delays clinical use. Several DNA-based tumor approaches have been studied, including evaluating altered gene copy number, aberrant methylation of genes, and identification of specific genetic mutations. Gene copy number is a general term that encompasses gene amplification (gene copy increase), ploidy, and allelic loss (i.e., loss of heterozygosity or LOH). Loss of heterozygosity involves measurement of microsatellite markers, which are polymorphic tandem repeats of short nucleotide sequences spread throughout the genome. These markers help identify areas where portions of a chromosome are deleted.[4] Recently, single nucleotide polymorphisms have also been used as markers of LOH,[5] which has been useful in predicting the progression of preneoplastic lesions into frank neoplasia.[6,7] In addition, specific chromosomal areas of LOH are associated with prognosis across different cancer sites.[8–11] Aneuploidy has been associated with solid cancer prognosis in select studies.[12] Though not part of the staging parameters for breast cancer, her2 status (as determined by fluorescent *in situ* hybridization) is a prognostic marker and a target that directs clinical treatment with trastuzumab.[13,14] There is data to support the role of gene copy number in determining the prognosis of nonsmall-cell lung cancer patients treated with epidermal growth factor receptor (EGFR)-tyrosine kinase inhibitors.[15] Thus, gene copy number may be one area that is ripe for integration into staging schema in the coming years. Gene methylation involves the presence of DNA methyltransferase catalyzing the addition of a methyl group from S-adenosylmethionine covalently to the cytosine ring. Selective growth advantage may result from aberrant DNA methylation, particularly with the methylation of promoter regions leading to subsequent gene expression silencing. The genes *p16*, *Rb*, *PTEN*, and the *retinoic acid receptor beta* are commonly inactivated through this mechanism. Effects of methylation on cancer prognosis and staging are being explored currently.[16] Mutations of *p53*, *Rb*, *ras*, and other cell cycle, growth factor, or apoptotic pathway genes have been associated variably with the prognosis of solid tumors and may provide therapeutic targets.[17,18] A number of drugs and vaccines now in development target the effects of these mutations on their downstream pathways. A specific instance where mutations may have clinical impact is the recent discovery of mutations in the adenosine triphosphate (ATP)-binding pocket of EGFR gene. These mutations are associated with response to EGFR-tyrosine kinase inhibitor drugs in patients with advanced stage nonsmall lung cancer patients.[19,20] The ability to link pharmacologic response to specific mutations is more likely to result in incorporation of specific tumor mutations into classification and prognostic schema.

GENETIC POLYMORPHISMS IN CANCER PROGNOSIS AND PHARMACOGENETICS

Polymorphisms in genes involved in xenobiotic and chemotherapeutic drug metabolism, DNA repair, cell cycle, and stromal invasion pathways may be associated with survival outcomes of cancer patients. Polymorphic variants can alter messenger-ribonucleic acid (mRNA) or protein expression levels, and posttranslational modification of proteins. This research also focuses on phamacogenetics that could lead to improved prediction of drug response, prognosis, and individualized therapy. Polymorphisms of chemotherapy metabolizing genes or transporters may affect the disposition of the drug, compromising or enhancing either drug efficacy or drug toxicity. For example, platinum chemotherapy is conjugated by the glutathione s-transferase (GST) family of Phase II xenobiotic metabolism enzymes; taxanes and vinorelbine are metabolized primarily in the liver by CYP3A enzymes (CYP3A4 and CYP3A5); and gemcitabine is metabolized by cytidine deaminase. The *GST* polymorphisms have been associated variably with solid-tumor prognosis.[21–25] *UGT1A7* (UDP-glucuronosyltransferase) and *UGT1A9* polymorphisms may predict response and toxicity in colorectal cancer patients treated with capecitabine/irinotecan.[26] Pharmacogenetics may play an expanding role in the determination of specific therapies, as evidenced by the discovery of severe neutropenia from irinotecan that is associated with a genetic variant of *UGT1A1*,[27] resulting in recent changes to the irinotecan prescribing information and US Food and Drug Administration (FDA) approval of a DNA diagnostic test. Despite these successes, pharmacogenetic variants are more likely to alter treatment preferences than TNM (see Glossary) staging classification systems.

The DNA repair may play dual roles in cancer prognosis. Efficient DNA repair may decrease the number of somatic mutations and tumor aggressiveness, and may therefore be beneficial for survival. In contrast, an alternate theory suggests that efficient DNA repair will prevent the effective mechanism by which platinum drugs or radiation function, and decrease treatment efficiency. Studies suggest that DNA repair polymorphisms associated with altered DNA repair capacities may be associated with the prognosis of several solid tumors.[28–30] Polymorphisms of genes involved in other pathways, including matrix metalloproteinases (MMPs), angiogenesis (vascular endothelial growth factor, VEGF), inflammatory pathways (interleukins), and oxidative stress defense pathways, may also be prognostic across solid-tumor sites.[31–36]

Positive associations between genetic polymorphisms and cancer prognosis require confirmation in larger samples. Variation in frequency of genetic alleles across ethnicities further increases the complexity of these associations. Genetic variants will not be incorporated into clinical prognostic schema until larger observational and prospective clinical studies are performed. Technology allowing large-scale numbers of polymorphisms to be genotyped inexpensively will pave the way to such studies. Large-scale recruitment of cancer patients is also needed, along with uniform methods of tracking clinical outcomes. The resulting studies will likely change clinical outcome if we can identify alternative therapies directed at specific genetic variants.

RNA Prognostic Factors

Gene expression profiling is the use of high-throughput technologies to assay the RNA expressed in cells. Significant roles for gene expression profiling have been identified in solid tumors including breast cancer, melanoma, and lymphoma. Bittner et al.[37] identified a molecularly distinct melanoma with poor prognosis. Improved correlations with survival are found with the incorporation of gene profiling results into standard clinical prognostic indices for diffuse B-cell and follicular lymphomas.[38,39] In breast cancer, a gene expression signature strongly predicted breast cancer survival.[40] In addition, the prognostic data obtained from gene expression profiling are reproducible when using other techniques, such as quantitative reverse-transcriptase PCR.[41] The ability to better differentiate early stage cancers into individuals at high or low risk of recurrence could revolutionize classification systems.

Results from gene expression profiling from multiinstitutional or cooperative groups and the use of multiple cross-validation techniques[42] have significantly improved the quality of research studies in this area. Nonetheless, there are unresolved issues in incorporating RNA-based data into classification systems. First, samples will have to be collected and prepared differently from current standard practice since fresh frozen tissue is needed for most RNA-based studies. Second, increased costs for such analysis must be weighed against incremental benefit to patients. The cost and reliance of specialized technologies has led to attempts at reducing gene expression profiling results into evaluating smaller gene expression subsets that would still retain predictive power.[43] However, there may be benefits in evaluating patterns of gene expression rather than individual genes. Because of the multitude of biologic pathways involved, the expression of individual genes may not be strongly predictive of prognosis. Finding a balance between all of the above factors will be key to incorporating this technology into standard clinical use.

Protein-Based Prognostic Factors

A number of serum proteins, such as CA125 (ovarian cancer), PSA (prostate cancer), carcinoembryonic antigen (CEA) (colon cancer), and lactate dehydrogenase (LDH) (lymphomas) have been evaluated as prognostic factors. However, we will focus on advances in proteomics, the study of the proteome. The proteome is a collection of all the proteins expressed from the genome in all isoforms, polymorphisms, and post-translational modifications. Unlike genomic studies, proteomics, which quantitatively and qualitatively assesses protein expression patterns, protein interactions, and protein pathways, provides a dynamic picture of normal and abnormal cellular physiology.[44] Much of cancer proteomics focuses on the discovery of biomarkers for cancer diagnosis, prognosis, staging, recurrence, early detection, and response to therapy.[45] Meanwhile, the concept of biomarkers has expanded from a single measurement to signature patterns/profiles relevant to a large number of protein expressions.[46] For cancer, it is unlikely that any single biomarker will be a sufficient indicator; instead, multiple markers that function as the signature patterns/profiles will be necessary to achieve high predictive potential.[47]

A key feature of all state-of-art proteomic technologies is to enable the collection of hundreds or thousands of data points relevant to proteins or peptides from one sample and one measurement. Given the extreme complexity, several complementary technologies are currently applied for cancer proteomics because no single instrument or technology could cover all aspect of proteomics.[45,48] The development of tissue and protein arrays has also provided high-throughput quantitative tools with which to validate the clinical utility of biomarkers identified through discovery-based studies.[49] However, most of the recent progress in proteomics has been driven by the breakthrough advances in mass spectrometry (MS) technology, which revolutionized protein identification and increased sensitivity by several orders of magnitude.[50] Advances in MS have made it possible to rapidly generate complex proteomic profiles from clinical samples, and powerful bioinformatics tools have been developed to analyze these massive data sets.[51]

Potential candidates of biomarkers have been found in a variety of solid tumors.[52–56] Although proteomics has established itself as a valuable tool for basic cancer research, the application of proteomic technologies is still far from clinical application. A major obstacle in translating proteomic findings into clinical practice has been the lack of validation in large clinical trials. The identification of proteins *per se* is not sufficient to understand biological function because most proteins are post-translationally modified. Currently, no clinical integration of proteomic technology into prognostic classification systems has taken place. The promise of phosphoproteomics, or of glycoproteomics, which enables the study of important physiological post-translational modifications of proteins, may transform our understanding of the function of proteins. In this setting, specific markers that tightly reflect cancer biology (and therefore biologic behavior) may be on the horizon.

Detection of Occult Tumor Cells as Prognostic Factors

Occult tumor cells can be detected in the circulation or in specific tissues, such as regional lymph nodes. Identification of circulating tumor cells may be through direct extraction of intact tumor cells, or through detection of tumor-specific circulating DNA. Specific antibodies against tumor-specific components, such as MART-1 in melanoma[57] or cytokeratin in carcinomas[58] can be used also to identify the tumor cells. Reverse transcriptase PCR assays, tumor cell enrichment procedures, and utilization of multiple tumor markers expressed in disseminated cells, have all advanced technology in this field. A recent study found that the number of circulating tumor cells before treatment is an independent predictor of progression-free survival and overall survival in patients with metastatic breast cancer.[59] Circulating tumor-specific DNA is being evaluated as a monitor of hormone adjuvant therapy in breast cancer.[60]

Detection of micrometastases using PCR techniques may supplement standard staining with hematoxylin and eosin (or even immunohistochemisty) in regional lymph node biopsies. Large studies with recently completed accrual are evaluating the role of these techniques in breast and lung cancers (American College of Surgeons Oncology Group studies, Z0010 and Z0040). In some cases, the goal has been to combine sentinel lymph node biopsy with detection of occult metastases, while others are evaluating micrometastases in bone marrow aspirates, bronchoalveolar lavages, and in other tissues samples. Results from the larger multi-institutional studies are forthcoming, though a recent meta-analysis showed added value to evaluating breast micrometastasis.[61]

We are on the brink of the integration of molecular prognostic factors into practice. Bioinformatics will form one cornerstone of this process, as huge amounts of molecular information become available per sample. The DNA, RNA, protein, and cell-based samples are the key to understanding how cancer metastasizes and spreads, and this will translate into improved molecularly based prognostic tools. Massive recruiting efforts in addition to the uniform tracking of clinical outcomes are needed.

BARRIERS TO INTEGRATION INTO CLINICAL PRACTICE AND METHODS TO OVERCOME SUCH BARRIERS

Four interrelated factors describe the barriers to improved integration of molecular prognostic factors into clinical practice: (1) lack of definitive studies or confirmatory studies; (2) lack of ability to deal with large comparisons; (3) problems with data pooling; and (4) infrastructure support. Each will be dealt with separately.

Lack of Definitive or Confirmatory Studies

There are few definitive studies of molecular prognostic factors because of a lack of uniformity within the cancer population, a lack of independence of prognostic factors, and studies of small sample size, all of which affect the reproducibility of results. Many studies are compromised by types of samples (primary and recurrent diseases are combined), variations in primary site (mixing anatomic subsites in addition to histologic subtypes), lack of robust clinical outcome data, and different methodologic platforms. Results of prognostic studies are dependent on evaluating a broad spectrum of patients. Yet, too wide a spectrum may dilute a strong effect within a subgroup of patients. For example, if the prognostic effect of a molecular variable is seen primarily in lung adenocarcinomas because of specific adenocarcinoma-related pathways, then inclusion of other types of nonsmall lung cancers (i.e., large cell and squamous cell cancers) could dilute a true association. In addition, molecular factors may be related directly to pathophysiologic changes. If these pathophysiologic processes were associated with specific environmental factors (e.g., smoking) or genetic factors (e.g., race or ethnicity), then evaluation of a specific subset of patients not associated with this genetic or environmental association would lead to discrepant results. If, as a result of broad sample selection, a study has a relatively small proportion of patients evaluable for a true molecular prognostic factor, that factor may not show statistical significance. For example, response to EGFR tyrosine kinase inhibitors is significantly higher in nonsmoking women of East Asian descent with adenocarcinoma histology. Studies with different percentages of nonsmokers and women, different ethnic, or histologic distributions may yield conflicting conclusions on the role of molecular characteristics of EGFR.

In oncology, there is an additional layer of complexity associated with prognosis: tumors that can acquire new genetic events over time. Thus, a prognostic factor may become irrelevant in the face of a new somatic change. One example is that of a secondary (acquired) resistance EGFR mutation in nonsmall cell lung cancer in individuals who have demonstrated an activating mutation in EGFR associated with response to EGFR-tyrosine kinase inhibitors.[62] On the benefit side, identifying biomarkers that can detect secondary resistance to therapy may allow earlier individualization of drug therapies. Although many molecular prognostic studies utilize a convenient case series, newer prognostic studies are being assessed from clinical trials, where the samples are well defined and homogeneous. However, not all prognostic markers can be evaluated through clinical trials. Certain tumors remain relatively rare, and not all clinical studies collect tissue and blood specimens suitable for specific molecular analyses identified after the initiation of the clinical study. Coordinated, well-designed, prospective large-scale efforts are still needed.

Lack of independence of prognostic factors that stems from the natural biology of cancer can lead to difficult choices of interrelated molecular factors that should be analyzed. Mutations and germline polymorphisms may lead to specific changes in gene expression levels and activity that result in protein expression changes, followed by secondary signaling changes, and multiple feedback loops. In rare instances, a single mutational change may lead to all the secondary changes. In most cases, the initial events are not definable or are multifactorial. How then to approach such complex interactions and signaling pathways? The answer lies in the proposed role of the identified prognostic factor. If the prognostic factor is being used to identify new biological targets through hypothesis generation, then it is the preponderance of information that is important. Are biomarkers downstream of the prognostic factor related to outcomes also? Are there alternative biologic explanations for the proposed prognostic factor that can also act as targets? In this setting, the interdependency of prognostic factors across a specific pathway may be beneficial rather than detrimental. Thus, the identification of novel pathways may lead to new biological targets. However, if the goal is to identify patients with molecularly identified poorer prognosis so that these patients can be offered entry into experimental protocols, then one would want molecular prognostic factors that are robust enough across multiple subsets of well-defined patient populations to be useful clinically. In addition, a balance must be struck between ease of measurement (e.g., genotyping) and specificity of result (e.g., gene expression array predicting metastatic potential).

The high cost of microarray technology, combined with the logistical problems associated with collecting a large series of representative cases has led to the modest sample sizes, even for multi-institutional studies of molecular prognosis. In addition, these studies have rarely tried to evaluate molecular prognostic variables from different tissues, such as comparing the additional benefit of classifying prognosis through DNA, RNA, and protein profiling simultaneously. Part of the problem stems from multiple comparisons, discussed below.

Large Numbers of Comparisons

The greater the number of comparisons, the greater is the probability of a statistically significant chance finding. The usual standard of performing "corrections" of the p value (i.e., setting the p value at a more stringent threshold of significance) is not desirable, given the extreme conservative nature of these corrections and the high likelihood of missing true associations. A number of approaches have been taken to deal with these massive numbers of comparisons in modestly sized sample sets, including Bayesian and nonparametric approaches and cluster analyses.[63–65] As more datasets are available and cross-validation approaches are developed, it may be easier to understand and accept the different modeling approaches undertaken. Prospective validation of such models is key to proving that multiple comparisons are not driving spurious associations with prognosis. Further, in specific instances, patterns across microarray results have been found to be prognostic, and these patterns may be easier to incorporate into the clinical setting, when compared with hundreds or thousands of microarray variables individually.

Problems with Data and Sample Pooling

One method of gathering a large number of samples has been through the pooling of data and samples. Cancer Consortiums have formed in lung, breast, prostate, colon cancers, and lymphomas, to name a few. Most of these consortia have data and sample pooling as a top priority. Yet, there are often basic problems with heterogeneity of samples, outcomes and sample data collection methods, determination of clinical prognostic variables, and missing information. Most molecular prognostic studies collect clinical prognostic variables in addition to performing specifically hypothesized molecular analysis. Thus, data pooling is often inadequate for analysis. In such circumstances, several steps are needed to achieve the goal of pooling: (1) cross-validation across platforms must take place if individual laboratories use different molecular techniques; (2) investigators must agree on the priority list of biomarkers to assess; (3) funding must be obtained to move this research forward. In addition, there may be specific problems that cannot be overcome, such as when samples from patients who have died since were collected in such a means as to preclude specific molecular analyses. There have been notable exceptions to the problem of direct pooling of data. In the evaluation of genetic polymorphisms, it is relatively cost-efficient to genotype large numbers of samples, the technology for genotyping is readily available, and there is known consistency among multiple genotyping technology platforms. Additional exceptions can be found with microarray analyses, such as gene expression profiling, that utilize common technology platforms driven by the availability of a limited number of platforms (until recently). In the future, discussion among research groups, either informally or in formal groups, such as consortia, may lay the groundwork for common assessments in prospective evaluations of molecular prognostic factors.

In addition to these issues, a number of practical problems surface. Ownership of pooled information must be decided on prior to pooling. In general, there should be incentive for individual investigators to volunteer their samples or data for such analyses. The current reward systems at most academic institutions do no recognize this form of collaborative work sufficiently. Thus, investigators face the prospect of sharing information with potential current and future competitors for grants and funding. In the optimal setting, a system of rewarding individual collaborators for such work should be developed. Nonetheless, the individual consortia have managed to work through the issue of ownership through careful negotiations among its members. Explicit statements of goals and manifests by these consortia also help to make these processes transparent. The barriers increase when data pooling involves partnering with industry, but are not insurmountable.

Another issue that is relevant to the use of large repositories of human biological materials (HBM) is that the current system for the protection of human subjects may be ill-equipped to address the ethical issues arising from such studies. Although regulatory reform will probably take some time, institutions and their institutional review boards (IRBs) should begin to act now to familiarize themselves with such projects and begin educational and policy strategies for informed consent and assessment of risk and benefit arising from such studies so that they may be conducted as effectively as possible.[66]

Infrastructure Support

Since we have identified the need for large sample sizes to properly evaluate multiple molecular prognostic factors in a definitive fashion, an infrastructure for such a process must be developed. This is an opportunity for a leadership position to be taken by governmental agencies, academic institutions, and the private sector to support such research. There are several ways for agencies to support these endeavors: (1) provide or allocate specific funding for such efforts; (2) acknowledge, recognize, and reward individual investigators and their teams who collaborate in such projects; (3) develop core statements of principles and fairness for which such collaborations must adhere to; (4) provide forums for facilitating discussion of such collaborative efforts; (5) facilitate investigators and IRBs in obtaining appropriate approval for studies. Examples of such infrastructure building include the NCI Pipeline for Systemic Biomarker Discovery, the NCI Early Detection Research Network in the United States, and various IARC committees in Europe. Further, networks have formed among governmental and academic institutions (e.g., the NIH Pharmacogenetics Research Network) with the goal of large-scale evaluation of patients systematically.

Summary of Barriers to Integration

Integration of prognostic markers into prognostic classifications is analogous, in many ways, to new drug development (Fig. 6.3). Unfortunately, most molecular prognostic

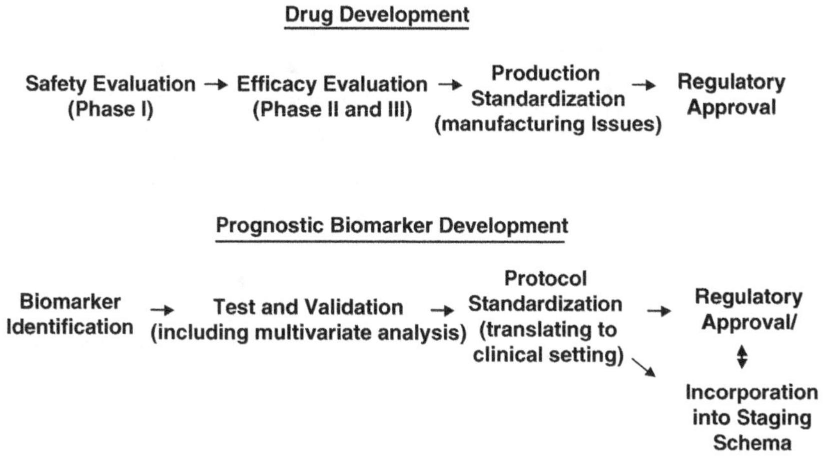

Drug Development

Safety Evaluation → Efficacy Evaluation → Production → Regulatory
(Phase I)   (Phase II and III)   Standardization   Approval
                                             (manufacturing Issues)

Prognostic Biomarker Development

                                          Protocol
Biomarker   →   Test and Validation   →   Standardization   →   Regulatory
Identification (including multivariate analysis) (translating to   Approval/
                                          clinical setting)   ↕

                                                             Incorporation
                                                             into Staging
                                                             Schema

FIGURE 6.3   Comparison between drug and prognostic biomarker development.

variables are still undergoing testing and validation. Implementation also requires standardization of techniques to measure these biologic variables, as key to regulatory approval. Regulatory approval is needed in order to use molecular prognostic factors in the clinical setting, a necessary and parallel step to incorporation into prognostic systems.

CONCLUSION

There are great expectations that molecular characteristics will be incorporated into future prognostic systems. Depending on the biology of the specific tumor site and the available targeted therapies, it is likely that biomarkers will be integrated to variable extent and under different scenarios. Figure 6.4 illustrates the possible ways for integration into traditional clinicopathologic prognostic schema. Scenario A has molecular biomarkers completely replacing clinical criteria, likely a rare and extreme event, limited to very specific tumor sites. Scenario B uses molecular markers to identify a very specific subset of patients who have distinct prognosis and targeted therapies available. In this instance, the molecular marker so strongly identifies a subgroup that no further clinical information is needed to further characterize this subset. An example of this is the BCR-ABL translocation in CML. In Scenario C, molecular markers are used to further prognosticate after clinicopathologic variables have been used to classify patients into traditional. One example is when specific molecular profiles further differentiates prognosis in early stage, but not late stage, cancers. Finally, Scenario D describes the circumstance where molecular characteristics are fully integrated into the prognostic system. In this instance, specific molecular characteristics of the tumor would form part of the definition of tumor staging while other molecular markers found in occult metastases help define nodal

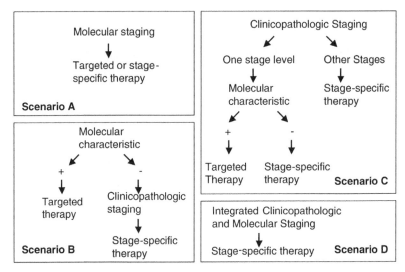

FIGURE 6.4 Possible integration strategies of molecular prognostic factors into standard clinicopathologic staging schema.

or metastasis staging. Thus, though possible in specific circumstances, molecular classification would unlikely replace clinical classification, but serve as an adjunct to clinical classification.

Methological issues as addressed above continue to pose challenges. These issues relate to multiple comparisons, sample and patient heterogeneity. In order to incorporate molecular characteristics into prognostic systems, the evidence will have to be strong, through large observational studies that will record multiple molecular parameters rather than a single molecular characteristic. Alternatively, clinical trials of targeted therapy are needed in molecularly distinct subgroups. There will be a need to compare across different categories of molecular factors, such as comparing DNA, RNA, and protein-based characteristics concurrently with each other and with clinical variables. The exploratory nature of microarray technology may identify smaller subsets of these molecular characteristics suitable for clinical use in the community setting. Finally, there will be emphasis on identifying molecular characteristics that are cost-efficient to implement. Hopefully, as these new technologies are adapted for clinical use, standardization across technologies will occur in addition to declining expenses.

With the completion of the human genome project, the emerging "omics" era has the potential to revolutionize disease diagnosis and management.[67] Evolving technologies have great potential in improving clinical prognostication. Our ability to evaluate the simultaneous influence of complex factors and infer information of value to cancer treatment is rapidly growing. The use of microarray technology opens new perspectives and brings the simultaneous identification of numerous DNA alterations at a grip, while microarrays or proteomic technologies help us to read the molecular signature (thousands of genes and proteins) of an individual patient's tumor. This is the promise of the future that eagerly awaits us.

REFERENCES

1. Green MR: Targeting targeted therapy. *N Engl J Med* 350:2191–2193, 2004.
2. Lehmann F, Lacombe D, Therasse P, et al.: Integration of Translational Research in the European Organization for Research and Treatment of Cancer Research (EORTC) Clinical Trial Cooperative Group Mechanisms. *J Transl Med* 1:2, 2003.
3. Mrozek K, Heerema NA, Bloomfield CD: Cytogenetics in acute leukemia. *Blood Rev* 18:115–136, 2004.
4. Tomlinson IP, Lambros MB, Roylance RR: Loss of heterozygosity analysis: practically and conceptually flawed? *Genes Chromosomes Cancer* 34:349–353, 2002.
5. Zhao X, Li C, Paez JG, et al.: An integrated view of copy number and allelic alterations in the cancer genome using single nucleotide polymorphism arrays. *Cancer Res* 64:3060–3071, 2004.
6. Jiang WW, Fujii H, Shirai T, et al.: Accumulative increase of loss of heterozygosity from leukoplakia to foci of early cancerization in leukoplakia of the oral cavity. *Cancer* 92:2349–2356, 2001.
7. Reid BJ, Blount PL, Rabinovitch PS: Biomarkers in Barrett's esophagus. *Gastrointest Endosc Clin N Am* 13:369–397, 2003.
8. Chang SC, Lin JK, Lin TC, et al.: Loss of heterozygosity: an independent prognostic factor of colorectal cancer. *World J Gastroenterol* 11:778–784, 2005.
9. Fenoglio-Preiser CM, Wang J, Stemmermann GN, et al.: TP53 and gastric carcinoma: a review. *Hum Mutat* 21:258–270, 2003.
10. Marsit CJ, Hasegawa M, Hirao T, et al.: Loss of heterozygosity of chromosome 3p21 is associated with mutant TP53 and better patient survival in non-small-cell lung cancer. *Cancer Res* 64:8702–8707, 2004.
11. Takita J, Hayashi Y, Yokota J: Loss of heterozygosity in neuroblastomas—an overview. *Eur J Cancer* 33:1971–1973, 1997.
12. Rajagopalan H, Lengauer C: Aneuploidy and cancer. *Nature (London)* 432:338–341, 2004.
13. Press MF, Bernstein L, Thomas PA, et al.: HER-2/neu gene amplification characterized by fluorescence in situ hybridization: poor prognosis in node-negative breast carcinomas. *J Clin Oncol* 15:2894–2904, 1997.
14. Slamon DJ, Leyland-Jones B, Shak S, et al.: Use of chemotherapy plus a monoclonal antibody against HER2 for metastatic breast cancer that overexpresses HER2. *N Engl J Med* 344:783–792, 2001.
15. Cappuzzo F, Varella-Garcia M, Shigematsu H, et al.: Increased HER2 gene copy number is associated with response to gefitinib therapy in epidermal growth factor receptor-positive non-small-cell lung cancer patients. *J Clin Oncol* 23:5007–5018, 2005.
16. Esteller M: CpG island hypermethylation and tumor suppressor genes: a booming present, a brighter future. *Oncogene* 21:5427–5440, 2002.
17. Partridge M, Gaballah K, Huang X: Molecular markers for diagnosis and prognosis. *Cancer Metastasis Rev* 24:71–85, 2005.
18. Vousden KH, Prives C: P53 and prognosis: new insights and further complexity. *Cell* 120:7–10, 2005.
19. Lynch TJ, Bell DW, Sordella R, et al.: Activating mutations in the epidermal growth factor receptor underlying responsiveness of non-small-cell lung cancer to gefitinib. *N Engl J Med* 350:2129–2139, 2004.

20. Paez JG, Janne PA, Lee JC, et al.: EGFR mutations in lung cancer: correlation with clinical response to gefitinib therapy. *Science* 304:1497–1500, 2004.

21. DeMichele A, Aplenc R, Botbyl J, et al.: Drug-metabolizing enzyme polymorphisms predict clinical outcome in a node-positive breast cancer cohort. *J Clin Oncol* 23:5552–5559, 2005.

22. Lee JM, Wu MT, Lee YC, et al.: Association of GSTP1 polymorphism and survival for esophageal cancer. *Clin Cancer Res* 11:4749–4753, 2005.

23. Okcu MF, Selvan M, Wang LE, et al.: Glutathione S-transferase polymorphisms and survival in primary malignant glioma. *Clin Cancer Res* 10:2618–2625, 2004.

24. Stoehlmacher J, Park DJ, Zhang W, et al.: Association between glutathione S-transferase P1, T1, and M1 genetic polymorphism and survival of patients with metastatic colorectal cancer. *J Natl Cancer Inst* 94:936–942, 2002.

25. Sweeney C, Nazar-Stewart V, Stapleton PL, et al.: Glutathione S-transferase M1, T1, and P1 polymorphisms and survival among lung cancer patients. *Cancer Epidemiol Biomarkers Prev* 12:527–533, 2003.

26. Carlini LE, Meropol NJ, Bever J, et al.: UGT1A7 and UGT1A9 polymorphisms predict response and toxicity in colorectal cancer patients treated with capecitabine/irinotecan. *Clin Cancer Res* 11:1226–1236, 2005.

27. Innocenti F, Undevia SD, Iyer L, et al.: Genetic variants in the UDP-glucuronosyltransferase 1A1 gene predict the risk of severe neutropenia of irinotecan. *J Clin Oncol* 22:1382–1388, 2004.

28. Gu J, Zhao H, Dinney CP, et al.: Nucleotide excision repair gene polymorphisms and recurrence after treatment for superficial bladder cancer. *Clin Cancer Res* 11:1408–1415, 2005.

29. Gurubhagavatula S, Liu G, Park S, et al.: XPD and XRCC1 genetic polymorphisms are prognostic factors in advanced non-small-cell lung cancer patients treated with platinum chemotherapy. *J Clin Oncol* 22:2594–2601, 2004.

30. Liu D, O'Day SJ, Yang D, et al.: Impact of gene polymorphisms on clinical outcome for stage IV melanoma patients treated with biochemotherapy: an exploratory study. *Clin Cancer Res* 11:1237–1246, 2005.

31. Ambrosone CB, Ahn J, Singh KK, et al.: Polymorphisms in genes related to oxidative stress (MPO, MnSOD, CAT) and survival after treatment for breast cancer. *Cancer Res* 65:1105–1111, 2005.

32. Graziano F, Ruzzo A, Santini D, et al.: Prognostic role of interleukin-1beta gene and interleukin-1 receptor antagonist gene polymorphisms in patients with advanced gastric cancer. *J Clin Oncol* 23:2339–2345, 2005.

33. Lai HC, Chu CM, Lin YW, et al.: Matrix metalloproteinase 1 gene polymorphism as a prognostic predictor of invasive cervical cancer. *Gynecol Oncol* 96:314–319, 2005.

34. Lu H, Shu XO, Cui Y, et al.: Association of genetic polymorphisms in the VEGF gene with breast cancer survival. *Cancer Res* 65:5015–5019, 2005.

35. Shin A, Cai Q, Shu XO, et al.: Genetic polymorphisms in the matrix metalloproteinase 12 gene (MMP12) and breast cancer risk and survival: the Shanghai Breast Cancer Study. *Breast Cancer Res* 7:R506–R512, 2005.

36. Zinzindohoue F, Lecomte T, Ferraz JM, et al.: Prognostic significance of MMP-1 and MMP-3 functional promoter polymorphisms in colorectal cancer. *Clin Cancer Res* 11:594–599, 2005.

37. Bittner M: A window on the dynamics of biological switches. *Nat Biotechnol* 23:183–184, 2005.

38. Dave SS, Wright G, Tan B, et al.: Prediction of survival in follicular lymphoma based on molecular features of tumor-infiltrating immune cells. *N Engl J Med* 351:2159–2169, 2004.

39. Rosenwald A, Wright G, Chan WC, et al.: The use of molecular profiling to predict survival after chemotherapy for diffuse large-B-cell lymphoma. *N Engl J Med* 346:1937–1947, 2002.

40. van de Vijver MJ, He YD, van't Veer LJ, et al.: A gene-expression signature as a predictor of survival in breast cancer. *N Engl J Med* 347:1999–2009, 2002.

41. Espinosa E, Vara JA, Redondo A, et al.: Breast Cancer Prognosis Determined by Gene Expression Profiling: A Quantitative Reverse Transcriptase Polymerase Chain Reaction Study. *J Clin Oncol* 23:7278–7285, 2005.

42. Feng Z, Prentice R, Srivastava S: Research issues and strategies for genomic and proteomic biomarker discovery and validation: a statistical perspective. *Pharmacogenomics* 5:709–719, 2004.

43. Lossos IS, Czerwinski DK, Alizadeh AA, et al.: Prediction of survival in diffuse large-B-cell lymphoma based on the expression of six genes. *N Engl J Med* 350:1828–1837, 2004.

44. Rai AJ, Chan DW: Cancer proteomics: Serum diagnostics for tumor marker discovery. *Ann N Y Acad Sci* 1022:286–294, 2004.

45. Kolch W, Mischak H, Pitt AR: The molecular make-up of a tumour: proteomics in cancer research. *Clin Sci (London)* 108:369–383, 2005.

46. Hanash S: Disease proteomics. *Nature (London)* 422:226–232, 2003.

47. Bischoff R, Luider TM: Methodological advances in the discovery of protein and peptide disease markers. *J Chromatogr B Analyt Technol Biomed Life Sci* 803:27–40, 2004.

48. Graham DR, Elliott ST, Van Eyk JE: Broad-based proteomic strategies: a practical guide to proteomics and functional screening. *J Physiol* 563:1–9, 2005.

49. Ornstein DK, Petricoin EF, 3rd: Proteomics to diagnose human tumors and provide prognostic information. *Oncology* (Williston Park) 18:521–529; discussion 529–532, 2004.

50. Conrads TP, Hood BL, Issaq HJ, et al.: Proteomic patterns as a diagnostic tool for early-stage cancer: a review of its progress to a clinically relevant tool. *Mol Diagn* 8:77–85, 2004.

51. Thadikkaran L, Siegenthaler MA, Crettaz D, et al.: Recent advances in blood-related proteomics. *Proteomics* 5:3019–3034, 2005.

52. Chen R, Pan S, Brentnall TA, et al.: Proteomic profiling of pancreatic cancer for biomarker discovery. *Mol Cell Proteomics* 4:523–533, 2005.

53. Conrads TP, Fusaro VA, Ross S, et al.: High-resolution serum proteomic features for ovarian cancer detection. *Endocr Relat Cancer* 11:163–178, 2004.

54. Goggins M: Molecular markers of early pancreatic cancer. *J Clin Oncol* 23:4524–4531, 2005.

55. Meyerson M, Carbone D: Genomic and proteomic profiling of lung cancers: lung cancer classification in the age of targeted therapy. *J Clin Oncol* 23:3219–3226, 2005.

56. Somiari RI, Somiari S, Russell S, et al.: Proteomics of breast carcinoma. *J Chromatogr B Analyt Technol Biomed Life Sci* 815:215–225, 2005.

57. Palmieri G, Ascierto PA, Perrone F, et al.: Prognostic value of circulating melanoma cells detected by reverse transcriptase-polymerase chain reaction. *J Clin Oncol* 21:767–773, 2003.

58. Muller V, Stahmann N, Riethdorf S, et al.: Circulating tumor cells in breast cancer: correlation to bone marrow micrometastases, heterogeneous response to systemic therapy and low proliferative activity. *Clin Cancer Res* 11:3678–3685, 2005.

59. Cristofanilli M, Budd GT, Ellis MJ, et al.: Circulating tumor cells, disease progression, and survival in metastatic breast cancer. *N Engl J Med* 351:781–791, 2004.

60. Fiegl H, Millinger S, Mueller-Holzner E, et al.: Circulating tumor-specific DNA: a marker for monitoring efficacy of adjuvant therapy in cancer patients. *Cancer Res* 65:1141–1145, 2005.

61. Braun S, Vogl FD, Naume B, et al.: A pooled analysis of bone marrow micrometastasis in breast cancer. *N Engl J Med* 353:793–802, 2005.

62. Kobayashi S, Boggon TJ, Dayaram T, et al.: EGFR mutation and resistance of non-small-cell lung cancer to gefitinib. *N Engl J Med* 352:786–792, 2005.

63. Gu CC, Rao DC, Stormo G, et al.: Role of gene expression microarray analysis in finding complex disease genes. *Genet Epidemiol* 23:37–56, 2002.

64. Shannon W, Culverhouse R, Duncan J: Analyzing microarray data using cluster analysis. *Pharmacogenomics* 4:41–52, 2003.

65. Yang D, Zakharkin SO, Page GP, et al.: Applications of Bayesian statistical methods in microarray data analysis. *Am J Pharmacogenomics* 4:53–62, 2004.

66. Meslin EM, Quaid KA: Ethical issues in the collection, storage, and research use of human biological materials. *J Lab Clin Med* 144:229–234: discussion 226, 2004.

67. Espina V, Dettloff KA, Cowherd S, et al.: Use of proteomic analysis to monitor responses to biological therapies. *Expert Opin Biol Ther* 4:83–93, 2004.

PROGNOSTIC FACTORS IN SPECIFIC CANCERS

HEAD AND NECK TUMORS

CHAPTER 7

Oral Cavity, Pharynx, and Larynx Cancer

JEAN BOURHIS

Cancers of the oral cavity, pharynx, and larynx have an annual worldwide incidence of ~500,000 new cases. Most commonly presenting in males and in those older than 50 years, their causation is profoundly linked to lifestyle exposure to tobacco and alcohol.[1] The predominant histology is squamous cell carcinoma (SCCHN), a locally aggressive tumor with a tendency to metastasize to cervical lymph nodes and/or retropharyngeal nodes. This risk varies according to anatomic site, being highest in the hypopharynx followed by the oropharynx and supraglottic larynx (generally equivalent), the oral cavity, and rarely the glottis except in locally advanced disease (notably T4-category). In presentations with large and/or numerous lymph node involvement, the risk of distant metastasis is markedly increased.[1] The main cause of failure is uncontrolled disease in the primary and regional lymph nodes, whereas other factors, such as the relatively high probability of a subsequent second primary cancer, the occurrence of distant metastases, and associated comorbidities also contribute to the relatively poor outcome.[2]

Assessment entails a complete history and physical examination including panendoscopy under general anesthesia to evaluate primary tumor extent and to exclude potential second primary tumors. The latter are not infrequent due to their common causality in the oral cavity, pharynx, larynx, esophagus, or bronchus. Depending on the anatomic region, investigations should focus on imaging of the primary site and the cervical nodes with contrast enhanced magnetic resonance imaging (MRI) and/or computed tomography (CT). Thoracic CT is generally indicated in advanced locoregional disease to exclude pulmonary metastases.

Early stage tumors are usually managed by a single modality with either surgery, external beam radiotherapy, or brachytherapy. For more locally advanced cases, a combined approach with surgery and postoperative radiotherapy (radiochemotherapy in

Prognostic Factors in Cancer, *Third Edition*, edited by Mary K. Gospodarowicz, Brian O'Sullivan, and Leslie H. Sobin.
Copyright © 2006 John Wiley & Sons, Inc.

high-risk patients) can be used. In some subsites, even if still operable (e.g., tonsil), and in nonoperable patients, radiotherapy is the treatment of choice. Improvements in delivery methods, such as altered fractionation, have been shown to increase locoregional control.[3] Intensity modulated radiotherapy (IMRT) is now used more frequently to ameliorate damage to salivary tissues because of the ability to treat more selective target volumes.[4] The benefits of chemotherapy are being increasingly recognized in both resectable and unresectable disease.[5–7] The value of adding chemotherapy to radiotherapy in several settings has been confirmed in a meta-analysis,[5] where the addition of chemotherapy was associated with a survival advantage of 4% at 5 years, most pronounced with the use of concomitant chemoradiotherapy.[5] Chemotherapy may also be employed for metastatic disease, though its value is considered palliative.

The most important prognostic factor remains the anatomic extent of disease, according to the TNM classification.[8] Anatomic location (larynx better prognosis than hypopharynx), as well as tumor extension into soft tissues, bone, and/or cartilage[2] are additional determinants of tumor control and survival.[2] Involvement of lymph nodes remains a strong negative prognostic factor.[9] From a large series of mucosal cancers, 5-year survival rates are ~90% for stage I disease, 75% for stage II, 60% for stage III, 30% for stage IVA, 25% for stage IVB, and <4% for stage IVC disease.[9] Deeply infiltrating tumors also carry a poorer prognosis than exophytic ones. Regarding tumor site specifically, a review of a series of 5161 successive cases showed 5-year overall survival rates of 30% for oral cavity, 14% for oropharynx, 12% for hypopharynx, and 40% for larynx cancer.[10] In addition, tumors with the highest association with combined alcohol and tobacco abuse (i.e., hypopharyngeal and sugraglottic) generally have a worse prognosis because of comorbidities (e.g., liver disease and second cancers) compared to disease where smoking is the only etiologic factor (e.g., glottic cancer).[9] To date, no convincing data are available as to the prognostic significance of tumor differentiation (well vs. poorly differentiated).

The interplay between host and environment related prognostic factors is important, especially in light of common underlying tumor causality. While these tumors tend to be more prevalent in less affluent communities, there is also the substantial influence of host comorbidity on the ability to tolerate intensive treatment. Survival rates are thus dependent on performance status, nutritional status, age, and the presence of comorbidity, such as cardiovascular, liver, or cerebrovascular disease.[2,11] In addition, the quality of treatment also affects outcome including how radiotherapy is delivered at the population level[12] or in the ability of a surgeon to achieve clear resection margins—though the latter is greatly confounded by the extent and complexity of disease presentation. For patients who undergo surgery, prognostic factors for recurrence include positive pathological margins, involvement of three or more nodes, the level of lymph node (i.e., lower neck level IV[13]) and, importantly, extracapsular nodal extension by tumor. These risks factors justify increased intensification of adjuvant treatment by combining postoperative radiochemotherapy.[6] In the case of negative histologic margins, the application of molecular tumor markers could represent a new prognostic tool to help guide adjuvant therapy in the future.[14]

Among the new and promising molecular prognostic factors, hyperexpression of epidermal growth-factor receptor (EGFR) has been shown to correlate with tumor size and stage, and appears to correlate with unfavorable outcomes: poorer survival, shorter disease-free interval, and higher recurrence rates after irradiation.[15] Other factors including plasma or imaging markers of hypoxia (osteopontin, PET-F18miso)[16–18] have been studied. Many other prognostic markers have been proposed including p53, Ki67, P16, tumor cell kinetics, hemoglobin level, and DNA profiling. These factors await further validation before they can be utilized and applied clinically.[19]

Ongoing improvement in the therapeutic ratio by further increasing tumor control without increasing treatment toxicity remains a major objective in the management of head and neck SCC. Judicious patient selection based on prognostic profiles and potentially combining targeted treatments may result in reduced loco-regional treatment toxicity.[20] A corollary to this improvement in loco-regional control is the significant emerging challenge of a changing natural history and pattern of disease relapse manifested by distant metastasis (see Summary Table).

Prognostic Factors in Oral Cavity, Pharynx, and Larynx Cancer

Prognostic Factors	Tumor Related	Host Related	Environment Related
Essential	T category N category M category Anatomic subsite	Performance status	

Additional	Resection margin
	Number of
	  involved nodes
	Extracapsular
	  nodal extension
	Perineural, lympho-
	  vascular invasion
	Tumor hypoxia
		Comorbidities
		Age
			Radiation dose
			Overall treatment time
			Quality of surgery and
			  radiotherapy

New and promising	EGFR expression Surgical molecular margins Osteopontin DNA profiling		

Sources:
• ESMO guidelines for management of SCC of the head and neck 2005.
http://www.esmo.org/reference/referenceGuidelines/pdf/new_pdf/ESMO_16_SCCHN.pdf.
• National Cancer Institute: Lip and Oral Cavity (PDQ®): Treatment Guidelines 2005.
http://www.cancer.gov/cancertopics/pdq/treatment/lip-and-oral-cavity/healthprofessional/.
• NCCN Clinical Practice Guidelines in Oncology: Head and Neck Cancer 2005.
http://www.nccn.org/professionals/physician_gls/PDF/head-and-neck.pdf.

REFERENCES

1. Kowalski LP, Carvalho AL: Natural history of untreated head and neck cancer. *Eur J Cancer* 36:1032–1037, 2000.
2. Baatenburg de Jong RJ, Hermans J, Molenaar J, et al.: Prediction of survival in patients with head and neck cancer. *Head Neck* 23:718–724, 2001.

3. Overgaard J, Hansen HS, Specht L, et al.: Five compared with six fractions per week of conventional radiotherapy of squamous-cell carcinoma of head and neck: DAHANCA 6 and 7 randomised controlled trial. *Lancet* 362:933–940, 2003.

4. Lin A, Kim HM, Terrell JE, et al.: Quality of life after parotid-sparing IMRT for head-and-neck cancer: a prospective longitudinal study. *Int J Radiat Oncol Biol Phys* 57:61–70, 2003.

5. Pignon JP, Bourhis J, Domenge C, et al.: Chemotherapy added to locoregional treatment for head and neck squamous-cell carcinoma: three meta-analyses of updated individual data. MACH-NC Collaborative Group. Meta-Analysis of Chemotherapy on Head and Neck Cancer. *Lancet* 355:949–955, 2000.

6. Bernier J, Domenge C, Ozsahin M, et al.: Postoperative irradiation with or without concomitant chemotherapy for locally advanced head and neck cancer. *N Engl J Med* 350:1945–1952, 2004.

7. Cooper JS, Pajak TF, Forastiere AA, et al.: Postoperative concurrent radiotherapy and chemotherapy for high-risk squamous-cell carcinoma of the head and neck. *N Engl J Med* 350:1937–1944, 2004.

8. Sobin L, Wittekind C: *TNM Classification of Malignant Tumours* (6th ed.). New York, Wiley-Liss, 2002.

9. Iro H, Waldfahrer F: Evaluation of the newly updated TNM classification of head and neck carcinoma with data from 3247 patients. *Cancer* 83:2201–2207, 1998.

10. Lefebvre J-L LE, Kara A: *Oral cavity, pharynx and larynx cancer* (2nd ed.). New York. Wiley-Liss, 2001.

11. Borggreven PA, Kuik DJ, Quak JJ, et al.: Comorbid condition as a prognostic factor for complications in major surgery of the oral cavity and oropharynx with microvascular soft tissue reconstruction. *Head Neck* 25:808–815, 2003.

12. Groome PA, O'Sullivan B, Mackillop WJ, et al.: Compromised Local Control due to Treatment Interruptions and Late Treatment Breaks in Early Glottic Cancer: A Population-Based Outcomes Study Supporting the Need for Intensified Treatment Schedules. *Int J Radiat Oncol Biol Phys* 64:1002–1012, 2006.

13. Kowalski LP, Bagietto R, Lara JR, et al.: Prognostic significance of the distribution of neck node metastasis from oral carcinoma. *Head Neck* 22:207–214, 2000.

14. Temam S, Casiraghi O, Lahaye JB, et al.: Tetranucleotide microsatellite instability in surgical margins for prediction of local recurrence of head and neck squamous cell carcinoma. *Clin Cancer Res* 10:4022–4028, 2004.

15. Bentzen SM, Atasoy BM, Daley FM, et al.: Epidermal growth factor receptor expression in pretreatment biopsies from head and neck squamous cell carcinoma as a predictive factor for a benefit from accelerated radiation therapy in a randomized controlled trial. *J Clin Oncol* 23:5560–5567, 2005.

16. Nordsmark M, Bentzen SM, Rudat V, et al.: Prognostic value of tumor oxygenation in 397 head and neck tumors after primary radiation therapy. An international multi-center study. *Radiother Oncol* 77:18–24, 2005.

17. Overgaard J, Eriksen JG, Nordsmark M, et al.: Plasma osteopontin, hypoxia, and response to the hypoxia sensitiser nimorazole in radiotherapy of head and neck cancer: results from the DAHANCA 5 randomised double-blind placebo-controlled trial. *Lancet Oncol* 6:757–764, 2005.

18. Hicks RJ, Rischin D, Fisher R, et al.: Utility of FMISO PET in advanced head and neck cancer treated with chemoradiation incorporating a hypoxia-targeting chemotherapy agent. *Eur J Nucl Med Mol Imaging* 2005.

19. Quon H, Liu FF, Cummings BJ: Potential molecular prognostic markers in head and neck squamous cell carcinomas. *Head Neck* 23:147–159, 2001.

20. Bonner JA, Harari PM, Giralt J, Azarnia N, Shin DM, Cohen RB, Jones CU, Sur R, Raben D, Jassem J. Ove R, Kies MS, Baselga J, Youssoufian H, Amellal N, Rowinsky EK, Ang KK: Phase III study of high dose radiation with or without cetuximab in the treatment of locoregionally advanced squamous cell cancer of the head and neck (SCCHN). *New Eng J Med* 2006.

CHAPTER 8

Paranasal Sinus Cancer

JOHN N. WALDRON

Paranasal sinus cancer (PSC) is rare and represents <5% of all head and neck malignancy. The majority arise from the maxillary sinus (70–80%), with the remainder from the ethmoid sinus (10–20%), and the sphenoid or frontal sinuses are exceptionally rare primary sites. Squamous cell carcinoma accounts for 60–75% of cases with adenocarcinomas, adenoid cystic carcinomas, and undifferentiated carcinomas accounting for the other 25–40%. Treatment is complicated by the close proximity of these tumors to critical neurovascular anatomy. Treatment guidelines and recent reviews for cancers arising in the ethmoid and maxillary sinuses exist.[1–4] However, the outcome of patients presenting with PSC is unsatisfactory and most centers report 5-year cause specific survival rates of 40–50%.[5,6] Death is often due to failure to control local disease.

Patient assessment entails a complete history and physical examination. Imaging with contrast enhanced computerized tomography (CT) of head and neck, and/or magnetic resonance imaging (MRI), which has a particular advantage in differentiating overt tumor from the frequent presence of retained mucous and inflammatory tissue in the sinuses. Chest X-ray (or chest CT in patients with advanced loco-regional disease) should be performed. Attention to pathology confirmation is essential given the potential for many rare malignant histologies to originate in the paranasal sinuses in addition to the carcinomas referred to in this chapter. Management in a multidisciplinary setting is encouraged with input from plastic surgery, dentistry, speech pathology, and nutritional support services.

Anatomic disease extent is the most important prognostic factor.[7,8] Squamous cell and adenocarcinomas have similar outcomes once stage is taken into account. Adenoid cystic cancers will often demonstrate superior initial local control compared to squamous carcinomas, but have a propensity to recur many years after the original diagnosis and to develop distant metastasis (usually in lung) even if the primary is controlled.[8] Undifferentiated tumors, which are considered to have the worst prognosis, often

Prognostic Factors in Cancer, Third Edition, edited by Mary K. Gospodarowicz,
Brian O'Sullivan, and Leslie H. Sobin.
Copyright © 2006 John Wiley & Sons, Inc.

present with a rapidly expanding primary site and propensity to failure at distant metastatic sites.[9] Better prognosis for younger and female patients has been reported.[7,10] Performance status as a predictor of outcome is likely related to the ability to tolerate radical treatment.

Presenting symptoms of PSC include pain, facial swelling, nasal obstruction, nasal discharge or epistaxis, and oral cavity symptoms. Masticator space, skull base, or orbital involvement can cause trismus, cranial neuropathies, and diplopia. Facial erythema and induration suggest involvement of the overlying skin, while proptosis suggests gross orbital involvement. Malignant adenopathy in the neck is documented in 10–15% of patients at presentation.

Treatment usually consists of a combination or sequence of surgery, radiation, and chemotherapy. In general, early stage tumors are managed by surgical resection or primary radiation. For more advanced tumors, a combined modality approach with radical surgical resection followed by radiation is advised. Inoperable tumors are managed by radiation alone. Chemotherapy is often utilized in combination with radiation though the rarity of these tumors has meant that randomized trial data are not available in contrast to many other head and neck cancers. The establishment of clear surgical margins and the delivery of higher doses of radiation over shorter overall treatment times has been associated with better outcome.[7] However outcome assessments associated with the different available treatment approaches are subject to selection bias. In fact multivariate analyses of outcome in contemporary series has failed to identify treatment approach as an independent predictor of outcome.[5,10,11] Therefore, intensive radiotherapy approaches with concurrent chemotherapy or complete surgical removal and adjuvant radiotherapy remain reasonable recommendations in the absence of level I evidence. If patients present with or develop distant metastasis, there is no curative treatment available and best supportive care is indicated.

Dulguerov et al.[10] noted an improvement in outcome over the past four decades. These improvements are likely related to advances in CT and MR imaging and treatment techniques that in turn have resulted in changes in treatment selection and the accuracy with which treatment can be administered.[12] Advanced surgical techniques now permit complete resection more often than was possible two decades ago. High-precision intensity modulated radiation therapy (IMRT) permits optimal radiation delivery and sparing of normal tissues thus reducing toxicity and allowing dose escalation.[13,14] The use of concurrent chemotherapy holds promise based on other head and neck cancers.[15]

Since the prospect of randomized clinical trials in this disease is remote, it remains critical that patient groups within Phase I and II clinical trials be uniformly staged and described to facilitate comparison. Controversies remain regarding the relative roles of surgery and radiotherapy as the predominant treatments for a given scenario, and the precise place of adjuvant treatments in patients treated with surgery, and the role of chemotherapy in combination with radiotherapy. Whatever the specifics of the treatment approach the management of these rare tumors remains complex and when appropriate patients should be referred to centers with the necessary expertise to offer aggressive state-of-the art treatment.

■■■■■■■ SUMMARY TABLE

Prognostic Factors in Paranasal Sinus Cancer

Prognostic Factors	Tumor Related	Host Related	Environment Related
Essential	T category N category M category		
Additional	Histopathological subtype	Age Gender Performance status	Radiation dose Total time of treatment Clear surgical margins
New and promising			High precision dose escalation radiation Concurrent cytotoxic or biologic therapies Ideal integration with advanced surgical techniques

Sources:
• Head and Neck Cancer In: Practice Guidelines in Oncology: National Comprehensive Cancer Network 2005. http://www.nccn.org/professionals/physician_gls/PDF/head-and-neck.pdf.
• Paranasal Sinus Cancer Treatment Guidelines: National Cancer Institute http://www.cancer.gov/ cancertopics/types/head-and-neck/ 2005.

REFERENCES

1. Head and Neck Cancer, Practice Guidelines in Oncology: National Comprehensive Cancer Network. http://www.nccn.org Accessed 2005.

2. Paranasal Sinus Cancer Treatment Guidelines: National Cancer Institute. http://cancer. gov Accessed 2005.

3. Costantino PD, Murphy MR, Moche JA: Cancer of the Nasal Vestibule, Nasal Cavity, and Paranasal Sinus—Surgical Management, in Harrison LB, Sessions RB, Hong WK (eds.): *Head and Neck Cancer—A Multidisciplinary Approach* (2nd ed.). Philadelphia, Lippinncott Williams and Wilkins, 2005, pp. 455–479.

4. Parsons JT, Kies MS: Cancer of the Nasal Vestibule, Nasal Cavity, and Paranasal Sinus— Radiation Therapy and Chemotherapy Management, in Harrison LB, Sessions RB,

Hong WK (eds.): *Head and Neck Cancer—A Mulitdisciplinary Approach* (2nd ed.). Philadelphia, Lippinncott Williams and Wilkins, 2005, pp. 480–528.

5. Katz TS, Mendenhall WM, Morris CG, et al.: Malignant tumors of the nasal cavity and paranasal sinuses. *Head Neck* 24:821–829, 2002.

6. Porceddu S, Martin J, Shanker G, et al.: Paranasal sinus tumors: Peter MacCallum Cancer Institute experience. *Head Neck* 26:322–330, 2004.

7. Waldron JN, Witterick I: Paranasal Sinus Cancer, in Gospodarowicz MK, Henson DE, Hutter RVP, et al. (eds.): *Prognostic Factors in Cancer* (2nd ed.). New York, Wiley-Liss, 2001, pp. 167–182.

8. Waldron J, Witterick I: Paranasal sinus cancer: caveats and controversies. *World J Surg* 27:849–855, 2003.

9. Kim BS, Vongtama R, Juillard G: Sinonasal undifferentiated carcinoma: case series and literature review. *Am J Otolaryngol* 25:162–166, 2004.

10. Dulguerov P, Jacobsen MS, Allal AS, et al.: Nasal and paranasal sinus carcinoma: are we making progress? A series of 220 patients and a systematic review. *Cancer* 92:3012–3029, 2001.

11. Waldron JN, O'Sullivan B, Gullane P, et al.: Carcinoma of the maxillary antrum: a retrospective analysis of 110 cases. *Radiother Oncol* 57:167–173, 2000.

12. Loevner LA, Sonners AI: Imaging of neoplasms of the paranasal sinuses. *Neuroimaging Clin N Am* 14:625–646, 2004.

13. Claus F, Boterberg T, Ost P, et al.: Short term toxicity profile for 32 sinonasal cancer patients treated with IMRT. Can we avoid dry eye syndrome? *Radiother Oncol* 64:205–208, 2002.

14. O'Daniel JC, Dong L, Kuban DA, et al.: The delivery of IMRT with a single physical modulator for multiple fields: a feasibility study for paranasal sinus cancer. *Int J Radiat Oncol Biol Phys* 58:876–887, 2004.

15. Cooper JS, Ang KK: Concomitant chemotherapy and radiation therapy certainly improves local control. *Int J Radiat Oncol Biol Phys* 61:7–9, 2005.

CHAPTER 9

Nasopharyngeal Cancer

JOSEPH WEE and ENG HUAT TAN

Nasopharyngeal Cancer (NPC) is rare in the West, but is the commonest head and neck cancer in the endemic regions of South China and Southeast Asia (incidence between 16 and 21 per 100,000 males),[1] with intermediate incidence rates (~6 per 100,000 males) in areas around the Mediterranean basin and in the arctic regions affecting the Inuits.

In the nonendemic regions, the etiology of NPC is closely related to smoking, and the histological type—the keratinizing form of squamous cell cancers (SCC) is in common with the other head and neck cancers. In the endemic regions, there is an association with the Epstein–Barr virus (EBV) and the consumption of salted fish.[2,3]

Patients typically present with neck masses, unilateral hearing loss, tinnitus, epistaxis, and cranial nerve palsies. Staging investigations should include history, physical examination, nasopharyngeal examination and biopsy, dental evaluation, as well as cross-sectional imaging of the primary and neck regions (preferably magnetic resonance imaging, MRI), and a metastatic screen including chest X-ray, hemogram, and chemistry panel.[2–4] Any clinical or laboratory suspicion of distant spread or the presence of advanced nodal disease (N2-3) would warrant a more thorough distant work up (imaging of the chest, liver, and bones).[3,4] Positron emission tomographic (PET) imaging appears promising and a recent study suggests that PET is more accurate and sensitive than conventional workup for N and M staging.[5]

High-dose radiotherapy (RT)[2–4] is the main stay of treatment and results in overall 5-year cure rates of ~60%.[6] Surgery, where feasible, is reserved for residual or recurrent nodal disease.[2–4] The addition of radiosensitizing chemotherapy concurrently during RT has been shown to improve overall survival in four recent randomized trials.[7] Two of these trials had an adjuvant component following chemo-RT. Hence, combined modality using a concurrent chemoradiotherapy schedule has become the standard of care for those with stage III/IV locally advanced disease.[2–4,7]

Prognostic Factors in Cancer, Third Edition, edited by Mary K. Gospodarowicz, Brian O'Sullivan, and Leslie H. Sobin.
Copyright © 2006 John Wiley & Sons, Inc.

Cross-sectional imaging is critical to ensure that there is adequacy of tumor coverage, especially in late T stage disease and early results with intensity modulated radiotherapy (IMRT)[8] appear to support this. The hazard rate for local failure is increased by 3.3% for each day of interruption[6] and the role of accelerated radiotherapy with or without concurrent chemotherapy[9,10] is under investigation. Brachytherapy[4] and stereotactic boosts[10] may enhance local control.

Patients who have completed primary treatment for NPC should be followed up with initial 1–3 monthly physical examinations as well as annual imaging and thyroid function screens.[4] For those that recur at the primary site, reirradiation or salvage surgery may be considered. A neck dissection should be considered for those with nodal recurrence.[2–4]

The mainstay of treatment for patients with disseminated disease is platinum-based chemotherapy.[4] The advent of newer cytotoxics have expanded the armamentarium of therapeutic agents available.[11]

Prognosis is closely related to the stage at presentation.[2,4] The role of the histological subtype is controversial. Some retrospective reviews suggest that patients with WHO Type I (keratinized scc) do not fare as well as those with the non-keratinized (WHO Type II) or undifferentiated (WHO Type III) forms of NPC,[4,6] while others show no difference.[4] Primary tumor volume delineated on CT[6,12] is currently being investigated as a prognosticator for local control. Quantification of plasma EBV DNA appears to be useful for monitoring patients with NPC and predicting the outcome of treatment.[13–15] However, it is still uncertain whether the use of this biomarker can complement the current TNM stage classification.

Patients with disseminated NPC also differ significantly in prognostic outcome. However, relatively fewer studies have been done to address this issue.[16–18] The presence of distant metastases at initial diagnosis, shorter metastasis-free interval, and older age were significant independent predictors for a poorer outcome.[6] Ong et al. found that in addition to these variables, the presence of lung metastasis, anemia, and poor performance status were additional independently significant negative prognostic factors for survival.[16] However, age at diagnosis did not predict for survival in this study. A numerical scoring system based on these six factors was able to divide patients with disseminated NPC into three prognostic groups with significantly different median survival times. This prognostic index score has been validated in a separate cohort of patients with disseminated NPC.[18] This simple score may prove useful as a method to prognosticate and stratify patients as well as to promote consistent reporting among clinical trials in metastatic NPC.

■■■■■■■■ **SUMMARY TABLE**

Prognostic Factors in Nasopharyngeal Cancer

Prognostic Factors	Tumor Related	Host Related	Environment Related
Essential[2–4]	T category N category M category		
Additional	WHO Histologic type	Age Performance status Comorbidity	High-dose radiation boost Experienced team for chemotherapy support and salvage diagnosis and retreatment
New and promising	EBV DNA Tumor volume on CT		Functional imaging (e.g., PET) Overall RT treatment time

Sources:
• British Columbia Cancer Agency Cancer Management Guidelines: Head and Neck Cancer 2003. http://www.bccancer.bc.ca/HPI/CancerManagementGuidelines/HeadnNeck/start.htm.
• NCCN Clinical Practice Guidelines in Oncology: Head and Neck Cancer USA, 2005. http://www.nccn.org/professionals/physician_gls/PDF/head-and-neck.pdf.

REFERENCES

1. A Seow, Koh WP, Chia KS, et al.: Trends in Cancer Incidence in Singapore 1968–2002. Singapore Cancer Registry, Report No. 6, 2004.

2. National Cancer Institute: Nasopharyngeal Cancer (PDQ®): Treatment Guidelines. USA 2005. http://www.cancer.gov/cancertopics/pdq/treatment/nasopharyngeal/health professional/.

3. British Columbia Cancer Agency Cancer Management Guidelines: Head and Neck Cancer. Canada 2003. http://www.bccancer.bc.ca/HPI/CancerManagementGuidelines/HeadnNeck/start.htm.

4. NCCN Clinical Practice Guidelines in Oncology: Head and Neck Cancer. USA 2005. http://www.nccn.org/professionals/physician_gls/PDF/head-and-neck.pdf.

5. Chan JT, Chan SC, Yen TC, et al.: Nasopharyngeal carcinoma staging by (18)F-fluorodeoxyglucose positron emission tomography. *Int J Radiat Oncol Biol Phys* 62:501–507, 2005.

6. O'Sullivan B, Chong VF: Nasopharyngeal Carcinoma, in Gospodarowicz MK, Henson DE, Hutter RVP, et al. (eds.): UICC Prognostic factors in Cancer, 2nd ed. New York, Wiley, 2001.

7. Program in Evidence-Based Care: Practice Guidelines and Evidence Based Summaries—Head & Neck Cancer Site Gp *http://www.cancercare.on.ca/index_headAndneckCancer guidelines.htm Cancer Care Ontario*, 2005.

8. Teo PM, Ma BB, Chan AT: Radiotherapy for nasopharyngeal carcinoma—transition from two-dimensional to three-dimensional methods. *Radiother Oncol* 73:163–172, 2004.

9. Lee, A.W.: Preliminary Results of a Prospective Randomized Study (NPC-9902 Trial) on the Therapeutic Gain by Concurrent Chemotherapy and/or Accelerated Fractionation for Locally-Advanced Nasopharyngeal Carcinoma. East West Symposium on Nasopharyngeal Carcinoma. Toronto, Canada, 2005 (personal communication).

10. Le QT, Tate D, Koong A, et al.: Improved local control with stereotactic radiosurgical boost in patients with nasopharyngeal carcinoma. *Int J Radiat Oncol Biol Phys* 56:1046–1054, 2003.

11. Agulnik M, Siu LL: State-of-the-art management of nasopharyngeal carcinoma: current and future directions. *Br J Cancer* 92:799–806, 2005.

12. Chen MK, Chen TH, Liu JP, et al.: Better prediction of prognosis for patients with nasopharyngeal carcinoma using primary tumor volume. *Cancer* 100:2160–2166, 2004.

13. Lin JC, Wang WY, Chen KY, et al.: Quantification of plasma Epstein-Barr virus DNA in patients with advanced nasopharyngeal carcinoma. *N Engl J Med* 350:2461–2470, 2004.

14. Chan AT, Lo YMD, Zee B, et al.: Plasma Epstein–Barr virus DNA and residual disease after radiotherapy for undifferentiated nasopharyngeal carcinoma. *J Natl Cancer Inst* 94:1614–1619, 2002.

15. Hong RL, Lin CY, Ting LL, et al.: Comparison of clinical and molecular surveillance in patients with advanced nasopharyngeal carcinoma after primary therapy: the potential role of quantitative analysis of circulating Epstein–Barr virus DNA. *Cancer* 100:1429–1437, 2004.

16. Ong YK, Heng DM, Chung B, et al.: Design of a prognostic index score for metastatic nasopharyngeal carcinoma. *Eur J Cancer* 39:1535–1541, 2003.

17. Teo PM, Kwan WH, Lee WY, et al.: Prognosticators determining survival subsequent to distant metastasis from nasopharyngeal carcinoma. *Cancer* 77:2423–2431, 1996.

18. Toh CK, Heng D, Ong YK, et al.: Validation of a new prognostic index score for disseminated nasopharyngeal carcinoma. *Br J Cancer* 92:1382–1387, 2005.

CHAPTER 10

Salivary Gland Cancer

ADAM S. GARDEN

The major glands include the parotid, submandibular and sublingual glands, while hundreds of minor glands are dispersed throughout the upper aerodigestive tract. Salivary gland malignancies account for 1–2% of all head and neck cancers. The parotid glands are the most common site for a salivary gland neoplasm, followed by the submandibular glands. The wide range of biologic behavior and varied histopathologic subtypes complicate the diagnosis, management algorithms, assessment of prognosis, as well as published outcomes, which largely relates to the heterogeneity of reported series with respect to treatments and even era of analysis.

Mucoepidermoid carcinomas are the most common cancers of the parotid gland (comprising 25–50%) followed by adenocarcinoma (including salivary ductal and terminal ductal carcinomas), and adenoid cystic carcinoma (10%). Most of the remainder include malignant mixed tumors (carcinoma expleomorphic adenoma), and acinic cell carcinoma.[1] In contrast, adenoid cystic carcinoma is the most common malignancy of the submandibular and minor glands approximating 50% of cancers, followed by the mucoepidermoid subtype.[2,3]

The most common presentation is with an asymptomatic mass;[1] palpable cervical lymph nodes, facial nerve palsy, deep fixation, and rapid tumor enlargement are significant parameters indicative of malignancy.[4] Pain is uncommon, but an ominous finding as is facial nerve involvement or less commonly hypoglossal nerve involvement.

These cancers often spread along nerves, and attention to neurotropic findings is important. Computerized tomography (CT), or especially magnetic resonance imaging (MRI) to assess perineural spread to the skull base are important to plan management. Fine-needle aspiration for diagnosis may be helpful,[5] particularly in the assessment of recurrence, but remains controversial because of concern regarding accuracy. Chest and bone imaging may be considered because of the tendency to metastasize to these locations.[5]

Prognostic Factors in Cancer, Third Edition, edited by Mary K. Gospodarowicz, Brian O'Sullivan, and Leslie H. Sobin.

Surgery is the most usual treatment approach with the extent determined by the amount and location of disease. Elective neck dissection is generally considered unnecessary, but the location of the major glands readily lend themselves to sampling of adjacent nodal levels at the resection. Risk factors for neck metastasis include histological subtype (i.e., adenocarcinoma, undifferentiated carcinoma, high-grade mucoepidermoid carcinoma, squamous cell carcinoma, and salivary duct carcinoma), higher T category, and a severe desmoplastic tumor reaction.[6] Postoperative adjuvant radiation is indicated in selective situations; examples include the setting of high tumor grade, perineural invasion, inadequate resection margins, multiple involved lymph nodes, extraglandular or soft tissue extension, or when there is concern that the resection was inadequate.[7] The latter indication is common when the deep lobe of the parotid is involved, or when facial nerve conservation (recommended whenever possible) has been accomplished. Radiotherapy alone is recommended for inoperable cases,[8] and advocates for neutron radiation have reported efficacy.[5] Chemotherapy for distant metastases and recurrent disease is problematic since response rates are lower than expected with other head and neck malignancies though experience with these more common cancers has led to its use with radiotherapy in locally advanced salivary cancers.[9] In general, the reported outcomes of patients with salivary gland malignancies are fair, with long-term survival rates ranging from ~40–70%.[5,7] Studies have demonstrated improved results in more recent decades attributed to the increasing use of adjuvant radiation for advanced cases.[5] Submandibular and minor salivary gland malignancies tend to fare worse than parotid malignancies,[5] but this is more likely due to other prognostic factors (see below). Studies from Memorial Sloan Kettering Cancer Center suggest differences in outcomes for differing glands are no longer apparent when stage is considered in the analyses.

Stage, and specifically T category, is consistently prognostic for disease specific survival and overall survival. Predominant criteria in the current T-categorization include primary tumor size and extraparenchymal extension. Histologic grade is also a highly significant predictor, with 10-year survival rates for high- versus low-grade lesions ranging from 20 versus 50% and 40 versus 80% in two recent series.[10,11] High grade tends to predict local aggressiveness, and hence radiation is recommended for such disease. High grade also predicts for distant failure approaching 40% compared to an overall salivary malignancy metastasis rate of ~25%.[11] Other prognostic features have less significance or are components of stage and grade and are reported with varying consistency in different series. For example, older age, male gender, perineural invasion, pathologic nodal involvement (uncommon), or extraglandular extension all tend to be associated with lower survival rates.[9,10,12]

Adenoid cystic carcinoma tends to be associated with a worse prognosis due to its quite unique and well-earned reputation for demonstrating high rates of perineural spread with a notorious infiltrative character that challenges the ability to achieve clear surgical margins. When large nerves are invaded, the 5-year survival rates are appreciably different, ranging from 92% with no invasion, to 82% in cases identified microscopically, to 61% in cases of clinical perineural invasion.[13] Irrespective of grade, adenoid cystic carcinoma has rates of distant spread of ~33%.[13] This entity is also known for late local and distant recurrences, sometimes exceeding 10 years from original diagnosis.

There is great interest in determining microscopic and molecular markers as prognosticators for these diseases. Aneuploidy, high proliferation (often correlated with high Ki-67 staging), p53 mutations, the presence of HER2/neu, VEGF expression and certain mucins have been identified as potential markers of poor prognosis.[14–20]

Useful randomized trials are unlikely to be undertaken for these uncommon tumors, especially since outcomes are only poor for a subgroup with high grade or high stage disease, and the unusually long natural history presents a challenge to the randomized trial process. However, current directions include studying the biology of the disease to determine if there are subgroups that may benefit from a molecular targeted approach.[20]

■■■■■■■ **SUMMARY TABLE**

Prognostic Factors in Salivary Gland Cancer

Prognostic Factors	Tumor Related	Host Related	Environment Related
Essential	T category N category M category Histologic grade Histologic subtype		
Additional	Resection margin Perineural invasion, particularly cranial nerve involvement	Age Gender	Postoperative radiation Neutron radiation
New and promising	Ploidy Ki-67 *P53* HER2/neu Mucin production		

Source:
• Head and Neck Cancer: Salivary Gland Tumors. Practice Guidelines in Oncology: National Comprehensive Cancer Network.
http://www.nccn.org v1. Accessed 2005.

REFERENCES

1. Terhaard CH, Lubsen H, Van der Tweel I, et al.: Salivary gland carcinoma: independent prognostic factors for locoregional control, distant metastases, and overall survival: results of the Dutch head and neck oncology cooperative group. *Head Neck* 26:681–692; discussion 692–683, 2004.

2. Bhattacharyya N: Survival and prognosis for cancer of the submandibular gland. *J Oral Maxillofac Surg* 62:427–430, 2004.

3. Storey MR, Garden AS, Morrison WH, et al.: Postoperative radiotherapy for malignant tumors of the submandibular gland. *Int J Radiat Oncol Biol Phys* 51:952–958, 2001.

4. Wong DS: Signs and symptoms of malignant parotid tumours: an objective assessment. *J R Coll Surg Edinb* 46:91–95, 2001.

5. Eisele DW, Kleinberg LR: Management of malignant salivary gland tumors, in Harrison LB, Sessions RB, Hong WK (ed.): *Head and neck cancer: a multidisciplinary approach.* 2nd ed. Philadelphia, Lippincott Williams & Wilkins, 2004, pp. 620–651.

6. Regis De Brito Santos I, Kowalski LP, Cavalcante De Araujo V, et al.: Multivariate analysis of risk factors for neck metastases in surgically treated parotid carcinomas. *Arch Otolaryngol Head Neck Surg* 127:56–60, 2001.

7. Mendenhall WM, Riggs CE, Cassisi NJ: Cancers of the head and neck: Section 2, Treatment of head and neck cancers, in DeVita Jr V, Helman S, Rosenberg S (eds.): *Principles and Practice of Oncology.* 7th ed. Philadelphia, Lippincott Williams & Wilkins, 2005, pp. 662–732.

8. Mendenhall WM, Morris CG, Amdur RJ, et al.: Radiotherapy alone or combined with surgery for salivary gland carcinoma. *Cancer* 103:2544–2550, 2005.

9. Hocwald E, Korkmaz H, Yoo GH, et al.: Prognostic factors in major salivary gland cancer. *Laryngoscope* 111:1434–1439, 2001.

10. Harbo G, Bundgaard T, Pedersen D, et al.: Prognostic indicators for malignant tumours of the parotid gland. *Clin Otolaryngol Allied Sci* 27:512–516, 2002.

11. Kokemueller H, Swennen G, Brueggemann N, et al.: Epithelial malignancies of the salivary glands: clinical experience of a single institution – a review. *Int J Oral Maxillofac Surg* 33:423–432, 2004.

12. Pohar S, Gay H, Rosenbaum P, et al.: Malignant parotid tumors: presentation, clinical/pathologic prognostic factors, and treatment outcomes. *Int J Radiat Oncol Biol Phys* 61:112–118, 2005.

13. Mendenhall WM, Morris CG, Amdur RJ, et al.: Radiotherapy alone or combined with surgery for adenoid cystic carcinoma of the head and neck. *Head Neck* 26:154–162, 2004.

14. Enamorado I, Lakhani R, Korkmaz H, et al.: Correlation of histopathological variants, cellular DNA content, and clinical outcome in adenoid cystic carcinoma of the salivary glands. *Otolaryngol Head Neck Surg* 131:646–650, 2004.

15. Jaehne M, Roeser K, Jaekel T, et al.: Clinical and immunohistologic typing of salivary duct carcinoma: a report of 50 cases. *Cancer* 103:2526–2533, 2005.

16. Lim JJ, Kang S, Lee MR, et al.: Expression of vascular endothelial growth factor in salivary gland carcinomas and its relation to p53, Ki-67 and prognosis. *J Oral Pathol Med* 32:552–561, 2003.

17. Nguyen LH, Black MJ, Hier M, et al.: HER2/neu and Ki-67 as prognostic indicators in mucoepidermoid carcinoma of salivary glands. *J Otolaryngol* 32:328–331, 2003.

18. Norberg-Spaak L, Dardick I, Ledin T: Adenoid cystic carcinoma: use of cell proliferation, BCL-2 expression, histologic grade, and clinical stage as predictors of clinical outcome. *Head Neck* 22:489–497, 2000.

19. Alos L, Lujan B, Castillo M, et al.: Expression of membrane-bound mucins (MUC1 and MUC4) and secreted mucins (MUC2, MUC5AC, MUC5B, MUC6 and MUC7) in mucoepidermoid carcinomas of salivary glands. *Am J Surg Pathol* 29:806–813, 2005.

20. Glisson B, Colevas AD, Haddad R, et al.: HER2 expression in salivary gland carcinomas: dependence on histological subtype. *Clin Cancer Res* 10:944–946, 2004.

CHAPTER 11

Thyroid Cancer

JAMES D. BRIERLEY and SYLVIA L. ASA

Thyroid cancer is uncommon, but generally associated with a favorable prognosis. Papillary and follicular (differentiated) tumors account for 94%, medullary for 4%, and poorly differentiated (insular) and anaplastic for 2%. The 10-year survival rates for papillary and follicular cancers are 95%, and for medullary 75%. Anaplastic thyroid carcinoma has very poor prognosis (<5% survival) with a median survival typically <4 months.[1] Insular carcinomas exhibit a behavior intermediate between differentiated and anaplastic carcinoma.

Presentation with distant metastatic disease is extremely rare, other than for anaplastic histology. Patients typically present with a thyroid mass and sometimes cervical node involvement. Occasionally symptoms from recurrent laryngeal nerve or tracheal and esophageal involvement are present. Anaplastic cancer is characterized by rapidly growing neck mass, pain, and respiratory distress and other stigmata of local invasion.

Patient assessment should include a complete history identifying any associated risk factors, especially previous radiation exposure, family history, and symptoms of local and/or regional spread, physical examination, thyroid function tests, cervical ultrasound, and fine needle aspiration cytology. Surgical resection or lobectomy may be required to establish the diagnosis if cytology is inconclusive.[1–3]

Surgery is the mainstay of treatment with adjuvant radioactive iodine (RAI) commonly used in papillary and follicular cancers. Adjuvant external beam radiation therapy is sometimes recommended in tumors with extrathyroidal extension, especially in older patients. All patients with tumors >1–1.5 cm may be treated with thyroidectomy[4] and radioactive iodine (RAI).[1–3,5] However, patients under 45 years of age with tumors <4 cm and no additional adverse prognostic features may be treated without RAI[1,2,6] and even by lobectomy and isthmusectomy alone.[7] Differentiated thyroid cancer is not chemosensitive and distant metastases are frequently treated with RAI.

Prognostic Factors in Cancer, Third Edition, edited by Mary K. Gospodarowicz, Brian O'Sullivan, and Leslie H. Sobin.

Chemotherapy with doxorubicin, cisplatin, or taxanes has been used in the management of anaplastic thyroid cancers with minimal success.[1]

The main prognostic factors include: histologic type, anatomic disease size and extent, and patient age.[4,8] Tumors >4 cm often exhibit extrathyroid extension and are associated with worse outcome. Extrathyroid tumor extension predicts locoregional and distant failure and cancer death. Multifocality has been associated with both locoregional and distant recurrence and increased mortality.[4,5] Hurthle cell carcinoma, a variant of follicular carcinoma, presents with more extensive disease and has a worse response to RAI therapy. Tall cell or columnar variants of papillary thyroid carcinoma, and tumors with vascular and lymphatic invasion all have a more aggressive course. Insular carcinoma predicts more aggressive behavior and a worse response to RAI.[9–12] The prognostic impact of lymph node involvement is uncertain, but probably predicts increased risk of neck recurrence, especially if there is extranodal invasion. Metastatic disease is associated with a markedly decreased survival. The exception is young patients with metastatic lung disease that may have an excellent prognosis if there are diffuse lung metastases that take up radioiodine evident on ^{131}I imaging, but are not detectable by X-ray.[13] An aneuploid DNA profile may be prognostic in papillary tumors. Ras or beta-catenin mutations, p27 downregulation or cyclin D1 upregulation, erbB-2 expression, and nm23-H1 immunoreactivity may be of prognostic value. Inactivating point mutations of p53 are more commonly seen in poorly differentiated and anaplastic tumors.[4]

In areas where goiter is endemic, higher mortality is observed, likely reflecting higher incidence of the follicular and anaplastic histologies and/or later detection.[14] Large-scale prophylactic iodinization in Switzerland and Paraguay has resulted in decreased follicular and anaplastic histologies with a resultant fall in population age-adjusted mortality.

Medullary thyroid cancers are derived from the parafollicular cells and are familial in 20–25% of cases either as part of the multiple endocrine neoplasia syndrome (MEN 2A or 2B) or in isolation (familial type). Any past survival advantage observed in MEN associated cases may have been due to earlier diagnosis secondary to screening. Although presenting at an earlier age, patients with MEN 2B have more advanced disease and poorer survival than those with MEN 2A.[11,15] Different sites of the RET oncogene mutation are associated with differences in morphology, but not prognosis.[4,16] Younger age, and female gender, are favorable prognostic indicators. Lymph node involvement and extrathyroid extension influence survival adversely. Patients with familial disease should have prophylactic thyroidectomy at an early age,[17] but if this is not performed and disease is identified, a total thyroidectomy with central node dissection is indicated. Bilateral neck dissection may be required in disease >1 cm, otherwise central nodal dissection is likely sufficient.[16] The most important predictive factor for survival is biochemical cure after surgery.[4] A decrease in the calcitonin level with time may indicate progression to poor differentiation. Carcinoembryonic antigen (CEA) has also been used as a marker for disease, with a short CEA doubling time being associated with rapidly progressive disease.[4]

Anaplastic thyroid carcinoma has a dismal prognosis presenting as advanced stage disease with median survival typically <4 months. Younger patients with small tumors

(<5 cm), no extrathyroidal invasion, and no lymph node involvement appear to have a better prognosis as does the rare patient in whom a complete surgical resection is possible. Management is surgical resection in the rare situations where this is possible. Otherwise, radiation alone or in combination with chemotherapy provides the mainstay of therapy.[1]

The main controversy in the management of patients with differentiated thyroid cancer is the definition of low-risk patients who do not require total thyroidectomy and radioactive iodine and can be adequately managed by lobectomy alone.[1–4,6]

■■■■■ **SUMMARY TABLES**

Prognostic Factors in Thyroid Carcinoma of Follicular Cell Derivation

Prognostic Factors	Tumor Related	Host Related	Environment Related
Essential	T category M category	Age	
Additional	N category Site of metastases	Gender	Endemic goiter
New and promising	Molecular profile		

Prognostic Factors in Medullary Thyroid Carcinoma

Prognostic Factors	Tumor Related	Host Related	Environment Related
Essential	T category N category M category		
Additional	Genetic Syndrome MEN 2B	Age Gender	
New and promising			

REFERENCES

1. Sherman S, et al.: Thyroid carcinoma, in practice guidelines in oncology. National Comprehensive Cancer Network. www.nccn.org Accessed 2005.

2. AACE: AACE/AAES medical/surgical guidelines for clinical practice: management of thyroid carcinoma. American Association of Clinical Endocrinologists. American College of Endocrinology. *Endocr Pract* 7:202–220, 2001.

3. British Thyroid Association, Guidelines for the management of thyroid cancer in adults. Royal College of Physicians: London, UK. 2002, pp. 1–70.

4. Baloch ZW, LiVolsi VA: Prognostic factors in well-differentiated follicular-derived carcinoma and medullary thyroid carcinoma. *Thyroid* 11:637–645, 2001.

5. Mazzaferri EL, Kloos RT: Clinical review 128: Current approaches to primary therapy for papillary and follicular thyroid cancer. *J Clin Endocrinol Metab* 86:1447–1463, 2001.

6. Dean DS, Hay ID: Prognostic indicators in differentiated thyroid carcinoma. *Cancer Control* 7:229–239, 2000.

7. Shaha AR: Implications of prognostic factors and risk groups in the management of differentiated thyroid cancer. *Laryngoscope* 114:393–402, 2004.

8. Carling T, Udelsman R: Cancer of the endocrine system, in DeVita V, Hellman S, Rosenberg S (eds.): *Cancer principles and practice of oncology*, Philadelphia, Lippincott Williams and Wilkins, 2005.

9. Pellegriti G, et al.: Long-term outcome of patients with insular carcinoma of the thyroid: the insular histotype is an independent predictor of poor prognosis. *Cancer* 95:2076–2085, 2002.

10. Akslen LA, LiVolsi VA: Prognostic significance of histologic grading compared with subclassification of papillary thyroid carcinoma. *Cancer* 88:1902–1908, 2000.

11. Volante M, et al.: Poorly differentiated carcinomas of the thyroid with trabecular, insular, and solid patterns: a clinicopathologic study of 183 patients. *Cancer* 100:950–957, 2004.

12. Nishida T, Katayama S, Tsujimoto M: The clinicopathological significance of histologic vascular invasion in differentiated thyroid carcinoma. *Am J Surg* 183:80–86, 2002.

13. Shoup M, et al.: Prognostic indicators of outcomes in patients with distant metastases from differentiated thyroid carcinoma. *J Am Coll Surg* 197:191–197, 2003.

14. Gyory F, et al.: Differentiated thyroid cancer and outcome in iodine deficiency. *Eur J Surg Oncol* 30:325–331, 2004.

15. Kebebew E, Clark OH: Medullary thyroid cancer. *Curr Treat Options Oncol* 1:359–367, 2000.

16. Randolph GW, Maniar D: Medullary carcinoma of the thyroid. *Cancer Control* 7:253–261, 2000.

17. Brandi ML, et al.: Consensus: Guidelines for diagnosis and therapy of MEN type 1 and type 2. *J Clin Endocrinol Metab* 86:5658–5671, 2001.

DIGESTIVE SYSTEM TUMORS

CHAPTER 12

Esophageal Cancer

HUBERT J. STEIN and BURKHARD H. VON RAHDEN

Esophageal adenocarcinomas (ACs) are rapidly increasing in incidence in the Western World, now clearly outnumbering the formerly prevailing squamous cell cancers (SCC). In comparison, esophageal SCCs still predominate in the Eastern World.[1] Esophageal ACs are known to be related to gastroesophageal reflux and arise predominantly in the lower third of the esophagus from underlying specialized intestinal metaplasia, the so-called Barrett's esophagus.[2] In contrast, SCCs arise throughout the esophagus, with tobacco and alcohol intake regarded as the main risk factors. Prognosis is related to both the histological type and anatomical location.[3] Esophageal ACs fare more favorably, proximally located SCCs have a worse prognosis.

The main prognostic factors are related to the anatomic extent of disease according to the TNM staging system.[4] Long-term survival is only feasible where complete surgical resection has been achieved. Preoperative estimation of the T and N category is critical in order to tailor therapeutic strategies, because the clinical T category is the major determinant of surgical resectability. Locally limited tumors (T1-2) are approached with primary resection. Radical esophagectomy may represent overtreatment in T1a disease, that is, tumors limited to the mucosa, and equivalent prognosis may be achievable with limited surgical or endoscopic resection.[5] Advanced T3-4 tumors are increasingly managed with neoadjuvant therapies with the aim of rendering tumors surgically resectable.[6] Depth of invasion (pT-category) is also an important predictor of survival, with pT1-2 tumors exhibiting a much more favorable prognosis than pT3-4 tumors.[7] In contrast, tumor length *per se* is not an independent prognostic factor. Lymphatic vessel invasion is a prognostic factor in both SCCs[8] and ACs.[9]

Both the presence and number of involved lymph node metastases are strongly prognostic after R0-resection.[5] However, long-term survival following extensive lymphadenectomy is still possible in selected cases with a limited number of involved regional lymph nodes. Tumor spread to distant lymph nodes is currently classified as

Prognostic Factors in Cancer, Third Edition, edited by Mary K. Gospodarowicz, Brian O'Sullivan, and Leslie H. Sobin.
Copyright © 2006 John Wiley & Sons, Inc.

M1a or M_{1LYH},[4] for example, abdominal/celiac nodal mestastases from a cervical/ supracarinal primary or cervical node involvement from a distal esophageal primary. This category is considered to have an intermediate prognosis; faring worse than pN1 status, but better compared to the setting of hematogenous metastases to distant organs (M1b).[7]

The presence of systemic metastases, both macroscopic and microscopic tumor deposits, is associated with a median survival of <6 months.[5] In contrast, the prognostic role of individual tumor cells, or tumor-cell deposits detected in the bone marrow, lymph nodes, or blood, remains controversial.[10] The response to neoadjuvant treatment is increasingly acknowledged as a favorable prognostic factor, as a subset will be amenable to curative subsequent surgical resection.[6]

The quality of treatment and, in particular, the quality of surgery also have a crucial impact on survival, due mostly to the continuous advancement of therapeutic management and improved surgical techniques that have decreased both surgical morbidity and mortality.[1,3] The incidence of surgical complications, such as anastomotic leak, vocal cord paralysis, or chylothorax, which are at least in part attributable to these technical aspects, are also prognostic for compromised long-term survival.[11] Surrogates for surgical quality include hospital-volume (annual case load per institution) and surgeon-volume (annual number of cases per surgeon). The frequency of a complete, residual-tumor free resection (R0) thus reflects both a tumor-related prognostic factor, quality of the surgical technique, as well as optimal patient selection.[7,12]

A vast variety of potential new and promising molecular prognostic factors in esophageal cancer are being investigated. These include mutations in tumor suppressor genes (p53, p21), amplification of oncogenes (hst-1, int-2), overexpression of cell cycle associated molecules (Ki-67, Cyclin D1), intercellular adhesion molecules (cadherins, integrins, CD-44, IgCAMs, selectins), growth factors (VEGF, TGF-α, FGF-3) and growth factor receptors (EGF-R, c-erbB2/ HER2/neu), expression of tumor-associated proteases and protease inhibitors (uPA, dThdPase, MMP-2, MMP-7, MT1-MMP) and chemokines (MCP-1, MIF, CD147), the ploidy, DNA distribution pattern and the number of nucleolar organizer regions.[13-15]

■■■■■■■■ **SUMMARY TABLE**

Prognostic Factors in Esophageal Cancer

Prognostic Factor	Tumor Related	Host Related	Environment Related
Essential	T category N category M category Histologic type R status		Quality of Treatment Surgical Quality Hospital-volume Surgeon-volume
Additional	Localization Lymphatic invasion Response to neoadjuvant treatment	Gender Age	
New and promising	Isolated tumor cells Tumor suppressor genes Cyclin D1, Ki 67 VEGF		

Sources:
• ESMO Minimum Clinical Recommendations for diagnosis, treatment and follow-up of esophageal cancer http://annonc.oupjournals.org/cgi/reprint/16/suppl_1/i26.
• NCCN Clinical Practice Guidelines in Oncology: Esophageal Cancer. http://www.nccn.org/ professionals/ physician_gls/PDF/esophageal.pdf.

REFERENCES

1. Siewert JR, von Rahden B, Stein H: Current status of esophageal cancer – West versus East : The European point of view. *Esophagus* 1:147–159, 2004.

2. Spechler SJ: Clinical practice. Barrett's Esophagus. *N Engl J Med* 346:836–842, 2002.

3. Siewert JR, Stein HJ, von Rahden BH: Multimodal treatment of gastrointestinal tract tumors: consequences for surgery. *World J Surg* 29:940–948, 2005.

4. Sobin LH, Wittekind Ch: *UICC: TNM Classification of malignant tumors.* 6th ed. New York, Wiley-Liss, 2002.

5. Stein HJ, Feith M, Brücher et al.: Early esophageal cancer: pattern of lymphatic spread and prognostic factors for long-term survival after surgical resection. *Ann Surg* 242:566–573, 2005.

6. Brücher BL, Stein HJ, Zimmermann F, et al.: Responders benefit from neoadjuvant radiochemotherapy in esophageal squamous cell carcinoma: results of a prospective phase-II trial. *Eur J Surg Oncol* 30:963–971, 2004.

7. Stein HJ, Feith M: Cancer of the esophagus. In Gospodarowicz MK, Henson DE, Hutter RVP et al. (eds.): *Prognostic Factors in Cancer*, 2nd ed. New York, Wiley-Liss, 2001.

8. Brücher BL, Stein HJ, Werner M, et al.: Lymphatic vessel invasion is an independent prognostic factor in patients with a primary resected tumor with esophageal squamous cell carcinoma. *Cancer* 92:2228–2233, 2001.

9. von Rahden BH, Stein HJ, Feith M, et al.: Lymphatic vessel invasion as a prognostic factor in patients with primary resected adenocarcinomas of the esophagogastric junction. *J Clin Oncol* 23:874–879, 2005.

10. Jiao X, Krasna MJ: Clinical significance of micrometastasis in lung and esophageal cancer: a new paradigm in thoracic oncology. *Ann Thorac Surg* 74:278–284, 2002.

11. Rizk NP, Bach PB, Schrag D, et al.: The impact of complications on outcomes after resection for esophageal and gastroesophageal junction carcinoma. *J Am Coll Surg* 2005, 198:42–50, 2004.

12. Birkmeyer JD, Stukel TA, Siewers AE, et al.: Surgeon volume and operative mortality in the United States. *N Engl J Med* 2005;349:2117–2127, 2003.

13. von Rahden BH, Stein HJ, Puhringer F, et al.: Coexpression of cyclooxygenases (COX-1, COX-2) and vascular endothelial growth factors (VEGF-A, VEGF-C) in esophageal adenocarcinoma. *Cancer Res* 65:5038–5044, 2005.

14. Zhu SC, Li R, Wang YX, et al.: Impact of simultaneous assay, the PCNA, cyclinD1, and DNA content with specimens before and after preoperative radiotherapy on prognosis of esophageal cancer-possible incorporation into clinical TNM staging system. *World J Gastroenterol* 11:3823–3829, 2005.

15. Matsumoto M, Furihata M, Kurabayashi A, et al.: Prognostic significance of serine 392 phosphorylation in overexpressed p53 protein in human esophageal squamous cell carcinoma. *Oncology* 67:143–150, 2004.

CHAPTER 13

Gastric Cancer

J.H.J.M. VAN KRIEKEN and CORNELIS J.H. VAN DE VELDE

Although the incidence of gastric cancer is decreasing worldwide, the prognosis is still generally poor. Insight in the pathogenesis (the role of *Helicobacter pylori* and Epstein–Barr virus, EBV) and molecular genetics (p53 or ras mutations)[1] of this tumor has increased. Important new data now exist on the role of local surgery, extended lymphadenectomy, and chemotherapy.[2] Outcome is clearly dependent on many factors, but complete surgical excision remains central. Since the diagnostic criteria for gastric cancer vary, this has led to differences in study populations, and therefore reported outcomes. This may partially explain the higher incidence and better prognosis of gastric cancer in regions, such as Japan.

Histological typing and grading is based on the World Health Organization (WHO) international histological classification. The two most common types are tubular and signet-ring-cell carcinoma. Epstein–Barr virus is associated with some cases of gastric cancer and this forms a separate category.[3] Grading is of limited value.[4] In addition there are two classification schemes based on growth patterns: the Ming (expanding and infiltrating) and the Laurén (diffuse and intestinal). More recently, the Goseki classification[5] was introduced with good reproducibility, which gives additional prognostic information on the degree of tubular differentiation and intracellular mucin production. Histological typing is recommended to recognize rare types with special features.

The stage according to the TNM (see Glossary) classification[6] remains the key prognostic factor. The presence of positive peritoneal washings can be assessed preoperatively and signifies a very poor prognosis.[7] The number of positive lymph nodes is also important, but often <15 nodes are found, especially when a D1 resection is performed.[8] Other prognostic measures include metastatic lymph node ratio[9] and extracapsular spread.[10] The presence of lymphovascular invasion is an independent prognostic factor.[11]

Radical surgery is the mainstay of treatment options and the only chance for cure. Long-term follow up after limited (D1) and extended lymph node dissection (D2)

Prognostic Factors in Cancer, *Third Edition*, edited by Mary K. Gospodarowicz, Brian O'Sullivan, and Leslie H. Sobin.
Copyright © 2006 John Wiley & Sons, Inc.

demonstrated no decrease in relapse rates nor improvement in survival by D2 dissection.[12] Extended lymph node dissection was even potentially harmful in terms of increased morbidity and hospital mortality, however, dedicated, high volume centers in Western Europe and Japan now report low operative morbidity and mortality, the latter <5% for extended lymph node dissections in selected patients.[13] The additional benefit of pancreatico-splenectomy to remove lymph node stations 10 and 11 is very small.[14] Subgroup analysis shows a significant survival benefit for D2 dissections, hence an over D1 (or D1+) lymphadenectomy may be considered.

The value of additional treatment by chemoradiotherapy after D0 and D1 lymph node dissections has been demonstrated, with a progressive improvement in locoregional control and survival.[2] Different histological types (intestinal vs. diffuse type) show different biological behavior reflected in altered recurrence patterns that will influence the choice for optimizing neoadjuvant strategies. Locoregional treatment for gastric cancer will meet its optimum between best possible radical surgery with acceptable toxicity and individualized neoadjuvant treatment with modern conformal radiotherapy and radiosensitizing chemotherapy.[13,14] Promising results from genomic profiling and from nomograms that predict disease-specific survival may help discriminate between patients at higher risk of relapse.[1,15]

In the era of genomics, several approaches have been shown to be of potential value, such as comparative genomic hybridization array.[16] Single factors associated with growth control, invasion, and metastasis are increasingly being recognized. Examples include the epidermal growth factor[17] EpCAM,[18] and microvascular index.[19]

The factors tabulated generally reflect survival outcome. Other endpoints may have direct bearing on the treatment to be given for alternative endpoints, but may not independently influence survival.

▆▆▆▆▆▆ SUMMARY TABLE

Prognostic Factors in Gastric Cancer

Prognostic Factors	Tumor Related	Host Related	Environment Related
Essential	Histologic type T category N category M category		
Additional	Resection margin Goseki classification Venous invasion N-ratio Positive peritoneal cytology		D2 Resection
New and promising	EpCAM-expression EGFr-expression Proliferative index Microvessel density		Chemotherapy

Sources:
• NCCN Clinical Practice Guidelines in Oncology:Gastric Cancer 2004.
http://www.nccn.org/ professionals/physician_gls/PDF/gastric.pdf.
• ESMO Minimum Clinical Recommendations for diagnosis, treatment and follow-up of gastric cancer 2005.
http://annonc.oupjournals.org/cgi/reprint/16/suppl_1/i22.

REFERENCES

1. Weiss MM, Kuipers EJ, Postma C, et al.: Genomic profiling of gastric cancer predicts lymph node status and survival. *Oncogene* 22:1872–1879, 2003.

2. Xiong HQ, Gunderson LL, Yao J, et al.: Chemoradiation for resectable gastric cancer. *Lancet Oncol* 4:498–505, 2003.

3. van Beek J, zur Hausen A, Klein Kranenbarg E, et al.: EBV-positive gastric adenocarcinomas: a distinct clinicopathologic entity with a low frequency of lymph node involvement. *J Clin Oncol* 22:664–670, 2004.

4. Inoue K, Nakane Y, Michiura T, et al.: Histopathological grading does not affect survival after R0 surgery for gastric cancer. *Eur J Surg Oncol* 28:633–636, 2002.

5. Fontana MG, La Pinta M, Moneghini D, et al.: Prognostic value of Goseki histological classification in adenocarcinoma of the cardia. *Br J Cancer* 88:401–405, 2003.

6. Sobin LH, Wittekind Ch: UICC: *TNM Classification of malignant tumors* (6th ed.), New York, Wiley-Liss, 2002.

7. Bentrem D, Wilton A, Mazumdar M, et al.: The value of peritoneal cytology as a preoperative predictor in patients with gastric carcinoma undergoing a curative resection. *Ann Surg Oncol* 12:347–353, 2005.

8. Cozzaglio L, Doci R, Celotti S, et al.: Gastric cancer: extent of lymph node dissection and requirements for a correct staging. *Tumori* 90:467–472, 2004.

9. Bando E, Yonemura Y, Taniguchi K, et al.: Outcome of ratio of lymph node metastasis in gastric carcinoma. *Ann Surg Oncol* 9:775–784, 2002.

10. Nakamura K, Ozaki N, Yamada T, et al.: Evaluation of prognostic significance in extracapsular spread of lymph node metastasis in patients with gastric cancer. *Surgery* 137: 511–517, 2005.

11. Hyung WJ, Lee JH, Choi SH, et al.: Prognostic impact of lymphatic and/or blood vessel invasion in patients with node-negative advanced gastric cancer. *Ann Surg Oncol* 9:562–567, 2002.

12. Hartgrink HH, van de Velde CJ: Status of extended lymph node dissection: locoregional control is the only way to survive gastric cancer. *J Surg Oncol* 90:153–165, 2005.

13. Petrelli NJ: The debate is over; it's time to move on. *J Clin Oncol* 22:2041–2042, 2004.

14. Jansen EP, Boot H, Verheij M, et al.: Optimal locoregional treatment in gastric cancer. *J Clin Oncol* 23:4509–4517, 2005.

15. Kattan MW, Karpeh MS, Mazumdar M, et al.: Postoperative nomogram for disease-specific survival after an R0 resection for gastric carcinoma. *J Clin Oncol* 21:3647–3650, 2003.

16. Suzuki S, Egami K, Sasajima K, et al.: Comparative study between DNA copy number aberrations determined by quantitative microsatellite analysis and clinical outcome in patients with stomach cancer. *Clin Cancer Res* 10:3013–3019, 2004.

17. Gamboa-Dominguez A, Dominguez-Fonseca C, Quintanilla-Martinez L, et al.: Epidermal growth factor receptor expression correlates with poor survival in gastric adenocarcinoma from Mexican patients: a multivariate analysis using a standardized immunohistochemical detection system. *Mod Pathol* 17:579–587, 2004.

18. Songun I, Litvinov SV, van de Velde CJ, et al.: Loss of Ep-CAM (CO17-1A) expression predicts survival in patients with gastric cancer. *Br J Cancer* 92:1767–1772, 2005.

19. Gong W, Wang L, Yao JC, et al.: Expression of activated signal transducer and activator of transcription 3 predicts expression of vascular endothelial growth factor in and angiogenic phenotype of human gastric cancer. *Clin Cancer Res* 11:1386–1393, 2005.

CHAPTER 14

Colorectal Cancer

CAROLYN C. COMPTON

Colorectal cancer is the third most common type of cancer and the third leading cause of cancer deaths in Western nations.[1] In the United States, at least 145,000 new cases and 56,000 deaths are expected in 2005. Approximately 62% of new cases will involve the colon and 38% involve the rectum. Etiological factors include diet and lifestyle, but in 20–30% there is an inherited predisposition. There are known genetic syndromes, such as familial polyposis coli (1%) and hereditary nonpolyposis colorectal cancer (HNPCC) (3%), but in the majority of cases there is no identifiable syndrome. The pathogenesis of colorectal cancer is now fairly well known. In the majority of colorectal cancer, two genetic pathways define the transition from normal colonic mucosa to adenomatous polyp to colorectal cancer via a multistep pathway. The commonest cause accounting for nearly 80% of sporadic colorectal cancers involves a mutation of the APC (adenomatous polyposis coli) gene, while ~15% involve the microsatellite instability (MSI)[2] pathway that is also involved in HNPCC.

Clinical presentation is typically a change in bowel habit, bleeding, abdominal pain, anorexia, weight loss, or obstructive symptoms. Evaluation should consist of history, including family history, examination including rectal exam, colonoscopy and biopsy, and imaging at least of the liver and chest. Routine bloodwork should be supplemented with carcinoembryonic antigen (CEA) levels. Given the high incidence of colorectal cancer especially in Western nations, slow growth of adenomatous polyps and transformation to invasive cancer, screening is warranted. Usually, individuals without a family history are recommended to commence screening colonoscopy at age 50.[1]

The standard management of patients with nonmetastatic colorectal cancer is surgical resection. This may be performed with laparoscopic assistance in colon cancer. In rectal cancer, total mesorectal excision with sharp dissection has been shown to result in superior outcome compared to older techniques.[3,4] In stage III colon cancer, adjuvant chemotherapy is standard. In stage II and III rectal cancer, adjuvant radiotherapy

Prognostic Factors in Cancer, Third Edition, edited by Mary K. Gospodarowicz, Brian O'Sullivan, and Leslie H. Sobin.

and chemotherapy is required. Adjuvant radiation may be preoperative or postoperative although there is increasing evidence in favor of preoperative radiotherapy.[5]

The strongest prognostic factor in newly diagnosed colorectal cancer is the stage or anatomic extent of disease.[5–8] The UICC-TNM[9] and American Joint Committee on Cancer (AJCC)[10] staging classifications are advocated for use in both clinical trials and practice. The expected 5-year survival by stage ranges from 85 to 90% in stage I, to 70 to 75% for stage II, 35 to 40% for stage III, and <5% for stage IV disease.[6,8] The presence of medullary carcinoma, intratumoral lymphocytes, and Crohn's-like lymphoid response implies improved prognosis, while high grade, lymphatic and venous invasion, infiltrating tumor border, perineural invasion, and tumor budding at the infiltrating edge of tumor all imply inferior prognosis.[11,12]

A clinical presentation with obstruction, perforation or peritonitis, presence of diabetes, elevated preoperative serum CEA, and thrombocytosis are associated with inferior outcomes. Poor quality of surgery, fewer than 13 lymph nodes removed or found in the surgical specimen,[13] inadequate surgical clearance in rectal cancer (tumor 1 mm or less from the circumferential resection margin), defects in the mesorectum down to muscle and the presence of postoperative residual disease are all associated with inferior outcomes.[3,12]

Poor performance status, distant metastasis, high-grade disease, anemia, elevated CEA, leucocytosis, and elevated LDH are associated with poor outcome in patients with unresectable, gross residual, and metastatic disease. In patients presenting with metastatic disease confined to one organ, liver or lung, curative-intent surgery can be performed with about a 30% chance of cure. Poor prognostic factors for successful surgical salvage of oligometastases include the disease-free interval of <1 year (>3 years is more favorable), synchronous presentation with the primary cancer, and more than one metastatic site.[11]

Numerous molecular factors have been associated with worse prognosis.[14–17] They include aneuploidy, deletion of chromosome 18q, elevated thymidylate synthase protein, and p53 (17p) deletion. There is also increasing evidence that targeting of growth factors, growth factor receptors and downstream pathways in patients with advanced colon cancer will result in improved outcomes. Bevacizumab, an endothelial growth factor antibody and cetuximab an endothelial growth factor-receptor antibody are two such examples. Whether they are of benefit in the adjuvant setting remains to be determined.[18] Retrospective analyses suggest that DNA indexes, angiogenesis, and genetic/biological markers such as loss of heterozygosity at chromosome 18, mutant TP53, and the presence of microsatellite instability may identify prognostic differences that could in future help with patient stratification and guide adjuvant therapy.[19]

■■■■■■■ **SUMMARY TABLE**

Prognostic Factors in Colorectal Cancer

Prognostic Factor	Tumor Related	Host Related	Environment Related
Essential	T category N category M category Venous/lymphatic invasion	Obstruction	Quality of surgery Quality of total mesorectal excision (rectal cancer)
Additional	Grade Peripheral tumor budding Tumor border configuration Perineural invasion Medullary type CEA Perforation	Thrombocytosis Diabetes mellitus	Number of lymph nodes in resection specimen
New and promising	Microsatellite instability LOH 18q status P53 DNA ploidy TGF-B1 type II receptor Thymidylate synthase polymorphism VEGF expression 20q copy number Karyotype Proliferation rate Metalloproteinase expression Gene expression profiles		

Sources:
• National Cancer Institute : Colon Cancer (PDQ®): Treatment Guidelines 2005.
http://www. cancer.gov/cancertopics/pdq/treatment/colon/healthprofessional/.
• NCCN Clinical Practice Guidelines in Oncology:Rectal Cancer 2005.
http://www.nccn.org/professionals/ physician_gls/PDF/rectal.pdf.
• American Society of Clinical Oncology Recommendations on Adjuvant Chemotherapy for Stage II Colon Cancer 2004.
http://www.asco.org/asco/downloads/JCO.2004.05.063v1.pdf.
• ESMO Minimum Clinical Recommendations for diagnosis, treatment and follow-up of colon cancer 2005.
http://annonc.oupjournals.org/cgi/reprint/16/suppl_1/i16.

REFERENCES

1. Colon Cancer Fact Sheet, in Society. AC (ed.), 2005.
2. Popat S, Hubner R, Houlston RS: Systematic review of microsatellite instability and colorectal cancer prognosis. *J Clin Oncol* 23:609–618, 2005.
3. Bokey EL, Chapuis PH, Dent OF, et al.: Surgical technique and survival in patients having a curative resection for colon cancer. *Dis Colon Rectum* 46:860–866, 2003.
4. Nelson H, Petrelli N, Carlin A, et al.: Guidelines 2000 for colon and rectal cancer surgery. *J Natl Cancer Inst* 93:583–596, 2001.
5. Gill S, Loprinzi CL, Sargent DJ, et al.: Pooled analysis of fluorouracil-based adjuvant therapy for stage II and III colon cancer: who benefits and by how much? *J Clin Oncol* 22:1797–1806, 2004.
6. Greene FL, Stewart AK, Norton HJ: New tumor-node-metastasis staging strategy for node-positive (stage III) rectal cancer: an analysis. *J Clin Oncol* 22:1778–1784, 2004.
7. Compton CC, Fielding LP, Burgart LJ, et al.: Prognostic factors in colorectal cancer. College of American Pathologists Consensus Statement 1999. *Arch Pathol Lab Med* 124:979–994, 2000.
8. Gunderson LL, Sargent DJ, Tepper JE, et al.: Impact of T and N stage and treatment on survival and relapse in adjuvant rectal cancer: a pooled analysis. *J Clin Oncol* 22: 1785–1796, 2004.
9. Sobin LH, Wittekind Ch: UICC: TNM Classification of malignant tumors (6th ed.). New York, Wiley-Liss, 2002.
10. AJCC Cancer Staging Manual. New York, Springer, 2002.
11. Stocchi L, Nelson H, Sargent DJ, et al.: Impact of surgical and pathologic variables in rectal cancer: a United States community and cooperative group report. *J Clin Oncol* 19:3895–3902, 2001.
12. Birbeck KF, Macklin CP, Tiffin NJ, et al.: Rates of circumferential resection margin involvement vary between surgeons and predict outcomes in rectal cancer surgery. *Ann Surg* 235:449–457, 2002.
13. Le Voyer TE, Sigurdson ER, Hanlon AL, et al.: Colon cancer survival is associated with increasing number of lymph nodes analyzed: a secondary survey of intergroup trial INT-0089. *J Clin Oncol* 21:2912–2919, 2003.
14. Garrity MM, Burgart LJ, Mahoney MR, et al.: Prognostic value of proliferation, apoptosis, defective DNA mismatch repair, and p53 overexpression in patients with resected Dukes' B2 or C colon cancer: a North Central Cancer Treatment Group Study. *J Clin Oncol* 22:1572–1582, 2004.
15. Diep CB, Thorstensen L, Meling GI, et al.: Genetic tumor markers with prognostic impact in Dukes' stages B and C colorectal cancer patients. *J Clin Oncol* 21:820–829, 2003.
16. Watanabe T, Wu TT, Catalano PJ, et al.: Molecular predictors of survival after adjuvant chemotherapy for colon cancer. *N Engl J Med* 344:1196–1206, 2001.
17. Eschrich S, Yang I, Bloom G, et al.: Molecular staging for survival prediction of colorectal cancer patients. *J Clin Oncol* 23:3526–3535, 2005.

18. Allegra C, Sargent DJ: Adjuvant therapy for colon cancer—the pace quickens. *N Engl J Med* 352:2746–2748, 2005.

19. Cascinu S, Georgoulias V, Kerr D, et al.: Colorectal cancer in the adjuvant setting: perspectives on treatment and the role of prognostic factors. *Ann Oncol* (14 Suppl) 2:ii25–29, 2003.

CHAPTER 15

Anal Cancer

BERNARD J. CUMMINGS

Cancers of the anal region are relatively uncommon although the incidence has been increasing over the past 30 years.[1] They are found most frequently in Western Europe and North America, where the incidence is ~0.5–1 per 100,000.[2] About 80% occur in the anal canal and 20% in the perianal skin. Anal canal cancers are more common in women, but perianal cancers occur with equal frequency in men and women.

The current World Health Organization (WHO) histological classification recommends the generic term anal squamous cell carcinoma for the various subtypes described in previous classifications, namely, basaloid (cloacogenic), large-cell keratinizing and large-cell non-keratinizing.[3] This grouping accounts for ~80% of anal canal cancers, the remainder being adenocarcinomas or, infrequently, small cell (anaplastic) cancers. Most perianal cancers are large-cell keratinizing squamous cell cancers.

Clinical examination and imaging, particularly computerized tomography (CT), are used to assess the extent of the primary cancer, the principal regional lymph node groups (perirectal, internal iliac, and inguinal for anal canal cancers, and inguinal for perianal cancers) and sites of metastases (most frequently external, common iliac and paraaortic nodes, liver, and lungs). Blood counts, liver, and renal function tests are necessary to assess potential tolerability of treatment. Risk factors for development of anal cancer, such as immunosuppression associated with medical treatment or human immunodeficiency virus (HIV) infection, which may affect treatment choices and prognosis, should be noted.[1,2]

The initial treatment for most anal canal squamous cell cancers should be based on radiation therapy rather than surgery.[2,4] Local excision is adequate treatment for small superficial well or moderately differentiated cancers that have not infiltrated the anal sphincters. Oncologic excision of most cancers necessitates abdominoperineal resection with permanent colostomy. Although there have been no randomized trial comparisons, there are no major differences in the survival rates in patients managed by surgery or by radiation with or without chemotherapy.[2] Overall 5-year survival rates average ~55–65%. However, the likelihood of retaining anorectal function after radiation-based treatment is ~60–70% overall.

Randomized trials have demonstrated superior cancer-specific survival rates, though not overall survival rates, and superior local control and colostomy-free survival rates in patients managed by radiation with concurrent 5-fluorouracil and mitomycin compared to the same dose and schedule of radiation alone.[2] In a further randomized trial, the combination with radiation of both 5-fluorouracil and mitomycin rather than 5-fluorouracil alone, resulted in better local control and cancer-specific survival rates, again without significant improvement in overall survival.[2] Several investigators have introduced cisplatin rather than mitomycin in combined modality schedules.[2,5] Radiation alone is effective for small tumors up to ~4 cm and is still preferred by some.[2,4]

Local excision is the most expedient treatment for perianal cancers if anal function can be preserved. Otherwise combined radiation and chemotherapy protocols similar to those for anal canal cancer are preferred.[2,6] Carcinoma residual or recurrence after completion of radiation or radiation and chemotherapy is associated with poor pelvic control and survival rates after attempted salvage surgery in some, but not all, series.[2] While anorectal function is fair to good in those whose cancer is eradicated by radiation-based treatment, up to ~5% of patients have significant toxicity that may require surgical management.[4] Consistently effective curative treatment for extrapelvic metastases has not yet been identified.

The most deleterious prognostic factor for survival is the presence of extra-pelvic metastases.[2] Survival following the diagnosis of such metastases is generally <12 months. When cancer is confined to the pelvis, the size of the primary tumor is the most useful indicator for survival and for local control and preservation of anorectal function.[7] Based on tabulation of published studies according to TNM categories,[8,9] the combination of radiation, 5-fluorouracil, and mitomycin resulted in 5-year survival rates of ~90% of cancers ≤2 cm in size (T1), 60–70% for tumors 2–5 cm (T2), 45–55% for larger (T3) or deeply invasive (T4) cancers, and 65–75% overall.[4] The corresponding local control rates (excluding salvage treatment) were ~90–100% (T1), 65–75% (T2), 40–55% (T3 or T4), and 60% overall.[4] In most studies, the 5-year survival rates for patients with regional node metastases were up to 20% lower than in node negative patients.[2,4] Adenocarcinomas have a somewhat lower survival rate than squamous cell cancers. Small-cell cancers often metastasize widely and have a poor prognosis.[2]

Advanced age and poor performance status carry a poor prognosis, but case selection affects many reports.[7] Women have a better prognosis in some series.[7] There are no identified tumor markers of consistent prognostic value.[7] In HIV-positive patients high viral load, low lymphocyte CD4+ counts and acquired immune deficiency syndrome (AIDS) have been prognostic of poor local tumor control and survival rates, and, in some series, of impaired tolerance of radiation and chemotherapy.[7]

An extensive review of nearly 50 reports on cytogenetic, flow cytometric, immunohistochemical, and other investigations suggested that these studies offered insights on cancer pathogenesis, but not guidance to prognosis of the individual or selection of treatment.[10] In recent large retrospective analyses, high intra- and peritumoral infiltrates of CD3+ and CD4+ lymphocytes were associated with poor survival rates in patients treated with chemoradiation,[11] and high thymidine phosphorylase cytoplasmic intensity and CD34 expression predicted improved disease-free survival in patients treated with radiation, 5-fluorouracil and mitomycin.[12] Although there is a strong correlation between the presence of certain types of human papilloma virus (HPV) and squamous cancers of the anal canal or perianal skin, no prognostic correlations have been identified.[1,13]

Ongoing randomized trials will determine whether the combination of 5-fluorouracil and cisplatin with radiation is more effective than the established standard of 5-fluorouracil, mitomycin, and radiation. Similarly, the roles of neoadjuvant and adjuvant chemotherapy are being evaluated. The most effective, and least toxic, radiation regimen is not yet determined, although advances in conformal radiation techniques have reduced the need for elective or toxicity-mandated interruptions in treatment.[4,14,15] The pathophysiology of late morbidity seen in some patients treated by combined modality treatment, especially deterioration in anorectal function, remains largely unexplained.[2] This functional deterioration is difficult to treat. The role of chemoradiation for anal adenocarcinoma is debated, although several small series suggest anorectal conservation is possible, and that chemoradiation is an alternative to the traditional treatment of radical surgery and colostomy.[16]

▀▀▀▀▀ SUMMARY TABLE

Prognostic Factors in Anal Cancer

Prognostic Factors	Tumor Related	Host Related	Environment Related
Essential	T category N category M category Histologic type		
Additional		Performance status HIV status	

New and promising	CD3 and CD4
	  lymphocytes in tumor
	CD34 expression
	Thymidine phosphorylase
	  cytoplasmic intensity		

Source:
• National Cancer Institute: Cancer (PDQ®): Treatment Guidelines; Anal Cancer 2005.
www.cancer.gov/cancertopics/pdq/treatment/anal/healthprofessional/

REFERENCES

1. Frisch M: On the etiology of anal squamous carcinoma. *Dan Med Bull* 49:194–209, 2002.
2. Cummings BJ, Swallow CJ, Ajani JA: Cancer of the Anal Region, in DeVita VT, Hellman S, Rosenberg SA (eds.): *Principles and Practice of Oncology, Cancer* 7th ed. Philadelphia, Lippincott, Williams and Wilkins, pp. 1125–1137, 2005.
3. Fenger C, Frisch M, Marti MC, et al.: Tumours of the anal canal, in Hamilton SR, Aaltonen LA (eds.): *Pathology and Genetics of Tumours of the Digestive System.* Lyon, IARC Press, 2000, pp. 145–155.
4. Cummings BJ, Brierley JD: Anal canal, in Perez CA, Brady LW, Halperin EC, et al. (eds.): *Principles and Practice of Radiation Oncology*, 4th ed. Philadelphia, Lippincott, Williams and Wilkins, 2003, pp. 1630–1648.
5. Hung A, Crane C, Delclos M, et al.: Cisplatin-based combined modality therapy for anal carcinoma: a wider therapeutic index. *Cancer* 97:1195–1202, 2003.
6. Bieri S, Allal AS, Kurtz JM: Sphincter-conserving treatment of carcinomas of the anal margin. *Acta Oncol* 40:29–33, 2001.
7. Cummings BJ: Anal Cancer, in Gospodarowicz MK, Henson DE, Hutter RV, et al. (eds.): *Prognostic Factors in Cancer*, 2nd ed. New York, Wiley-Liss, 2001, pp. 281–296.
8. Sobin LH, Wittekind C: *TNM Classification of Malignant Tumours*, 6th ed. New York, Wiley-Liss, 2002.
9. Greene FL, Page DL, Fleming D, et al.: *AJCC Cancer Staging Manual*, 6th ed. New York, Springer Publishers, 2002.
10. Fenger C: Prognostic factors in anal carcinoma. *Pathology* 34:573–578, 2002.
11. Grabenbauer GG, Lahmer G, Distel LV, et al.: Tumor infiltrating T-cells determine outcome in anal carcinoma. (abstr). *Proc Am Soc Ther Radiat Oncol, Int J Radiat Oncol Biol Phys* 63:S16, 2005.
12. Mawdsley S: Anal Cancer Trial Management Group: The role of biological molecular markers in predicting both response to treatment and clinical outcome in squamous cell carcinoma of the anus. (abstr) Proceedings of the 2004 Gastrointestinal Cancers Symposium: Current Status and Future Directions for Prevention and Management, 2004, p. 183.
13. Zbar AP, Fenger C, Efron J, et al.: The pathology and molecular biology of anal intraepithelial neoplasia: comparisons with cervical and vulvar intraepithelial carcinoma. *Int J Colorectal Dis* 17:203–215, 2002.
14. Wong CS, Tsang RW, Cummings BJ, et al.: Proliferation parameters in epidermoid carcinomas of the anal canal. *Radiother Oncol* 56:349–353, 2000.
15. Graf R, Wust P, Hildebrandt B, et al.: Impact of overall treatment time on local control of anal cancer treatment with radiochemotherapy 65:14–22, 2003.
16. Belkacemi Y, Berger C, Poortmans P, et al.: Management of anal canal adenocarcinoma: a large retrospective study from the Rare Cancer Network. *Int J Radiat Oncol Biol Phys* 56:1274–1283, 2003.

CHAPTER 16

Hepatocellular Carcinoma

DANIEL H. PALMER and PHILIP J. JOHNSON

Hepatocellular carcinoma (HCC) is the fifth commonest cancer in the world and the third commonest cause of cancer death. Although HCC occurs largely in patients with chronic liver disease, there is currently no evidence that screening high-risk groups influences overall survival.[1]

For most cancers, prognosis is predominantly related to tumor stage. However, the majority of HCCs arise in a cirrhotic liver, which itself contributes to prognosis and influences treatment options.[2] Thus, initial assessment is directed toward tumor staging and underlying liver function. Management requires a multidisciplinary approach between surgeon, interventional radiologist, and oncologist.

Surgery remains the only curative option, although resection in patients with cirrhosis should be reserved for those with well-preserved liver function. For patients with Child–Pugh class A cirrhosis, resection results in 5-year survival of 30–50%.[3] For patients with insufficient hepatic reserve to tolerate resection, but with small tumors meeting stringent criteria, transplantation can result in 5-year survival up to 75%.[4] For small lesions not suitable for resection or transplantation, local ablation (e.g., percutaneous ethanol injection, PEI; radio frequency ablation, RFA) is commonly used. Radio frequency ablation may be superior to PEI in terms of efficacy (4-year survival 74 vs. 57%) and need for fewer treatment sessions.[5]

The majority of patients are not candidates for surgery or ablation due to disease extent, vascular invasion and poor liver function. In selected patients, transarterial chemoembolisation may improve overall survival,[6] but is not suitable for those with portal vein involvement, Child C cirrhosis or extra-hepatic disease.

Systemic chemotherapy has no proven effect on overall survival and should be recommended only in the context of clinical trials. Tamoxifen has demonstrated no benefit in randomized controlled trials.[7]

Prognostic Factors in Cancer, Third Edition, edited by Mary K. Gospodarowicz,
Brian O'Sullivan, and Leslie H. Sobin.
Copyright © 2006 John Wiley & Sons, Inc.

Aside from transplantation, treatments do not positively (and may negatively) influence the underlying liver disease. For patients with HCC and advanced liver disease, the most appropriate treatment is symptom control.

A key prognostic factor for HCC is surgical resectability. Gross or microscopic residual disease is the most important adverse prognostic factor following resection. TNM remains a useful tool in predicting outcome in resected cases, but can only be applied once a patient has been deemed resectable, which has already taken into account tumor factors (e.g., size, morphology, portal vein involvement, extra-hepatic disease), host factors (e.g., hepatic reserve, performance status), and availability of surgical expertise and intensive care. T-category incorporates tumor size, morphology, and vascular invasion.[8] Large tumor size and multinodularity are independent predictors of a poor prognosis. Histological evidence of vascular invasion increases with tumor size, but is an independent prognostic factor; even large tumors have a good prognosis following resection in its absence. Portal vein thrombosis, evidence of macrovascular invasion, is an independent adverse prognostic factor.[2, 9–11] For patients undergoing transplantation, waiting time for a donor organ is an important prognostic factor, as well as size and number of tumors and vascular invasion.[4] Serum alpha-fetoprotein (AFP) is a tumor marker commonly used in the diagnosis and monitoring of HCC. It also has prognostic value, low-serum AFP being associated with longer survival, although this may be due to a higher proportion of such patients having tumors arising in a non-cirrhotic liver. Higher AFP levels and a faster rate of change are both associated with worse survival.[2,12]

An increasing number of studies, usually on small series of surgically resected cases, have identified other biomarkers with potential prognostic significance. Presence of variant estrogen receptor (ER) is an independent adverse prognostic factor (3-year survival 16 vs. 52%).[13] Others include markers of cell proliferation (e.g., PCNA, Ki-67); cell cycle regulatory proteins (e.g., cyclins A, D and E, p73); oncogenes (e.g., ras, c-myc, c-erbB2); tumor suppressor genes (e.g., p53, pRb); apoptosis-related factors (e.g., CD95 and its ligand); molecules associated with invasion and metastasis (e.g., adhesion molecules: E-cadherin, catenins, osteopontin; metalloproteinases); angiogenic factors (e.g., VEGF).[14] Validation in larger prospective studies is required. Genomic and proteomic expression profiles on blood or urine may allow easier accessibility than surgical resection specimens and allow application to a wider range of patients with HCC.[15]

Histological subtype and degree of differentiation do not have prognostic significance apart from the fibrolamellar variant, which typically occurs in younger patients without cirrhosis, allowing resection more frequently.[2]

For nonresectable patients, tumor size remains a key prognostic factor, with survival approaching 3 years for tumors <3 cm, but only 3 months for those >8 cm.[2] Larger tumors may exacerbate already deranged liver function, directly affecting survival and compromising treatment options. Tumor-related symptoms, evidence of liver failure (jaundice, ascites, encephalopathy), and poor performance status are associated with a poor prognosis.[2]

Apparent differences in survival between geographical regions are confounded by a number of factors including the aetiology of the underlying liver disease, and the time of diagnosis.[16] In particular, the use of screening may introduce a significant lead time bias.

Prognostic models for HCC are complex and should take account of tumor stage, degree of liver impairment, patient fitness, and treatment efficacy. The Okuda system was the first to be widely used that incorporated both tumor factors and liver function.[2] The measure of tumor size was crude (50% liver replacement) and the system appears to be best at identifying patients with advanced disease with very poor prognosis. Attempts to refine this system, based on retrospective studies using multivariate analyses of prognostic variables, by incorporating more detailed tumor information and liver function (e.g., CLIP and CUPI) probably share the same limitation.[17–18] The Barcelona group has proposed a staging classification incorporating treatment indication.[19] This system is a decision-making algorithm rather than a prognostic index.

For the majority of patients, the prognosis of HCC remains poor with treatments, to date, having little impact on overall survival. Nevertheless prognostication is important for patients to plan their affairs, for the physician to plan treatment, and for the clinical trialist to stratify appropriately.

▰▰▰ SUMMARY TABLE

Prognostic Factors in Hepatocellular Carcinoma

Prognostic Factors	Tumor Related	Host Related	Environment Related
Essential	Size Vascular invasion Portal vein thrombosis	Liver function	Geography (birth in high-incidence area)
Additional	Morphology (multifocal disease)	Performance status	Access to surgery/ transplantation
New and promising	p53 mutation Gene expression analysis		

Sources:
• National Cancer Institute: Liver Cancer (PDQ®): Treatment Guidelines National Cancer Institute: http://www.cancer.gov/cancertopics/pdq/treatment/bileduct/healthprofessional/.
• NCCN Clinical Practice Guidelines in Oncology: Hepatobiliary Cancer http://www.nccn.org/professionals/ physician_gls/PDF/hepatobiliary.pdf.

REFERENCES

1. Mok T, Zee B, Lau J, et al.: An intensive screening program detected high incidence of hepatocellular carcinoma (HCC) in hepatitis B virus carriers (HBVC) with abnormal alfa-fetoprotein (AFP) or abdominal ultrasongraphy (AUS). *J Clin Oncol* 2004 ASCO Annual Meeting Proceedings (Post-Meeting edition). 22 (14S) (July 15 Suppl), 4002, 2004.
2. Johnson PJ: Hepatocellular Carcinoma, in Gospodarowicz MK, Henson DE, Hutter RVP, et al. (eds.): *Prognostic Factors in Cancer*. 2nd ed. New York, Wiley-Liss, 2001.

3. Esnaola NF, Mirza N, Lauwers GY, et al.: Comparison of clinicopathologic characteristics and outcomes after resection in patients with hepatocellular carcinoma treated in the United States, France, and Japan. *Ann Surg* 238:711–719, 2003.

4. Llovet JM, Schwartz M, et al.: Resection and liver transplantation for hepatocellular carcinoma. *Semin Liver Dis* 25:181–200, 2005.

5. Shiina S, Teratani T, Obi S, et al.: A randomized controlled trial of radiofrequency ablation with ethanol injection for small hepatocellular carcinoma. *Gastroenterology* 129:122–130, 2005.

6. Llovet JM, Real MI, Montana X, et al.: Barcelona Liver Cancer Group. Arterial embolisation or chemoembolisation versus symptomatic treatment in patients with unresectable hepatocellular carcinoma: a randomised controlled trial. *Lancet* 359:1734–1739, 2002.

7. Perrone F, Gallo C, Daniele B, et al.: Cancer of Liver Italian Program (CLIP) Investigators. Tamoxifen in the treatment of hepatocellular carcinoma: 5-year results of the CLIP-1 multicentre randomised controlled trial. *Curr Pharm Des* 8:1013–1019, 2002.

8. Sobin LH, Wittekind Ch (eds.), UICC: *TNM Classification of malignant tumors.* 6th ed. New York, Wiley-Liss, 2002.

9. Huo TI, Lui WY, Wu JC, et al.: Deterioration of hepatic functional reserve in patients with hepatocellular carcinoma after resection: incidence, risk factors, and association with intrahepatic tumor recurrence. *World J Surg* 28:258–262, 2004.

10. Wayne JD, Lauwers GY, et al.: Preoperative predictors of survival after resection of small hepatocellular carcinomas. *Ann Surg* 235:722–730; discussion 730–731, 2002.

11. Poon RT, Ng IO, Fan ST, et al.: J. Clinicopathologic features of long-term survivors and disease-free survivors after resection of hepatocellular carcinoma: a study of a prospective cohort. *J Clin Oncol* 19:3037–3044, 2001.

12. Parasole R, Izzo F, Perrone F, et al.: Prognostic value of serum biological markers in patients with hepatocellular carcinoma. *Clin Cancer Res* 7:3504–3509, 2001.

13. Villa E, Moles A, Ferretti I, et al.: Natural history of inoperable hepatocellular carcinoma: estrogen receptors' status in the tumor is the strongest prognostic factor for survival. *Hepatology* 32:233–238, 2000.

14. Cui J, Dong BW, Liang P, et al.: Construction and clinical significance of a predictive system for prognosis of hepatocellular carcinoma. *World J Gastroenterol* 11:3027– 3033, 2005.

15. Lee JS, Thorgeirsson SS: Genome-scale profiling of gene expression in hepatocellular carcinoma: classification, survival prediction, and identification of therapeutic targets. *Gastroenterology* 127:S51–S515, 2004.

16. Sherman M: Hepatocellular carcinoma: epidemiology, risk factors, and screening. *Semin Liver Dis* 25:143–154, 2005.

17. Prospective validation of the CLIP score: a new prognostic system for patients with cirrhosis and hepatocellular carcinoma. The Cancer of the Liver Italian Program (CLIP) Investigators. *Hepatology* 31:840–845, 2000.

18. Leung TW, Tang AM, Zee B, et al.: Construction of the Chinese University Prognostic Index for hepatocellular carcinoma and comparison with the TNM staging system, the Okuda staging system, and the Cancer of the Liver Italian Program staging system: a study based on 926 patients. *Cancer* 94:1760–1769, 2002.

19. Llovet JM, Fuster J, Bruix J: Barcelona-Clinic Liver Cancer Group. The Barcelona approach: diagnosis, staging, and treatment of hepatocellular carcinoma. *Liver Transpl* 10:S115–S120, 2004.

CHAPTER 17

Extrahepatic Biliary Tract and the Ampulla of Vater Cancers

CHRISTIAN WITTEKIND

Cancers of the extrahepatic biliary tract (carcinomas of the gallbladder and the extrahepatic bile ducts) are uncommon as are cancers of the Ampulla of Vater. Each year ~7000 people in the United States are diagnosed with gallbladder carcinoma, which constitutes nearly two-thirds of the biliary tract cancers, and is the fifth most common gastrointestinal tract tumor. Prognosis is generally poor with curative resection rates between 10 and 30% in carcinomas of the gallbladder and extrahepatic bile ducts, but rises to 80% in carcinomas of the Ampulla of Vater. Five-year survival rates are ~15 and 30%, respectively.[1] Identification of prognostic factors remains difficult in these rare malignancies.

CARCINOMA OF THE GALLBLADDER

Gallbladder cancer is usually detected at pathologic examination following cholecystectomy for symptomatic gallstones. More advanced tumors are evaluated by means of ultrasound and computerized tomography (CT) scan. Ultrasound can suggest the correct diagnosis in 75% of cases, increasing to 90% of cases with CT, the latter also providing a better assessment of regional nodes or peritoneal spread. Magnetic resonance (MR) plus MR cholangiography is considered by some to be the ideal staging procedure.

Anatomic disease extent as reflected by the TNM classification[2] is not only strongly prognostic, but is also a tool for stratifying resectable (stage IIB (T1, T2, T3 N1M0), from nonresectable tumors (locally unresectable, stage III, or stage IV with distant metastasis)). It is unclear whether patients with advanced cancer should undergo more radical resection, since the 5-year survival rate is only 10% for stage II cancers, decreasing to <5% when regional lymph nodes are involved.

Prognostic Factors in Cancer, *Third Edition*, edited by Mary K. Gospodarowicz, Brian O'Sullivan, and Leslie H. Sobin.

Prognosis in Resectable Tumors

The success of tumor resection remains the most reliable prognostic factor. Patients with microscopic residual tumor (R1) or macroscopic residual tumor (R2) have a prognosis as dismal as those with nonresectable tumors. When confined to the mucosa (pT1apN0M0 = stage IA) 5-year survival rates of 86% can be achieved, dropping to 56% in pT1bpN0M0 = stage IB tumors. In cases with lymph node metastasis (pT1-3pN1M0 = stage IIB) the 5-year survival rate falls to <5%.[1] Small cell, undifferentiated and giant cell carcinomas fare worse compared to papillary carcinomas.[3] High-grade cancers (G3,G4) have a poorer prognosis than low-grade carcinomas (G1,G2).[1] Other factors (e.g., vascular invasion) are controversial. At present, no other new and promising molecular prognostic factors are available for clinical application.[1]

CARCINOMA OF THE BILE DUCT

The treatment of bile duct carcinomas near the confluence depends on tumor extent. Disease entirely below the confluence should undergo resection of the extrahepatic bile ducts, gallbladder, and lymph nodes. Tumors above the confluence may require resection of a lobe of the liver. Pancreatoduodenectomy (classical or pylorus-preserving) is the treatment of choice with resectability rates of 80%. Unresectable bile duct carcinoma is incurable. Relief of bile duct obstruction can be achieved by stenting, palliative radiotherapy, or more recently, photodynamic therapy where 2-year survival rates can ~10–20%.[4–11] Chemotherapy and/or radiotherapy have not been demonstrated to alter the prognosis either in the adjuvant setting or in the treatment of unresectable disease.

Prognosis in Resectable Tumors

Tumor located in the distal third of the bile duct as well as successful resection with minimal or no residual disease are favorable prognostic factors. Tumors confined to the bile duct (pT1pN0M0 = stage I) have a 5-year survival of 22%, compared to only 2% when lymph node metastases are present. Perineural invasion is associated with a poor prognosis.[6] Small-cell, undifferentiated, and giant-cell carcinomas are also unfavorable, but papillary carcinomas have a slightly better prognosis.[1] Patients with high grade (G3,G4) have a poorer prognosis than those with low grade carcinomas (G1,G2).[1]

Prognosis in Nonresectable Tumors

Clinical symptoms (weight loss, nausea, etc.), and signs, such as ascites and poor performance status, are unfavorable prognostic factors, although these have not been specifically integrated into a clinical or laboratory prognostic system.[1] Serum CEA or CA19-9 cannot be reliably used to estimate tumor bulk or distant metastasis.

The type of surgery and the experience of the center are further environmental factors of prognostic importance.[7–9] In experienced centers, 5-year survival rates between 30 and 40% are achievable.[9–11]

CARCINOMA OF THE AMPULLA OF VATER

Only patients undergoing an R0 resection have a chance of long-term survival. Among these patients, disease extent is again the most reliable prognostic factor, with carcinomas confined to the ampulla being the most favorable. The overall survival after R0 resection is ~50%.[12–16] For T1N0M0 tumors, some authors advocate localized treatment that might, in experienced hands, confer a better prognosis.[17] The 5-year survival is 45% for N0 disease and falls to 10% in N1 disease. Papillary carcinomas have a slightly better prognosis.[1]

Of the putative molecular factors, Bax expression was the only parameter that influenced prognosis in resected ampullary carcinoma.[18] K-ras mutations did not correlate with survival.[1] In tumors with overexpression of cyclin D1, survival rates were decreased.[17]

■■■■■■ SUMMARY TABLES

Prognostic Factors in Gallbladder Cancer*

Prognostic Factors	Tumor Related	Host Related	Environment Related
Essential	T category N category M category		
Additional	Histologic type Grade	Performance status	Treatment
New and promising			

Source:
• British Columbia Cancer Agency Cancer Management Guidelines: Gallbladder and Bile Ducts.
http://www.bccancer.bc.ca/HPI/CancerManagementGuidelines/Gastrointestinal/10.Gallbladder/default.htm.
* For R0 resected cancer.

Prognostic Factors in Extrahepatic Bile Duct Cancer*

Prognostic Factors	Tumor Related	Host Related	Environment Related
Essential	T category N category M category		
Additional	Location Histologic type Histologic grade Perineural invasion	Performance status Anaemia	Treatment
New and promising			

Source:
• National Cancer Institute: Bile Duct Cancer (PDQ®): Treatment Guidelines
http://www.cancer. gov/cancertopics/pdq/treatment/bileduct/healthprofessional/.
* For R0 resected cancer.

Prognostic Factors in Ampulla of Vater Cancer*

Prognostic Factors	Tumor Related	Host Related	Environment Related
Essential	T category N category M category		
Additional	Histologic type Histologic grade	Performance status	Treatment
New and promising	Cyclin D1 Bax		

* For R0 resected cancer.

REFERENCES

1. Henson DE, Ries LG, Albores-Saavedra J: Extrahepatic Biliary Tract and the Ampulla of Vater Cancers, in Gospodarowicz MK, Henson DE, Hutter RVP et al. (eds.): *Prognostic Factors in Cancer* 2nd ed. New York, Wiley-Liss, 2001.
2. UICC: in Sobin LH, Wittekind Ch (eds.): TNM Classification of malignant tumors. 6th ed. New York, Wiley-Liss, 2002.

3. Albores-Saavedra J, Tuck M, McLaren BK, et al.: Papillary carcinoma of the gallbladder: analysis on noninvasive and invasive types. *Arch Pathol Lab Med* 129:905–909, 2005.

4. Berr F, Wiedmann M, Tannapfel A, et al.: Photodynamic therapy for advanced bile duct cancer. Evidence for improved palliation and extended survival. *Hepatology* 31:291–298, 2000.

5. Witzigmann H, Berr F, Ringel U, et al.: Surgical and palliative management and outcome in 184 patients with cholangiocarcinoma – palliative photodynamic therapy plus stenting is comparable to R1/r2 resection. Submitted for publication in *Ann Surg*.

6. Silva MA, Tekin K, Aytekin F, et al.: Surgery for hilar cholangiocarcinoma; a 10 year experience of a tertiary referral centre in the UK. *Eur J Surg Oncol* 31:533–539, 2005.

7. Kawasaki S, Imamura H, Kobayashi A, et al.: Results of surgical resection for patients with hilar bile duct cancer: application of extended hepatectomy after biliary drainage and hemihepatic portal vein embolization. *Ann Surg* 224:628–638, 2003.

8. Jarnagin WR, Fong Y, DeMatteo RP, et al.: Staging, resectability, and outcome in 225 patients with hilar cholangiocarcinoma. *Surgery* 107:597–604, 2001.

9. Jang JY, Kim SW, Park DJ, et al.: Actual long-term outcome of extrahepatic bile duct cancer after surgical resection. *Ann Surg* 241:77–84, 2005.

10. Seyama Y, Kubota K, Sano K, et al.: Long-term outcome of extended hemihepatectomy for hilar bile duct cancer with no mortality and high survival rate. *Ann Surg* 238:73–83, 2003.

11. Kondo S, Hirano S, Ambo Y, et al.: Forty consecutive resections of hilar cholangiocarcinoma with no postoperative mortality and no positive ductal margins: results of a prospective study. *Ann Surg* 240:95–101, 2004.

12. Brown KM, Tompkins AJ, Yong S, et al.: Pancreatoduodenectomy is curative in the majority of patients with node-negative ampullary cancer. *Arch Surg* 140:529–532, 2005.

13. Wang CH, Mo LR, Lin RC, et al.: A survival predictive model in patients undergoing radical resection of ampullary adenocarcinoma. *Hepatogastroenterology* 51:1495–1499, 2004.

14. Todoroki T, Koike N, Morishita Y, et al.: Patterns and predictors of failure after curative resections of carcinoma of the ampulla of Vater. *Ann Surg Oncol* 10:1176–1183, 2003.

15. DeCastro SM, van Heek NT, Kuhlmann KF, et al.: Surgical management of neoplasms of the ampulla of Vater: local resection or pancreatoduodenectomy and prognostic factors for survival. *Surgery* 136:994–1002, 2004.

16. Tran TC, Vitale GC: Ampullary tumors: endoscopic versus operative management. *Surg Innov* 11:255–263, 2004.

17. Tomazic A, Pegan V, Ferlan-Marolt K, et al.: Cyclin d1 and bax influence the prognosis after pancreatoduodenectomy for periampullary adenocarcinoma. *Hepatogastroenterology* 51:1832–1837, 2004.

18. Santini FD, Tonini G, Vecchio FM, et al.: Prognostic value of Bax, Bcl-2, p53, and TUNEL staining in patients with radically resected ampullary carcinoma. *J Clin Pathol* 58:159–162, 2005.

CHAPTER 18

Pancreas Cancer

PAULA GHANEH and JOHN P. NEOPTOLEMOS

Pancreatic cancer is a highly lethal disease. It is the fourth to fifth leading cause of cancer-related death in the Western world. The latest estimates from IARC indicate there will currently be >230,000 new cases diagnosed and >225,000 deaths world-wide each year.[1] The lifetime risk of developing pancreatic cancer is 1% in developing countries, representing 3% of all cancers and 5% of cancer deaths.

The majority of patients present with advanced disease, with an associated median survival of 3–6 months and a dismal long-term survival of 0.4%. Only the 2.6–9% of patients who are suitable for resection demonstrate improved 5-year survival rates of 10–18%. This rises to 30% with the use of adjuvant 5-fluorouracil chemotherapy.[2]

Ductal adenocarcinomas represent 90% of pancreatic exocrine tumors. The pathogenesis follows a progression from squamous (transitional) metaplasia to the precancerous lesion, Pancreatic Intraepithelial Neoplasia (PanIN).[3] The molecular events involved in pancreatic cancer, such as activation of K-ras oncogene, and inactivation of tumor suppressor genes p16, p53 and SMAD4 have been identified in these early lesions and carcinoma *in situ*.

The classical presentation is with jaundice, weight loss, and back pain, but often the symptoms are vague in nature, including pain, fatigue, dyspepsia, and abdominal discomfort. Assessment should include testing serum markers, such as CA19.9, although this has relatively low specificity. Gold standard imaging is currently contrast enhanced computerized tomography (CE-CT). This modality achieves diagnostic rates of 97%, 90% accuracy for predicting unresectability and 80–85% for predicting resectability. Laparoscopy and laparoscopic ultrasound affect management in 15% of patients assessed by CE-CT.[4] Magnetic resonance imaging (MRI) may add further correlative anatomical information.[5,6]

Prognostic Factors in Cancer, Third Edition, edited by Mary K. Gospodarowicz, Brian O'Sullivan, and Leslie H. Sobin.
Copyright © 2006 John Wiley & Sons, Inc.

The most important determinant of survival in pancreatic cancer is performance status and surgical resectability. The median survival following surgical resection is ~11–20 months, with 5-year survival ranging from 7 to 25%. This compares to median survivals of 6–11 and 2–6 months in unresectable locally advanced and metastatic disease, respectively.[7,8] The classical Kausch–Whipple procedure and the pylorus preserving procedure are the main surgical approaches, although the type of surgical resection *per se* does not influence long-term outcome.[9] This being said, tumor subsite remains important, with body and tail lesions faring worse compared to those more commonly arising from the pancreatic head.

Radical lymph node resection versus classical resection has not demonstrated an advantage. The resection of locally advanced disease that may include en bloc resection of portal or superior mesenteric vein demonstrates superior survival compared to definitive chemoradiotherapy.[10]

Pathological staging is according to the UICC TNM classification.[11] The most important pathological prognostic indicators are lymph node involvement and tumor grade.[12] Resection margin status is also significant.

A meta-analysis of five randomized adjuvant trials has confirmed the survival advantage of adjuvant chemotherapy, with the use of 5-fluorouracil currently regarded as standard.[13] The role of adjuvant gemcitabine compared to both surgery alone and to 5-fluorouracil is being investigated in the ESPAC-3 study. The indications for both neoadjuvant and adjuvant chemoradiotherapy, especially in resection margin positive disease remains to be clarified.

The development of high-volume specialist centers is the main reason for the reduction in perioperative mortality during the last decade, with a clear correlation between higher caseload and lower surgical mortality demonstrated.[14,15]

Novel genetic markers, such as K-ras mutation, enhanced TGF-β isoform expression Bcl-x_L and increased VEGF expression, MMP-9:E-cadherin ratio >3.0 have been studied and represent new and promising molecular prognostic factors that have been demonstrated thus far to influence survival.[16] Some of these factors may be important in determining the indication for and response to future therapies.

The majority of patients with pancreatic cancer present with unresectable disease. High-dose opiate analgesia, intraoperative, percutaneous, and endoluminal endosonography (EUS) guided neurolytic coeliac plexus block (with success rates of up to 74–78%) and bilateral or unilateral thoracoscopic splanchnicectomy may be indicated to control pain.[17] Pancreatic exocrine insufficiency is treated with pancreatic enzyme supplements. Jaundice and duodenal obstruction can be relieved using stents or operative bypass.

Gemcitabine is the current standard chemotherapy in unresectable disease, improving long-term survival compared to supportive therapy alone. Encouraging results have also been demonstrated with the combination of gemcitabine and erlotinib and also with capecitabine. Combined chemoradiotherapy has not yet demonstrated superior results.

High CA19-9 levels have also been correlated with poor outcome. Positive peritoneal cytology demonstrates a trend toward decreased survival. The prognostic value of disseminated tumor cells has not yet been proven. In stage III or IV disease, an elevated C-reactive protein and leucocytosis are also negative prognostic factors.

Primary screening for pancreatic cancer is not applicable to the general population. Investigational secondary screening programs are in place for familial pancreatic cancer, certain familial cancer syndromes, and hereditary pancreatitis (*:europac@liv.ac.uk; http://www.liv.ac.uk/surgery/europac.html*). Currently, the best method for secondary screening is via endoluminal endosonography.[18–20]

████████ SUMMARY TABLE

Prognostic Factors in Pancreatic Cancer

Prognostic Factors	Tumor Related	Host Related	Environment Related
Essential	T category N category M category	Performance status	Treatment center with expertise and high case load
Additional	Location (head lesions better) Histologic type Grade Perineural invasion CA 19.9 Resection margins	Leucocytosis GGT CRP	
New and promising	K-ras mutation TGF-β isoform expression Bcl-x$_L$ expression VEGF, PD ECGF MMP-9:E-cadherin ratio >3.0, MMP7 Bax expression DPC4, S100A6, AKT2, MUC4		

Source:
• National Cancer Institute: Pancreatic Cancer (PDQ®): Treatment Guidelines 2005.
http://www.cancer.gov/cancertopics/pdq/treatment/pancreatic/healthprofessional/.
• ESMO Minimum Clinical Recommendations for diagnosis, treatment and follow-up of pancreatic cancer 2004.
http://annonc.oupjournals.org/cgi/reprint/16/suppl_1/i24.

REFERENCES

1. International Agency for Research on Cancer. [cited 2005 Sept.]; Available from: http://www.iarc.fr/.

2. Neoptolemos J, et al.: A randomised trial of chemoradiotherapy and chemotherapy after resection of pancreatic cancer. *N Eng J Med* 350:1200–1210, 2004.

3. Hruban RH, et al.: Pancreatic intraepithelial neoplasia: a new nomenclature and classification system for pancreatic duct lesions. *Am J Surg Pathol* 25:579–586, 2001.

4. Connor S, et al.: Serum CA19-9 measurement increases the effectiveness of staging laparoscopy in patients with suspected pancreatic malignancy. *Dig Surg* 22:80–85, 2005.

5. Phoa SS, et al.: Value of CT criteria in predicting survival in patients with potentially resectable pancreatic head carcinoma. *J Surg Oncol* 91:33–40, 2005.

6. Soriano A, et al.: Preoperative staging and tumour resectability assessment of pancreatic cancer: prospective study comparing endoscopic ultrasonography, helical computed tomography, magnetic resonance imaging and angiography. *Am J Gastroenterol* 99: 492–510, 2004.

7. Alexakis N, et al.: Current standards of surgery for pancreatic cancer. *Br J Surg* 91: 1410–1427, 2004.

8. Cleary SP, et al.: Prognostic factors in resected pancreatic adenocarcinoma: Analysis of actual 5-year survivors. *J Am Coll Surg* 198:722–731, 2004.

9. Seiler CA, et al.: Randomized clinical trial of pylorus-preserving duodenopancreatectomy versus classical Whipple resection-long term results. *Br J Surg* 92:547–556, 2005.

10. Yeo CJ, et al.: Pancreaticoduodenectomy with or without distal gastrectomy and extended retroperitoneal lymphadenectomy for periampullary adenocarcinoma, part 2: randomized controlled trial evaluating survival, morbidity, and mortality. *Ann Surg* 236:355–366; discussion 366–368, 2002.

11. *TNM Classification of Malignant Tumours*. 6th ed. Sobin LH, Wittekind Ch: New York, Wiley-Liss, 2002.

12. Neoptolemos JP, et al.: Influence of resection margins on survival for patients with pancreatic cancer treated by adjuvant chemoradiation and/or chemotherapy in the ESPAC-1 randomized controlled trial. *Ann of Surg* 234:758–768, 2001.

13. Stocken DD, et al.: Meta-analysis of randomised adjuvant therapy trials for pancreatic cancer. *Br J Cancer* 92:1372–1381, 2005.

14. Birkmeyer JD, et al.: Hospital volume and surgical mortality in the United States. *N Engl J Med* 346:1128–1137, 2002.

15. Guidelines for the management of patients with pancreatic cancer periampullary and ampullary carcinomas. *Gut* 54 (Suppl 5): vol. 16, 2005.

16. Garcea G, et al.: Molecular prognostic markers in pancreatic cancer: A systematic review. *Eur J Cancer* 41:2213–2236, 2005.

17. Wong G, et al.: Effect of neurolytic celiac plexus block on pain relief, quality of life, and survival in patients with unresectable pancreatic cancer. A randomised controlled trial. *JAMA* 291:1092–1099, 2004.

18. Howes N, et al.: Clinical and genetic characteristics of hereditary pancreatitis in Europe. *Clin Gastroenterol Hepatol* 2:252–261, 2004.

19. Klein AP, et al.: Prospective risk of pancreatic cancer in familial pancreatic cancer kindreds. *Cancer Res* 64:2634–2638, 2004.

20. Yan L, et al.: Molecular analysis to detect pancreatic ductal adenocarcinoma in high-risk groups. *Gastroenterology* 128:2124–2130, 2005.

LUNG AND PLEURAL TUMORS

CHAPTER 19

Lung Cancer

MICHAEL D. BRUNDAGE and WILLIAM J. MACKILLOP

Lung cancer is a group of heterogeneous clinical entities with common molecular and cellular origins, but with different accumulated genetic mutations with different clinical behaviors and prognoses. Lung cancers are the most common cause of cancer death in both males and females in North America.[1] A substantive amount of clinical and basic science research has focussed on prognostic factors in patients with lung cancer, and more than 100 prognostic factors pertaining to the tumor, the patient, or the environment having been reported; the reader is referred to more detailed descriptions of the breadth of this literature.[2,3]

The recognized clinical heterogeneity among lung cancer patients has led to the division of prognostic subgroups. The most important distinction is between small cell lung cancer (SCLC) and nonsmall cell lung cancer (NSCLC). The second is disease extent, or anatomical stage. NSCLC, is staged using the TNM classification;[4] SCLC as either limited or extensive disease.[4] Some advocate TNM (see Glossary) system for SCLC.[5] A comprehensive review of all prognostic factors is beyond the scope of this chapter, which focuses on those factors that have established clinical relevance to treatment guidelines for these common presentations.[2]

Most studies of NSCLC evaluate patients with resected disease, but few have addressed the prognosis based on preoperative information.[2] In patients with resectable disease, but who are inoperable for medical reasons and treated with radical radiotherapy,[1] T category, symptoms, performance status, and hemoglobin are significant predictors of survival. For patients undergoing resection, with recurrence rates of 20–85%,[4] the determination of prognosis is clinically relevant. Completely resected cases[5] with pT2pN0 disease are candidates for chemotherapy, whereas those with pN2 disease or positive resection margins (R1 cases) are candidates for radiotherapy with or without chemotherapy.[1,6] Controversy exists regarding the definition of TNM stage groupings, methods of anatomical staging (including the use of

Prognostic Factors in Cancer, Third Edition, edited by Mary K. Gospodarowicz, Brian O'Sullivan, and Leslie H. Sobin.

positron emission tomography (PET) scanning),[7–9] and the appropriate extent of mediastinal dissection,[1,3] among others.

The significance of cell type (large-cell undifferentiated, adenocarcinoma, or squamous cell) has been studied extensively. Studies show inconsistent evidence regarding the significance of adenocarcinoma compared to other NSCLC subtypes.[2] Bronchioalveolar cancer and carcinoid tumors constitute notable exceptions.[1] Many other tumor factors have been shown to have independent prognostic significance,[2] but are not utilized routinely for treatment decision making. These factors include histologic features, chemistry, and serum tumor markers, tumor proliferation, and cellular markers. Other molecular markers, include regulators of cellular growth (kRAS, RB, EGFr, erb-b2, MRP-1, HGF), of the metastatic cascade (TPA, Cyclin D-1, cathepsin), and of apoptosis (p53, bcl-2).[1–3,10] Patient-related characteristics predictive after complete surgical resection are less powerful in the setting of resected disease than in the advanced-disease setting. Thus, patient-related factors are generally not considered important for clinical decision making in this scenario, with the exception of comorbidities influencing medical operability and radiotherapy tolerance.[3,4]

The majority of studies consider both locally advanced (typically T4 or N3 or uresectable T3N2 cases) and metastatic NSCLC (M1 cases) under the term of "advanced" disease. The distinction between the two entities, however, is important for the consideration of particular subgroups of patients due to treatment decision-making implications.[1] Factors essential to decision making are stage, weight loss, and performance status, indicators of potential success with combined-modality loco-regional therapy.

Patients without systemic manifestations of illness, those patients with no substantial weight loss, and high performance status, have been shown to have higher survival rates following induction chemotherapy followed by radiotherapy, or concurrent chemo–radiotherapy. They have been shown to have better survival when treated with continuous hyperfractionated and accelerated radiotherapy (CHART) as compared to conventional fractionation, and with higher radiation dose. The role of surgery is currently being investigated, as is the role of combination chemo–radiotherapy in more symptomatic patients.[1] A subgroup of patients is that with cT3N0M0 disease, particularly when located in the superior pulmonary sulcus (Pancoast's tumor).[11]

In the setting of advanced (stage IV) disease, markers of functional impact, such as weight loss, performance status, symptom burden, and pretreatment quality of life, have been shown to have independent prognostic significance for median survival duration following systemic therapy. Chemotherapy itself, as an environment-related factor, is known to improve patients' median survival over best-supportive care alone in patients without substantial systemic manifestations of illness. More recent clinical trials research has been directed at finding chemotherapy regimens with higher response rates and/or lower toxicity.[1] Additional factors include markers relating to the extent of clinically detectable disease, hematological or biochemical markers associated with disease extent. In a large study of 2531 patients enrolled on a variety of clinical trials, Albain and colleagues[4] identified good performance status, female gender, and age >70 years as the most important factors for survival overall. Patient self-reported indices, such as quality of life scores and/or anxiety and depression measures, are new emerging prognostic factors.[2]

In the setting of small cell lung cancer (SCLC), stage is considered an essential factor since patients with limited disease generally receive loco-regional radiotherapy and prophylactic cranial radiotherapy in addition to chemotherapy,[1] and are considered potentially curable. The use of prophylactic cranial radiotherapy predicts for fewer central nervous system (CNS) recurrences compared to untreated patients, but has not been consistently shown to increase patients' median survival. The use of loco-regional radiotherapy, in contrast, has been clearly demonstrated to improve survival of limited stage patients. In addition, the timing of thoracic radiotherapy (early vs. late in relation to chemotherapy treatment[12]), and the use of altered fractionation strategies and/or higher doses of radiotherapy have been shown in some studies to increase patient survival. These issues, in addition to novel systemic therapeutic strategies, continue to be investigated in clinical trials.[1] Large studies of treated patient cohorts, have shown outcome in limited disease to be best predicted by good performance status, female sex, age <70 years, white race, normal serum lactate dehydrogenase (LDH), and concurrent chemo–radiotherapy. A normal serum LDH, multidrug chemotherapy, and a single metastatic lesion best predicted survival outcomes for patients with extensive disease.

■■■■■■ SUMMARY TABLES

Prognostic Factors in Surgically Resected NSCLC

Prognostic Factors	Tumor Related	Host Related	Environment Related
Essential	T Category N Category Extracapsular nodal extension Superior sulcus location Intrapulmonary metastasis	Weight loss Performance status	Resection margins Adequacy of mediastinal dissection
Additional	Histologic type Grade Vessel invasion Tumor size	Gender Age	Radiotherapy dose Adjuvant radiation
New and promising	Molecular/biologic markers	Quality of life Marital status	

Sources:
• NCCN Clinical Practice Guidelines in Oncology: Non-Small Cell Lung Cancer 2005.
http:// www.nccn.org/professionals/physician_gls/PDF/nscl.pdf.
• Program in Evidence-Based Care: Practice Guidelines and Evidence Based Summaries Lung Cancer Site Group 2003.
http://www.cancercare.on.ca/index_lungCancerguidelines.htm.

Prognostic Factors in Advanced[a] NSCLC

Prognostic Factors	Tumor Related	Host Related	Environment Related
Essential	Stage SVCO Solitary brain Solitary adrenal metastasis Number of sites	Weight loss Performance status	Chemoradiotherapy Chemotherapy
Additional	Number of metastatic sites Pleural effusion Liver metastases Hemoglobin LDH Albumin	Gender Symptom burden	
New and promising	Molecular/biologic markers	Quality of life Marital Status Anxiety/depression	

[a] Locally advanced or metastatic.

Prognostic Factors in SCLC

Prognostic Factors	Tumor Related	Host Related	Environment Related

Essential	Stage	Performance
		Status
		Age
		Comorbidity
			Chemotherapy
			Thoracic
			  radiotherapy
			Prophylactic
			  cranial RT

Additional	LDH Alkaline Phosphatase Cushing's syndrome M0 Mediastinal involvement M1 Number of sites bone or brain involvement WBC, Platelet count		
New and promising	Molecular/biologic markers		

Source:
• NCCN Clinical Practice Guidelines in Oncology: Small Cell Lung Cancer 2005.
http://www.nccn.org/professionals/physician_gls/PDF/sclc.pdf.

REFERENCES

1. Cameron R, Loehrer Sr, Thomas CR Jr: Neoplasms of the Mediastinum: in DeVita VT HS, Rosenberg SA, (eds.): *Cancer: Principles and Practice of Oncology*. 7th ed. Philidelphia: Lippincott-Raven; 2005, pp. 845–860.

2. Brundage MD, Davies D, Mackillop WJ: Prognostic factors in non-small cell lung cancer: a decade of progress. *Chest* 122:1037–1057, 2002.

3. Solan MJ, Werner-Wasik M. Prognostic factors in non-small cell lung cancer. *Semin Surg Oncol* 21:64–73, 2003.

4. Brundage MD, Mackillop WJ: Lung Cancer, in Gospodarowicz MK HD, Hutter RVP, O'Sullivan B, et al. (eds.): *Prognostic Factors in Cancer*. 2nd ed. New York, Wiley-Liss; pp. 351–370, 2001.

5. Wittekind Ch, Henson DE, et al.: TNM Supplement. *A commentary on uniform use*. 3rd ed. New York, Wiley-Liss, 2003.

6. Arriagada R, Le Pechoux C, Pignon JP: Resected non-small cell lung cancer: need for adjuvant lymph node treatment? From hope to reality. *Lung Cancer* 42:S57–S64, 2003.

7. Sihoe AD, Yim AP: Lung cancer staging. *J Surg Res* 117:92–106, 2004.

8. Schrevens L, Lorent N, Dooms C, et al.: The role of PET scan in diagnosis, staging, and management of non-small cell lung cancer. *Oncologist* 9:633–643, 2004.

9. Ukena D, Hellwig D: Value of FDG PET in the management of NSCLC. *Lung Cancer* 45:S75–S78, 2004.

10. O'Byrne KJ, Cox G, Swinson D, et al.: Towards a biological staging model for operable non-small cell lung cancer. *Lung Cancer* 34:S83–S89, 2001.

11. Kraut MJ, Vallieres E, Thomas CR Jr: Pancoast (superior sulcus) neoplasms. *Curr Probl Cancer* 27:81–104, 2003.

12. Fried DB, Morris DE, Poole C, et al.: Systematic review evaluating the timing of thoracic radiation therapy in combined modality therapy for limited-stage small-cell lung cancer. *J Clin Oncol* 22:4837–4845, 2004.

CHAPTER 20

Malignant Pleural Mesothelioma

NIRMAL K. VEERAMACHANENI and RICHARD J. BATTAFARANO

Approximately 2000–3000 cases of diffuse malignant pleural mesothelioma (DMPM) are diagnosed each year in the United States. While exposure to asbestos remains the leading risk factor for development of DMPM, 20% of patients have no prior history of asbestos exposure.[1] The natural history of DMPM is one of locoregional progression with development of distant metastasis. The presentation of the tumor is often insidious, and delay in diagnosis is common. Despite aggressive multimodality treatment, the median survival is poor ranging from 4–18 months.[1,2]

Mesotheliomas are classified into epithelial, sarcomatoid, desmoplastic, and biphasic types.[3] Epithelial type is the most common (50–57%) histology and is associated with the best prognosis. Biphasic (24–34%) and sarcomatoid histologies (16–19%) are associated with a poor prognosis, with essentially no 5-year survivors in the largest reported series. Desmoplastic mesothelioma, in which >50% of the tumor consists of dense hypocellular collagen, has a similarly poor prognosis with a median survival of 6 months. As such, some authors consider desmoplastic mesothelioma to be a variant of sarcomatoid mesothelioma. Accurate tissue diagnosis is essential because the prognosis is based heavily upon histologic typing.[4]

In order to obtain adequate tissue for pathologic examination, invasive measures, such as video assisted thoracoscopy, or open pleural biopsy, are required. Cervical mediastinoscopy provides access to the paratracheal and subcarinal lymph nodes for lymph node staging. Fine needle aspiration biopsies often do not yield adequate tissue to differentiate malignant pleural mesothelioma from metastatic adenocarcinoma to the pleura. The surgeon must be cognisant of the biopsy strategy, and orient the incisions to permit definitive resection of the biopsy site(s) at a later time. Combinations of computerized tomography (CT) and positron emission tomography (PET) imaging are useful in assessing locoregional and distant disease.[5,6] Magnetic

Prognostic Factors in Cancer, Third Edition, edited by Mary K. Gospodarowicz, Brian O'Sullivan, and Leslie H. Sobin.

resonance (MRI) is a useful adjunct to assess the degree of local involvement and suitability for resection.[7]

Combinations of surgery, radiation therapy, and chemotherapy have been attempted with varying success. Evidence is based mainly from nonrandomized studies with small sample sizes and over differing and lengthy time periods. In the setting of favorable histology, resectable disease and minimal comorbidities, complete surgical resection may be accomplished by extrapleural pneumonectomy.[8] A more limited resection, such as pleurectomy and decortication, may be offered if negative margins can be achieved.[9]

Adjuvant therapy using hyperthermic cisplatin-based chemotherapy at the time of pneumonectomy, photodynamic therapy to eradicate microscopic disease, and radiation treatment to the surgically resected field have been employed by various institutions with varying degrees of success.[10] Combination chemotherapy, particularly platinum-containing regimens in nonsurgical candidates continues to be actively studied. The best available data regarding prognostic variables are from large series of patients treated with aggressive surgical resection,[8] as well as collective reviews of phase II chemotherapy trials.[11]

To identify those most likely to benefit from aggressive therapy, considerable effort has focused on developing a universally accepted staging system.[12] Initial efforts by Butchart and Sugarbaker defined stage by local tumor invasion and resected margins, but these systems did not provide adequate prognostic information due to limitations of imaging modalities. The most recent TNM classification is a modification of the International Mesothelioma Interest Group system, and differentiates tumors by tumor size, lymph node involvement, and the presence of metastatic disease.[13] These different systems clearly indicate that microscopically positive resection margins (R1) confer a worse prognosis, as does the presence of involved subcarinal or mediastinal lymph nodes.[14] In many studies, no long-term survivors were reported in the presence of lymph node metastasis.[14,15] Due to the aggressive nature of this malignancy, careful patient selection is necessary both to identify those most likely to benefit from multimodality therapy, and to minimize treatment related morbidity and mortality.

The presence of chest pain suggests locally advanced disease not amenable to complete surgical extirpation and shorter median survival.[16] Eligibility criteria for aggressive surgical therapy by extrapleural pneumonectomy include Karnofsky performance score >70, and normal renal, hepatic and cardiac function.[11] Although the exact mechanism is unclear, the presence of thrombocytosis (platelet count $>400,000/\mu L$) or leukocytosis ($>8.3 \times 10E\ 9/L$) have been associated with a worse outcome.[2,16] Similarly, excessive weight loss is associated with worse outcome. Patients with advanced age have shorter median survival compared to younger patients and similarly, male gender is associated with worse outcome.[17]

There are a number of new and promising molecular prognostic factors being explored. These include karyotype abnormalities, such as high S-phase fraction, DNA aneuploidy; proliferation indices, cell cycle control processes, angiogenesis factors, and other factors affecting the extracellular matrix (e.g., high microvessel count and fibroblast growth factor-2).[17]

■■■■■■■ SUMMARY TABLE

Prognostic Factors in Malignant Pleural Mesothelioma

Prognostic Factors	Tumor Related	Host Related	Environment Related
Essential	Stage Histologic type		
Additional	Symptoms	Performance status Age Gender Weight loss	Multimodality therapy
New and promising	High S-phase fraction DNA aneuploidy Angiogenesis factors Fibroblast growth factor-2		

Sources:
• National Cancer Institute: Malignant Mesothelioma (PDQ®): Treatment Guidelines 2005.
http:// www.cancer.gov/cancertopics/pdq/treatment/malignantmesothelioma/healthprofessional/.
• ESMO Minimum Clinical Recommendations for diagnosis, treatment and follow-up of Malignant Pleural Mesothelioma 2004.
http://annonc.oupjournals.org/cgi/reprint/16/suppl_1/i32.

REFERENCES

1. Kukreja J, Jaklitsch MT, Wiener DC, et al.: Malignant pleural mesothelioma: overview of the North American and European experience. *Thorac Surg Clin* 14:435–445, 2004.

2. Steele JP, Klabatsa A, Fennell DA, et al: Prognostic factors in mesothelioma. *Lung Cancer* 49:S49–S52, 2005.

3. Travis WD CT, Corrin B, Shimosato Y, Brambilla E: Histological typing of Lung and Pleural Tumors. 3rd ed. Berlin, Springer, 1999.

4. Corson JM: Pathology of mesothelioma. *Thorac Surg Clin* 14:447–460, 2004.

5. Wang ZJ, Reddy GP, Gotway MB, et al.: Malignant pleural mesothelioma: evaluation with CT, MR imaging, and PET. *Radiographics* 24:105–119, 2004.

6. Flores RM, Akhurst T, Gonen M, et al.: Positron emission tomography defines metastatic disease but not locoregional disease in patients with malignant pleural mesothelioma. *J Thorac Cardiovasc Surg* 126:11–16, 2003.

7. Heelan R: Staging and response to therapy of malignant pleural mesothelioma. *Lung Cancer* 45:S59–S61, 2004.

8. Sugarbaker DJ, Jaklitsch MT, Bueno R, et al.: Prevention, early detection, and management of complications after 328 consecutive extrapleural pneumonectomies. *J Thorac Cardiovasc Surg* 128:138–146, 2004.

9. Rusch VW, Venkatraman ES: Important prognostic factors in patients with malignant pleural mesothelioma, managed surgically. *Ann Thorac Surg* 68:1799–1804, 1999.

10. Paul S, Neragi-Miandoab S, Jaklitsch MT: Preoperative assessment and therapeutic options for patients with malignant pleural mesothelioma. *Thorac Surg Clin* 14:505–516, ix, 2004.

11. Steele JP, Klabatsa A: Chemotherapy options and new advances in malignant pleural mesothelioma. *Ann Oncol* 16:345–351, 2005.

12. Van Schil P: Malignant pleural mesothelioma: staging systems. *Lung Cancer* 49:S45–S58, 2005.

13. Pleural Mesothelioma, AJCC Cancer Staging Manual. New York, Springer, 2002, pp. 205–209.

14. Sugarbaker DJ, Flores RM, Jaklitsch MT, et al.: Resection margins, extrapleural nodal status, and cell type determine postoperative long-term survival in trimodality therapy of malignant pleural mesothelioma: results in 183 patients. *J Thorac Cardiovasc Surg* 117:54–63; discussion 63–65, 1999.

15. Pilling JE, Stewart DJ, Martin-Ucar AE, et al.: The case for routine cervical mediastinoscopy prior to radical surgery for malignant pleural mesothelioma. *Eur J Cardiothorac Surg* 25:497–501, 2004.

16. Edwards JG, Abrams KR, Leverment JN, et al.: Prognostic factors for malignant mesothelioma in 142 patients: validation of CALGB and EORTC prognostic scoring systems. *Thorax* 55:731–735, 2000.

17. Burgers JA, Damhuis RA: Prognostic factors in malignant mesothelioma. *Lung Cancer* 45:S49–S54, 2004.

CHAPTER 21

Malignant Thymoma

ANDREA BEZJAK and DAVID G. PAYNE

Tumors of the thymus are rare, accounting for 15% of mediastinal tumors. Most thymomas are slow growing tumors with a long natural history. Recurrences can be seen decades after seemingly successful initial treatment. These issues have management implications with a lack of high-quality evidence to guide practice. Most evidence is based on case series of often heterogenous patient groups who were treated with a variety of modalities over a prolonged period of time.[1]

Stage is the most important prognostic factor. The most frequently used staging classification for thymomas originally comes from Masaoka[2] with the proposed UICC TNM classification[3] using similar criteria. The Masaoka stage is based on the degree of invasion of thymoma into surrounding tissues, as determined by imaging and/or at the time of resection and subsequent histopathological examination. Recent reports detail the distribution of cases, and the associated rates of recurrence and survival.[4,5] Another essential prognostic factor is pathologic subtype of thymoma. A number of pathologic classifications have been proposed, starting with the Bernatz classification of spindle cell thymomas, lymphocytic thymomas (both associated with excellent survival rates), epithelial, and mixed-cell types (associated with poorer rates of survival). Subsequent Marino–Muller–Hermelink classification, based on the degree of differentiation of the malignant cell toward a pattern corresponding to the thymic cortex or medulla, was confirmed to be of prognostic significance,[6] with medullary, mixed, and well-differentiated organoid tumors being associated with early stage thymomas. Histology and the Masaoka stage were independent predictors for overall ($p < 0.05$) and disease-free survival ($p < 0.004$, $p < 0.0001$). The current histologic classification is one developed by the World Health Organization (WHO); studies support its prognostic significance with 5- and 10-year survival rates as follows: 100% for types A and AB thymomas, 100% and 86% for type B1, 85% and 85% for B2, and 51% and 38% for B3, respectively.[7] The

Prognostic Factors in Cancer, Third Edition, edited by Mary K. Gospodarowicz, Brian O'Sullivan, and Leslie H. Sobin.

WHO histologic type was correlated with invasion into neighboring organs, recurrence rate, disease free survival, and overall survival.[4]

The mainstay of treatment of thymomas is surgery. The role of radiation in stage II completely resected thymomas is controversial, based on up to 40% local recurrence rates historically with surgery alone. However, more recent series of surgery alone have documented excellent local control.[8,9] Stage III thymomas are usually resected, followed by postoperative radiotherapy to reduce the risk of local relapse; doses of 40–50 Gy are used for microscopic disease, and 50–60 Gy for gross disease. This results in high rates of local control in the mediastinum, although a risk of pleural, pericardial, or lung parenchymal relapse remains and it is not clear if that can be mitigated by adjuvant treatment. Some authors advocate preoperative radiation of unresectable thymomas, and prophylactic pericardial or hemithoracic radiation to prevent relapses in those areas, but this remains controversial. The role of debulking surgery in unresectable stage III thymomas or resection of primary or metastatic deposits in stage IV thymomas is also unclear.[10] Chemotherapy is most commonly used to treat metastatic and/or recurrent disease, using a single drug (e.g., cisplatinum, prednisone) or more often multidrug combination. No regimen is widely accepted as standard. There is increasing interest in the use of induction chemotherapy prior to surgery and radiotherapy in advanced stage unresectable tumors, aiming to render the tumor resectable, and/or reduce the volume of normal lung at risk for subsequent radiation injury. Only Phase II studies have been performed, using a variety of regimens, usually containing platinum.

The amount of postoperative residual disease is an important prognostic factor, with 95% 5-year survival rates for completely resected disease, compared to 50% with subtotal resection.[11] Another series reported a 93% 5-year survival of patients with stages III and IV completely resected thymomas, versus 64.4% for patients with the same stages but subtotally resected.[12]

Other factors, that are prognostic in some series include

- Presence of paraneoplastic syndrome: In some (particularly older) series, myasthenia gravis has been identified as an adverse prognostic factor, due to increased perioperative mortality, however, with improved supportive care, it may actually be a favorable factor as it leads to an earlier diagnosis.[13]
- Tumor size: worse survival for large thymomas (<10 vs. ≥ 10 cm), e.g., 97% versus 72% 5-year survival.[7]

There are some newer promising molecular prognostic factors. Epidermal growth factor receptor has been found to be expressed in 28/37 patients with invasive thymomas;[14] c-KIT expression was more common in thymic carcinomas;[15] this may provide a therapeutic option that targets these receptors. Stage IV thymomas were found to have much higher expressions of Cten mRNA, and its expression was correlated with evidence of tumor progression.[16] Cten mRNA likely plays a role in focal adhesion, cell motility, and/or migration. Human homolog of rad17 gene (Hrad17) mRNA, which is implicated in cell checkpoint control, was found to be expressed at significantly higher levels in invasive thymomas (stages II–IV) than in stage I thymomas, and it was not present in normal thymus tissue. Diploid tumors had a significantly higher probability of survival as compared to aneuploid tumors.[17]

Future studies of molecular targets may offer new avenues of therapeutic approaches in thymomas.

■■■■■■■ SUMMARY TABLE

Prognostic Factors in Thymoma

Prognostic Factors	Tumor Related	Host Related	Environment Related
Essential	Cell type Clinical stage Metastases		
Additional	Size Paraneoplastic syndrome	Performance status Age	Access to care
New and promising	Aneuploidy EGFR p53 cKIT Cten mRNA		

Sources:
• National Cancer Institute: Thymoma (PDQ®): Treatment Guidelines 2003.
http://www.cancer. gov/cancertopics/pdq/treatment/malignant-thymoma/healthprofessional/.
• British Columbia Cancer Agency Cancer Management Guidelines: Thymoma 2001.
http://www.bccancer. bc.ca/HPI/CancerManagementGuidelines/Lung/Thymoma/default.htm.

REFERENCES

1. Payne D: Malignant Thymoma: in Gospodarowicz MK, Henson DE, Hutter RVP, et al. (eds.), *Prognostic Factors in Cancer*. 2nd ed., New York, Wiley-Liss, 2001, pp. 387–398.

2. Rena O, Papalia E, Maggi G, et al.: World Health Organization histologic classification: an independent prognostic factor in resected thymomas. *Lung Cancer* 50:59–66, 2005.

3. Wittekind Ch, Henson DE, et al.: *TNM Supplement. A commentary on uniform use*. 3rd ed. New York, Wiley-Liss, 2003.

4. Kondo K, Yoshizawa K, Tsuyuguchi M, et al.: WHO histologic classification is a prognostic indicator in thymoma. *Ann Thorac Surg* 77:1183–1188, 2004.

5. Sonobe M, Nakagawa M, Ichinose M, et al.: Thymoma: analysis of prognostic factors. *Jpn J Thor Cardiovasc Surg* 49:35–41, 2001.

6. Lardinois D, Rechsteiner R, Lang RH, et al.: Prognostic relevance of Masaoka and Muller-Hermelink classification in patients with thymic tumors. *Ann Thorac Surg* 69:1550–1555, 2000.

7. Nakagawa K, Asamura H, Matsuno Y, et al.: Thymoma: a clinicopathologic study based on the new World Health Organization classification. *J Thorac Cardiovasc Surg* 126: 1134–1140, 2003.

8. Mangi AA, Wright CD, Allan JS, et al.: Adjuvant radiation therapy for stage II thymoma. *Ann Thorac Surg* 74:1033–1037, 2002.

9. Singhal S, Shrager JB, Rosenthal DI, et al.: Comparison of stages I-II thymoma treated by complete resection with or without adjuvant radiation. *Ann Thorac Surg* 76:1635–1641, discussion 1641–1632, 2003.

10. Zhu G, He S, Fu X, et al.: Radiotherapy and prognostic factors for thymoma: a retrospective study of 175 patients. *Int J Radiat Oncol Biol Phys* 60:1113–1119, 2004.

11. Moore KH, McKenzie PR, Kennedy CW, et al.: Thymoma: trends over time. *Ann Thorac Surg* 72:203–207, 2001.

12. Kondo K, Monden Y: Therapy for thymic epithelial tumors: a clinical study of 1,320 patients from Japan. *Ann Thorac Surg* 76:878–884; discussion 884–875, 2003.

13. de Perrot M, Liu J, Bril V, et al.: Prognostic significance of thymomas in patients with myasthenia gravis. *Ann Thorac Surg* 74:1658–1662, 2002.

14. Henley JD, Koukoulis GK, Loehrer PJ Sr: Epidermal growth factor receptor expression in invasive thymoma. *J Cancer Res Clin Oncol* 128:167–170, 2002.

15. Henley JD, Cummings OW, Loehrer PJ Sr: Tyrosine kinase receptor expression in thymomas. *J Cancer Res Clin Oncol* 130:222–224, 2004.

16. Sasaki H, Yukiue H, Kobayashi Y, et al.: Cten mRNA expression is correlated with tumor progression in thymoma. *Tumour Biol* 24:271–274, 2003.

17. Gawrychowski J, Rokicki M, Gabriel A, et al.: Thymoma—the usefulness of some prognostic factors for diagnosis and surgical treatment. *Eur J Surg Oncol* 26:203–208, 2000.

BONE AND SOFT TISSUE TUMORS

CHAPTER 22

Osteosarcoma

HENRIK C. BAUER

Osteosarcoma accounts for one-third of the rare group of primary bone tumors. Osteosarcomas are of high-grade malignancy and 90% of patients have overt or occult metastatic disease at presentation.[1] There are also several extremely rare low-grade osteosarcoma variants, for example, parosteal osteosarcoma, which will not be addressed.

Osteosarcoma classically presents in adolescents, but there is a second peak in the seventh decade.[2] Occasionally, the disease is secondary to underlying bone disease, for example, Paget's disease, or previous treatment, for example, radiotherapy. Osteosarcomas mostly occur in the distal ends of long bones, but may occur in any bone. Multimodality treatment involves preoperative chemotherapy, resection of the primary tumor and metastases if present, and postoperative chemotherapy.

Patients with a solitary bone lesion, regardless of age, should be referred before biopsy to a center with complete facilities to deliver multimodality treatment. Staging includes X-ray and magnetic resonance imaging (MRI) of the entire involved bone, thoracic computerized tomography (CT), and isotope bone scan. Baseline blood chemistry, cardiac, renal function, and hearing are assessed and sperm banking should be considered. The diagnosis is based on biopsy performed at a sarcoma center, by fine or core needle or by surgical incision.[3] The histopathology must correlate with the clinical and radiological features, otherwise the diagnosis must be reassessed.

Long-term survival rates of 60–70% can be expected after multimodality treatment of patients without overt metastases.[1,4] Limb-sparing surgery is safe in >90% of patients, yielding local control rates of 95%, similar to those achieved after amputation. The efficacy of the preoperative chemotherapy and the quality of the surgical margin are the main prognostic factors for local tumor control. Pathological fracture is no longer considered a precluding factor for safe limb sparing surgery.[5] Since local recurrence is a major risk factor for metastatic disease,[6,7] radiotherapy may be indicated where anatomy prohibits surgical remission.[8] Reconstruction is based mostly on

Prognostic Factors in Cancer, Third Edition, edited by Mary K. Gospodarowicz, Brian O'Sullivan, and Leslie H. Sobin.

megaprosthesis, but also bone allografts, vascularized fibular grafts, and rotation plasty.[1] Long-term survivors of osteosarcoma have equivalent functional and quality of life outcomes, irrespective of whether undergoing amputation or limb sparing surgery.[9]

The extent of the disease is the most important tumor-related prognostic factor in osteosarcoma. Patients with lung metastases at presentation have a survival rate of only 20%, and the prognosis is even worse for those with skeletal or other metastases.[4,10] However, for patients with a minimal number of metastases (generally accepted as five or less) lung metastases who are rendered in complete surgical remission, the prognosis approaches that of patients without overt metastatic disease. Immunomagnetic detection of hematogenous micrometastases in peripheral blood and bone marrow may have prognostic implications.[11]

For patients with relapsed disease, the expected salvage rate is ~20%. Favorable prognostic factors are few lung metastases, >2-years disease-free interval, response to salvage chemotherapy, and complete surgical remission.[7,12] The prognosis for patients with metastases to nonpulmonary sites remains dismal.

Increasing tumor size is also a major adverse prognostic factor.[1,4] Tumor site is probably not *per se* of prognostic importance, but rather reflects tumor size and the ability to render a patient free of disease surgically.[13] Hence, tumors of the pelvis and axial skeleton are associated with a poorer outcome.

Other tumor related potential prognostic factors include abnormalities of the p53 or the retinoblastoma gene and different proto-oncogenes.[1] Overexpression of P-glycoprotein leading to multidrug resistance has been implicated as one mechanism for failure of chemotherapy. Cytogenetic analysis of osteosarcoma reveals complex karyotypic aberrations but no significant prognostic information has been gained to date. In a large, multicenter study TP53 mutations did not provide prognostic information.[14]

There is no apparent difference in outcome between preadolescents and young adults.[15] However, osteosarcoma presenting in the older age group is reported to have a worse prognosis, which may not be due to inherent disease differences, but rather that older patients do not receive, or do not tolerate, more intensive treatment. Specific treatment protocols for osteosarcoma patients older than 40 years should improve outcome, for example, Euroboss protocol by collaborative groups SSG, ISG, and COSS – http://www.ssg-org.net/.

There are several reports that female gender is a favorable prognostic factor, but its significance remains unclear.[16] Interestingly, Scandinavian females treated according to the ISG/SSG I protocol fared better than males, but there was no difference among Italian females (unpublished).

The most important treatment associated prognostic factor is multiagent chemotherapy. A three drug regimen of high-dose methotrexate, doxorubicin, and cisplatin has yielded survival rates of 60–70% in several studies.[1] Adding high-dose ifosfamide as a fourth drug has not been demonstrated to improve survival. The prognostic importance of escalating the chemotherapy dose intensity remains unclear.[1,17]

The extent of tumor necrosis after preoperative chemotherapy is a consistent prognostic factor. The different schemes of grading chemotherapy response entail problems of definition and reproducibility.[18] Regardless, the survival rate among "good" responders is ~75% and for "poor" responders 50%. Radiological methods, such as

MRI and position emission tomography (PET), used to assess tumor response are not sufficiently specific or sensitive to guide treatment.

The rationale for giving preoperative chemotherapy is to modify the postoperative treatment based on chemotherapy response to improve outcome for poor responders. This approach has largely been a failure.[1,4,16] In current chemotherapy regimens, preoperative drugs are continued also in "poor" responders postoperatively, but additional drugs are added that are not given to "good" responders.

Morbidity after multimodality treatment includes impaired heart or kidney function, impaired hearing, electrolyte disturbances, sterility, and complications after limb sparing surgery.[1] Follow up for 10 years is therefore appropriate.

There is a consensus among major international sarcoma groups that survival will not surpass 60% with current chemotherapeutic agents and that novel agents need to be developed. For example, Interferon[19] is now being assessed in a randomized trial performed by collaborative sarcoma groups in Europe and America "EURAMOS" (http://www.ctu.mrc.ac.uk/euramos/).

■■■■■■ **SUMMARY TABLE**

Prognostic Factors in High Grade Osteosarcoma

Prognostic Factors	Tumor Related	Host Related	Environment Related
Essential	T category Tumor size M1c category M1b category	Age	Tumor necrosis after preoperative chemotherapy Surgical remission[a] Management by multidisciplinary sarcoma team
Additional	Anatomical site ALP, LDH Local recurrence[b]	Gender Performance status	Local recurrence[b] Chemotherapy dose intensity
New and promising	P-glycoprotein Different oncogenes Hematogenous micrometastases		Interferon

[a] Refers to both primary tumor and metastases at diagnosis or at relapse.
[b] Local recurrence reflects both high-grade malignancy and treatment failure.

Sources:
• NCCN Clinical Practice Guidelines in Oncology: Bone Cancer 2005.
http://www.nccn.org/professionals/physician_gls/PDF/bone.pdf.
• ESMO Minimum Clinical Recommendations for diagnosis, treatment and follow-up of osteosarcoma 2005.
http://annonc.oupjournals.org/cgi/reprint/16/suppl_1/i71.

REFERENCES

1. Marina N, Gebhardt M, Teoit L, et al.: Biology and therapeutic advances for pediatric osteosarcoma. *Oncologist* 9:422–442, 2004.

2. Grimer RJ, Cannon SR, Taminiau AB, et al.: Osteosarcoma over the age of forty. *Eur J Cancer* 39:157–163, 2003.

3. Soderlund V, Skoog L, Kreicbergs A: Combined radiology and cytology in the diagnosis of bone lesions: a retrospective study of 370 cases. *Acta Orthop Scand* 75:492–499, 2004.

4. Bielack SS, Kempf-Bielack B, Delling G, et al.: Prognostic factors in high-grade osteosarcoma of the extremities or trunk: an analysis of 1,702 patients treated on neoadjuvant cooperative osteosarcoma study group protocols. *J Clin Oncol* 20:776–790, 2002.

5. Bacci G, Ferrari S, Longhi A: Nonmetastatic osteosarcoma of the extremity with pathological fracture at presentation: local and systemic control by amputation or limb salvage after preoperative chemotherapy. *Acta Orthop Scand* 74:449–454, 2004.

6. Rodriguez-Galindo C, Shah N, McCarville MB, et al.: Outcome after local recurrence of osteosarcoma: the St. Jude Children's Research Hospital experience (1970–2000). *Cancer* 100:1928–1935, 2004.

7. Kemp-Bielack B, Bielack SS, Jurgens H, et al.: Osteosarcoma relapse after combined modality therapy: an analysis of unselected patients in the Cooperative Osteosarcoma Study Group (COSS). *J Clin Oncol* 23:559–568, 2005.

8. DeLaney TF, Park L, Goldberg SI, et al.: in Munzenrider JE, Suit HD (eds.): Radiotherapy for local control of osteoarcoma. *Int J Radiat Oncol Biol Phys* 61:492–498, 2005.

9. Nagaranjan R, Clohisy DR, Negila JP: Function and quality-of-life of survivors of pelvic and lower extremity osteosarcoma and Ewing's sarcoma: the Childhood Cancer Survivor Study. *Br J Cancer* 91:1858–1865, 2004.

10. Mialou V, Philip T, Kalilfa C, et al.: Metastatic osteosarcoma at diagnosis. *Cancer* 104:1100–1109, 2005.

11. Bruland OS, Hoifodt H, Saeter G, et al.: Hematogenous micrometastases in osteosarcoma patients. *Clin Cancer Res* 11:4666–4673, 2005.

12. Hawkins DS, Arndt CA: Pattern of disease recurrence and prognostic factors in patients with osteosarcoma treated with contemporary chemotherapy. *Cancer* 98:2447–2456, 2003.

13. Donati D, Giacomini S, Gozzi E, et al.: Osteosarcoma of the pelvis. *Eur J Surg Oncol* 30:332–340, 2004.

14. Wunder JS, Gokgoz N, Parkes R: TP53 mutations and outcome in osteosarcoma: a prospective, multicenter study. *J Clin Oncol* 23:1483–1490, 2005.

15. Bacci G, Longhi A, Bertoni F, et al.: Primary high-grade osteosarcoma: comparison between preadolescent and older patients. *J Pediatr Hematol Oncol* 27:129–134, 2005.

16. Smeland S, Muller C, Alvegard TA: Scandinavian Sarcoma Group Osteosarcoma Study SSG VIII: prognostic factors for outcome and the role of replacement salvage chemotherapy for poor histological responders. *Eur J Cancer* 39:488–494, 2003.

17. Bacci G, Forni C, Ferrari S: Neoadjuvant chemotherapy for osteosarcoma of the extremity: intensification of preoperative treatment does not increase the rate of good histologic

response to the primary tumor or improve the final outcome. *J Pediatr Hematol Oncol* 25:845–853, 2003.

18. Bohling T, Bocchini P, Bertoni F, et al.: Diagnosis and tumor response in osteosarcoma and Ewing's sarcoma. *Acta Orthop Scand* 75:72–76, 2004.

19. Müller C, Smeland S, Bauer HCF, et al.: Interferon-α as the only adjuvant treatment in high-grade osteosarcoma: Long term follow up of the Karolinska Hospital series. *Acta Oncol* 44:475–480, 2005.

CHAPTER 23

Soft Tissue Sarcomas

BRIAN O'SULLIVAN and CHARLES N. CATTON

Soft tissue sarcomas (STS) are rare diseases for which surgery provides the mainstay of management. They comprise more than 40 histologies and may arise in any location. The STS typically infiltrate adjacent soft tissues and involvement of critical structures impacts local control rates.[1,2] Metastasis to the lung (limb, trunk, and head and neck sarcomas) or liver (intraabdominal sarcomas) is frequent; lymph node metastasis is uncommon.[1,2]

Assessment entails a complete history and physical examination. Depending on the anatomic region, investigations should focus on imaging of the primary site with contrast enhanced magnetic resonance imaging and/or computerized tomography (CT). Thoracic CT is always indicated in intermediate to high-grade tumors >5 cm with negative chest X-ray. Carefully planned tissue biopsy (core needle or incisional) is mandatory to establish grade and histologic subtype.[3] Expert molecular and cytogenetic analysis may be considered to differentiate subtypes, such as synovial, myxoid liposarcoma, clear cell, alveolar rhabdomyosarcoma, and dermatofibrosarcoma protruberans (DFSP).[2,4,5]

Randomized clinical trials have shown the efficacy of adjuvant therapies following gross tumor excision. Five-year local control rates exceeding 90% are anticipated in patients undergoing radical surgery or radiotherapy with conservative surgery.[2,6,7] Cytoreductive chemotherapy may be considered prior to surgery in borderline resectable tumors though this remains unproven. Patients with local recurrence or metastatic disease may be salvaged with retreatment; 20% 5-year survival has been observed following resection of metastasis in selected patients.[2] Chemotherapy may be employed for unresectable and metastatic sarcomas though its value is considered palliative.

The variability of sarcoma presentations permits a proportion of tumors to be managed by surgery alone. The problem is selecting cases without compromising control. In Scandinavia, a recent change to increased radiotherapy use for deep lesions

Prognostic Factors in Cancer, Third Edition, edited by Mary K. Gospodarowicz,
Brian O'Sullivan, and Leslie H. Sobin.
Copyright © 2006 John Wiley & Sons, Inc.

especially, was associated with a reduction in the amputation rate.[8] This change was also associated with improvement in local control and survival at the Karolinska Hospital in Stockholm, where radiotherapy is used more often than at other Scandinavian centers and is under study by the Scandinavian Sarcoma Group Registry.[8] These findings and additional evidence suggests that multidisciplinary pretreatment evaluation and management in specialized centers may be advantageous.[9,10]

Specific tumor related factors in untreated patients include stage, anatomic location, tumor size, histologic grade, and depth of invasion as primary determinants of overall survival.

Numerous multivariate analyses have shown histologic grade to be the best available predictor of biologic aggressiveness in STS.[3] Surprisingly, no consensus exists for the morphologic criteria to be applied in the grading process. Moreover, whether characterized by a two grade (high vs. low), three grade, or four grade system it remains a durable and consistent harbinger of outcome.

Although differences among the major anatomic sites are accepted,[2] prognosis is also associated with tumors at different subsites within the same anatomic structure. For example, there appears to be different prognosis for upper versus lower limb,[3] and proximal versus distal margin-positive extremity location fares worse following brachytherapy.[11]

Resection margin status has also been a very consistent prognostic factor, especially for local recurrence. Positive margins doubles the local recurrence risk and increases distant recurrence and disease-related death.[12] Positive resection margins may have different causes, some of which have no impact on local recurrence. The highest risk of local recurrence are caused by the following scenarios: (1) patients with prereferral unplanned excision and who have a positive margin on subsequent reexcision and (2) unanticipated positive margins occurring during primary sarcoma resection.[13]

Lymph node metastasis has been regarded as a particularly adverse finding in STS conferring similar risk to distant metastasis in the TNM stage classification. Recent information about isolated lymph node metastasis (as opposed to simultaneous distant metastasis) contradicts this view.[14,15] Indeed intensively treated isolated lymph node metastasis appear to have a prognosis similar to stage III lesions in the TNM system (i.e., those with high-grade, deep and lesions >5 cm).[15] The impact of this variable could be reconsidered in future editions of the staging system.

Molecular parameters investigated include mutations in p53 and mdm2, Ki-67 status, altered expression of the retinoblastoma gene product (pRb) in high-grade sarcomas,[2-4] although there is conflicting evidence for a relationship to the presence of SYT-SSX fusion transcripts in synovial sarcoma.[3,16] Evidence supporting the prognostic significance of alterations in pRb expression and p53/mdm2 status is also uncertain. The presence of t(17;22) translocation in DFSP may predict response to imatinib.[5] Tissue hypoxia, assessed in various ways including directly or by CA IX assessment, appears associated with the development of distant metastases independently from depth, size, and grade.[17]

Local recurrence is an outcome event in itself, but has often been described as a predictor for local control, function, and potentially survival. However, it is a problematic factor because of its potential for biological selection of adverse tumors and this knowledge is not known at the time the patient first presents for treatment.[3] Local recurrence may be due to inadequate initial treatment due to adverse anatomic factors, poor treatment quality, adverse biology, or a combination of factors.

Patients with neurofibromatosis 1 (NF1) are at significant risk of developing neurogenic sarcoma and a high proportion of these patients will develop distant metastases compared to patients with neurogenic sarcomas without NF1.[6] Age appears to have predictive value for overall survival.[18] Radiation induced sarcomas have a particularly adverse prognosis unrelated to the tumor-related characteristics of the new sarcoma and may be associated with a relative paucity of options within tissues previously irradiated.[19]

Finally, controversy exists about optimal treatment approaches for local disease including whether surgery alone is preferred. Local approaches have not been adequately compared against each other excepting one randomized trial comparing pre- versus postoperative radiotherapy that had identical cancer outcome, but different toxicity profiles for both approaches.[7] The role of systemic chemotherapy remains controversial, despite the absence of benefit in meta-analysis.[1,2,20] This is perpetuated by the weakness of some trials, the expectation of poor systemic outcome, and the potential for responses to chemotherapy when employed in induction schedules.

The factors tabulated generally reflect survival outcome. Other endpoints may have direct bearing on the treatment to be given for alternative endpoints, but may not independently influence survival. An example is envelopment or invasion of neurovascular structures $\pm$ bone, and which would directly influence the need for amputation, and therefore would be essential factors for an endpoint like limb preservation.

■■■■■■ **SUMMARY TABLES**

Prognostic Factors in Localized Soft Tissue Sarcomas

Prognostic Factors	Tumor Related	Host Related	Environment Related
Essential	Anatomic site Histologic type T category Grade Depth of invasion M category		
Additional	Resection margin	Neurofibromatosis 1 (NF 1) Radiation induced sarcomas Age	Quality of surgery and radiotherapy
New and promising	Ki-67 *p53* SYT-SSX fusion transcript EWS-FL11 fusion transcript Tumor hypoxia		

Sources:

• NCCN Clinical Practice Guidelines in Oncology: Sarcoma 2005.

http://www.nccn.org/professionals/physician_gls/PDF/sarcoma.pdf.

• ESMO Minimum Clinical Recommendations for diagnosis, treatment and follow-up of soft tissue sarcoma 2005.

http://annonc.oupjournals.org/cgi/reprint/16/suppl_1/i69.

Prognostic Factors in Metastatic Soft Tissue Sarcomas

Prognostic Factors	Tumor Related	Host Related	Environment Related
Essential	Interval between diagnosis and metastases Low tumor burden (size and number of metastases)		
Additional			Complete tumor excision
New and promising			

Sources:
- NCCN Clinical Practice Guidelines in Oncology: Sarcoma 2005.
http://www.nccn.org/professionals/physician_gls/PDF/sarcoma.pdf.
- National Cancer Institute: Sarcoma (PDQ®): Treatment Guidelines 2005.
http://www.cancer.gov/cancertopics/pdq/treatment/adult-soft-tissue-sarcoma/healthprofessional/.

REFERENCES

1. O'Sullivan B, Bell R, Bramwell V: Sarcomas of the soft tissues, in Souhami R, Tannock I, Hohenberger P, et al. (eds.): *Oxford Textbook of Oncology*. Oxford, Oxford University Press, 2002, pp. 2495–2523.

2. Brennan M, Singer S, Maki R, et al.: Sarcomas of Soft Tissue and Bone, in DeVita Jr V, Helman S, Rosenberg S (eds.): *Cancer. Principles and Practice of Oncology*. Philadelphia, Lippincott Williams and Wilkins, 2005, pp. 1581–1637.

3. O'Sullivan B, Pisters PW: Staging and prognostic factor evaluation in soft tissue sarcoma. *Surg Oncol Clin N Am* 12:333–353, 2003.

4. Borden E, Baker L, Bell R, et al.: Soft tissue sarcomas of adults: state of the translational science. *Clin Cancer Res* 9:1941–1956, 2003.

5. McArthur G, Demetri G, van Oosterom A, et al.: Molecular and clinical analysis of locally advanced dermatofibrosarcoma protuberans treated with imatinib: Imatinib Target Exploration Consortium Study B2225. *J Clin Oncol* 23:866–873, 2005.

6. Pisters P, O'Sullivan B, Pollack R: Soft Tissue Sarcoma, in Gospodarowicz MK, Henson DE, Hutter RVP, et al. (eds.): *Prognostic Factors in Cancer*. New York, Wiley-Liss, 2001, pp. 415–433.

7. O'Sullivan B, Davis A, Turcotte R, et al.: Preoperative versus postoperative radiotherapy in soft-tissue sarcoma of the limbs: a randomised trial. *Lancet* 359:2235–2241, 2002.

8. Bauer HCF, Alvegård TA, Berlin Ö, et al.: The Scandinavian Sarcoma Group Register 1986–2001. *Acta Orthop Scand Suppl* 311:8–10, 2004.

9. Clark M, Thomas J: Delay in referral to a specialist soft-tissue sarcoma unit. *Eur J Surg Oncol* 31:443–448, 2005.

10. Ray-Coquard I, Thiesse P, Ranchere-Vince D, et al.: Conformity to clinical practice guidelines, multidisciplinary management and outcome of treatment for soft tissue sarcomas. *Ann Oncol* 15:307–315, 2004.

11. Alektiar KM, Velasco J, Zelefsky MJ, et al.: Adjuvant radiotherapy for margin-positive high-grade soft tissue sarcoma of the extremity. *Int J Rad Oncol Biol Phys* 48:1051–1058, 2000.

12. Stojadinovic A, Leung DH, Hoos A, et al.: Analysis of the prognostic significance of microscopic margins in 2084 localized primary adult soft tissue sarcomas. *Ann Surg* 235:424–434, 2002.

13. Gerrand CH, Wunder JS, Kandel RA, et al.: Classification of positive margins after resection of soft-tissue sarcoma of the limb predicts the risk of local recurrence. *J Bone Joint Surg Br* 83:1149–1155, 2001.

14. Behranwala KA, A'Hern R, Omar AM, et al.: Prognosis of lymph node metastasis in soft tissue sarcoma. *Ann Surg Oncol* 11:714–719, 2004.

15. Riad S, Griffin AM, Liberman B, et al.: Lymph node metastasis in soft tissue sarcoma in an extremity. *Clin Orthop Relat Res* 426:129–134, 2004.

16. Guillou L, Benhattar J, Bonichon F, et al.: Histologic grade, but not SYT-SSX fusion type, is an important prognostic factor in patients with synovial sarcoma: a multicenter, retrospective analysis. *JCO* 22:4040–4050, 2004.

17. Maseide K, Kandel R, Bell R, et al.: *Clin Cancer Res*. Carbonic anhydrase IX as a marker for poor prognosis in soft tissue sarcoma. 10:4464–4471, 2004.

18. Strander H, Turesson I, Cavallin-Stahl E: A systematic overview of radiation therapy effects in soft tissue sarcomas. *Acta Oncol* 42:516–531, 2003.

19. Thijssens K, van Ginkel R, Suurmeijer A, et al.: Radiation-induced sarcoma: a challenge for the surgeon. *Ann Surg Oncol* 12:237–245, 2005.

20. Scoggins C, Pollock R: Extremity soft tissue sarcoma: evidence-based multidisciplinary management. *J Surg Oncol* 90:10–13, 2005.

CHAPTER 24

Gastrointestinal Stromal Tumors

STEFAN SLEIJFER and JAAP VERWEIJ

Gastrointestinal stromal tumors (GIST) belong to the group of soft-tissue sarcomas. These tumors are relatively rare with a yearly incidence of 10–15 cases per 1×10^6 persons. They predominantly arise in the digestive tract, mainly in the stomach or small intestine (90–95% of the cases), but can also develop from other sites, such as the omentum and retroperitoneum. Metastases occur predominantly within the peritoneal cavity and the liver. Dissemination to other sites, such as lymph nodes and lungs, is uncommon.[1,2]

Since the late 1990s, insight into the tumor pathophysiology of this entity has considerably improved. It was found that GISTs frequently overexpress the c-kit receptor.[1,2] In addition, it was found that GISTs harbor so-called gain-of-function mutations in the *c-kit* or *Platelet-derived Growth Factor-α receptor* (*PDGFRA*) genes in 85 and 5% of the cases, respectively.[1–3] Through these mutations, which can occur at several sites in these two genes, the receptors are constitutively activated, thereby leading to the malignant behavior of these tumors. The recognition that GIST tumor growth was driven by activated c-kit or PDGFRA prompted the search for treatments that target these two receptors. The advent of the tyrosine kinase inhibitor imatinib, which is highly effective in advanced disease, was therefore a major breakthrough,[4] particularly as other effective treatment options for advanced disease were not available.[2]

Assessment of patients presenting with GIST should include a complete history, inventory of comedication, plus physical and laboratory examination. Imaging with contrast enhanced computerized tomography (CT) of thorax and abdomen is required. [18F]2-Fluoro-2-deoxy-D-glucose positron emission tomography (FDG–PET) is considered a sensitive technique for establishing the extent of dissemination and is particularly useful when early assessment of an imatinib-induced response is necessary.[5] Tissue biopsy is mandatory to assess diagnosis. Expert molecular analysis is strongly recommended in order to establish whether there is a mutation in *c-kit* or *PDGFRA*,

Prognostic Factors in Cancer, Third Edition, edited by Mary K. Gospodarowicz, Brian O'Sullivan, and Leslie H. Sobin.
Copyright © 2006 John Wiley & Sons, Inc.

and if so, the exact site of mutation. Management in a multidisciplinary setting is required.

For patients with localized disease, surgery is the mainstay of treatment. However, 50% of the patients experience recurrent disease within 5 years following resection.[6] The most important prognostic factors for relapsed disease are tumor size and mitotic rate.[6-8] Based on these factors, a widely accepted classification system for defining the risk of aggressive behavior after resection has been established.[9] Other factors with prognostic significance include several particular DNA copy number alterations,[10] loss of p16 protein,[11] methylation of the *E-cadherin* gene[12] and the extent of tumor necrosis.[11] Controversy exists about the exact relevance of the presence of a *c-kit* mutation[8] and the precise mutational site in the *c-kit* gene,[13] whereas the microscopic margins of resection,[7] gender,[6,11] primary tumor site,[6,11] and age[11] have not been identified as independent prognostic factors.

The exact value of chemotherapy or radiotherapy as adjuvant treatments has never been assessed. However, it is highly unlikely that such strategies will be effective in this setting in view of their lack of activity against advanced GIST. Studies examining imatinib as adjuvant treatment after complete resection in certain risk groups are underway.

Until recently, there was no effective treatment available for patients with irresectable or metastatic GIST. Doxorubicin-based chemotherapy was the most frequently applied treatment, but yielded a 2-year overall survival of <20%.[14] The introduction of imatinib has dramatically improved the outcome of these patients. This compound yields a response rate exceeding 50%, a median progression-free survival of ~2 years, and a median overall survival exceeding 2.5 years.[14]

The most important factor predicting response and overall survival following imatinib treatment is the mutational status of the genes encoding c-kit and PDGFRA. Patients whose tumors harbor an exon 11 *c-kit* mutation, the most frequently occurring mutation, have a better outcome in terms of response and overall survival than patients with tumors expressing exon 9 *c-kit* mutations or no mutation at all.[15] In a phase III study comparing two doses of imatinib in advanced disease,[14] it was recently revealed that the higher dose of imatinib yielded a significant benefit over the lower dose in patients whose tumors express an exon 9 *c-kit* mutation in terms of progression-free survival. In patients with exon 11 *c-kit* mutated GISTs, there was no difference between the two tested doses, while wild-type *c-kit* harboring tumors actually did worse at the higher dose.[16] Therefore, the dose of imatinib should be tailored according to the mutational status of the tumor.

In the only phase III trial published to date,[14] presence of pulmonary metastases, initial low hemoglobin, and a small number of lesions were prognostic for progression within 3 months after treatment initiation.[17] Independent prognostic factors for progression or death after 3 months of treatment were a non-stomach primary site, low albumin before treatment, large size of lesions, and a low dose of imatinib.[17] Note, however, that correction for mutational site had not been performed yet in this analysis. For example, it can be anticipated that a non-stomach origin will fail to be an independent prognostic factor after correction for mutational status since *c-kit* mutations other than exon 11, which are associated with a less favorable outcome after imatinib therapy, are predominantly found in extra-gastric primary sites.[18] It warrants further investigations whether other factors potentially affecting the ultimate outcome of imatinib-treated GIST patients can serve as prognostic factors. Examples include over-expression of drug efflux pumps on GIST, which confers resistance against imatinib in preclinical models,[19] or activity of imatinib-metabolizing enzymes such as CYP3A4.[20]

In conclusion, GIST is one of the best examples of a tumor type in which advances in molecular biology have resulted in considerable improvements in the understanding of the pathogenesis, and consequently, in the treatment and clinical outcome of GIST patients. In addition, several prognostic factors for localized as well as advanced disease have been identified. It can be anticipated that further characterization of prognostic factors will lead to a more individualized treatment of patients presenting with GIST as a consequence of which the outcome of these patients will hopefully further improve.

■■■■■■ SUMMARY TABLES

Prognostic Factors in Localized Gastrointestinal Stromal Tumors

Prognostic Factors	Tumor Related	Host Related	Environment Related
Essential	Tumor size[a] Mitotic rate[a]		
Additional			Quality of surgery

New and promising	DNA copy
	  number changes
	Loss of p16 protein
	Extent of tumor necrosis
	Presence of c-kit mutation
	Mutational site in c-kit or
	  PDGFRA gene
			Application of adjuvant
			treatment

[a]Blay J.-Y., Bonvalot S, Casali P et al.: Consensus meeting for management of gastrointestinal stromal tumors. Report of the GIST Consensus Conference of 20–21 March 2004, under the auspices of ESMO. *Ann Oncol* 16: 566–578, 2005.

Prognostic Factors in Metastatic Gastrointestinal Stromal Tumors

Prognostic Factors	Tumor Related	Host Related	Environment Related
Essential			
Additional	Mutational site in c-kit or PDGFRA gene Presence of lung metastases Large tumor burden	Low hemoglobin Low albumin	
New and promising	Overexpression of drug-efflux pumps	Activity of imatinib-metabolizing enzymes	

REFERENCES

1. Corless CL, Fletcher JA, Heinrich MC: Biology of gastrointestinal stromal tumors. *J Clin Oncol* 22:3813–3825, 2004.

2. Joensuu H, Fletcher C, Dimitrijevic S, et al.: Management of malignant gastrointestinal stromal tumours. *Lancet Oncol* 3:655–664, 2002.

3. Heinrich MC, Corless CL, Duensing A, et al.: PDGFRA activating mutations in gastrointestinal stromal tumors. *Science* 299:708–710, 2003.

4. Joensuu H, Roberts PJ, Sarlomo-Rikala M, et al.: Effect of the tyrosine kinase inhibitor STI571 in a patient with a metastatic gastrointestinal stromal tumor. *N Engl J Med* 344: 1052–1056, 2001.

5. Stroobants S, Goeminne J, Seegers M, et al.: 18FDG-Positron emission tomography for the early prediction of response in advanced soft tissue sarcoma treated with imatinib mesylate (Glivec). *Eur J Cancer* 39:2012–2020, 2003.

6. Nilsson B, Bumming P, Meis-Kindblom JM, et al.: Gastrointestinal stromal tumors: the incidence, prevalence, clinical course, and prognostication in the preimatinib mesylate area. *Cancer* 103:821–829, 2005.

7. DeMatteo RP, Lewis JJ, Lueng D, et al.: Two hundred gastrointestinal stromal tumors. Recurrence patterns and prognostic factors for survival. *Ann Surg* 231:51–58, 2000.

8. Taniguchi M, Nishida T, Hirota S, et al.: Effect of c-kit mutation on prognosis of gastrointestinal stromal tumors. *Cancer Res* 59, 4297–4300, 1999.

9. Fletcher CDM, Berman JJ, Corless C, et al.: Diagnosis of gastrointestinal stromal tumors: a consensus approach. *Human Pathol* 33:459–465, 2002.

10. El-Rifai W, Sarlomo-Rikala M, Andersson LC, et al.: DNA sequence copy number changes in gastrointestinal stromal tumors: tumor progression and prognostic significance. *Cancer Res* 60:3899–3903, 2000.

11. Schneider-Stock R, Boltze C, Lasota J, et al.: Loss of p16 protein defines high-risk patients with gastrointestinal stromal tumors: a tissue microarray study. *Clin Cancer Res* 11, 638–645, 2005.

12. House MG, Guo M, Efron DT, et al.: Tumor suppressor gene hypermethylation as a predictor of gastric stromal tumor behavior. *J Gastrointest Surg* 7:1004–1014, 2003.

13. Miettinen M, El-Rifai W, Sobin L, Lasota J: Evaluation of malignancy and prognosis of gastrointestinal stromal tumors: a review. *Human Pathol* 33:478–483, 2002.

14. Verweij J, Casali PG, Zalcberg J, et al.: Progression-free survival in gastrointestinal stromal tumours with high-dose imatinib: randomised trial. *Lancet* 364:1127–1134, 2004.

15. Heinrich MC, Corless CL, Demetri G, et al.: Kinase mutations and imatinib responses in patients with metastatic gastrointestinal stromal tumors. *J Clin Oncol* 21:4342–4349, 2003.

16. Debiec-Rychter M: Oral presentation. EORTC Group Annual Meeting, 2005.

17. Van Glabbeke M, Verweij J, Casali PG, et al.: Initial and late resistance to imatinib (IM) in advanced gastrointestinal stromal tumors (GIST) are predicted by different prognostic factors: a European Organization for Research and Treatment of Cancer – Italian Sarcoma Group – Australasian Gastrointestinal Trials Group Study. *J Clin Oncol* 23:5795–5804, 2005.

18. Antonescu CR, Viale A, Sarran L, et al.: Gene expression in gastrointestinal stromal tumors is distinguished by KIT genotype and anatomic site. *Clin Cancer Res* 10:3282–3290, 2004.

19. Mahon FX, Belloc F, Lagarde V, et al.: MDR1 gene overexpression confers resistance to imatinib mesylate in leukemia cell line models. *Blood* 101:2368–2373, 2003.

20. O'Brien, Meinhardt P, Bond E, et al.: Effects of imatinib mesylate (STI571, Glivec) on the pharmacokinetics of simvastatin, a cytochrome p450 3A4 substrate, in patients with chronic myeloid leukaemia. *Br J Cancer* 89:1855–1859, 2003.

SKIN TUMORS

CHAPTER 25

Skin Cancer

MICHAEL POULSEN

Carcinomas of the skin comprise basal cell carcinoma (BCC), squamous cell carcinoma (SCC), and to a much lesser extent, Merkel cell carcinoma (MCC) and skin appendage tumors. Five-year survival rates are extremely high. However, 5-year survival is a deceptive endpoint for BCCs as patients relapse as late as 10–20 years. In SCC, survival decreases to 40% when nodal secondaries occur.[1] Merkel cell carcinoma has the poorest outcomes with an overall 5-year survival of 47%.[2]

A variety of treatments are used[3] including surgical excision, cryotherapy, electrodessication, radiotherapy, and Mohs surgery. Topical treatments (topical 5 fluorouracil or imiqimod) and photodynamic therapy have been used to treat some of the more favorable lesions. The TNM staging system[4] recognizes the importance of size as a prognostic factor. The majority of lesions fall into the T1N0M0 category. The surface dimension and the degree of infiltration should be determined. For tumors <1 cm, the local control with radiotherapy is 91–97%. The BCC lesions >2 cm treated with radiotherapy have worse outcomes[5] and with the infiltration beyond the subcutis (T4) disease-free survival is 50%.[1] Skin cancers involving cartilage and bone are less likely to be controlled with radiation treatment.

The presence of nodal disease is an infrequent occurrence, while MCC has a propensity for lymphatic spread.[6] The presence of nodal secondaries is a poor prognostic factor. For SCC, nodal disease is associated with a high recurrence rate of 34% and a disease specific survival of 61%.[7] The risk of recurrence is related to the number of nodes involved, as well as the presence of extranodal extension.[1] Nodal disease is a powerful prognostic factor for MCC.[6] The extent of disease in the parotid is also prognostic with increasing extent of parotid and cervical involvement associated with a poorer survival.[8] Recurrent skin carcinomas have poor control rates. Local control decreases with each episode of recurrence and salvage treatment.[1]

Prognostic Factors in Cancer, Third Edition, edited by Mary K. Gospodarowicz, Brian O'Sullivan, and Leslie H. Sobin.

The histologic subtype also provides prognostic information. Morphoeic, infiltrative, micronodular, and basi-squamous BCCs are associated with increased recurrence rates.[9] Recurrence is more likely with infiltrative and desmoplastic lesions and the risk of metastasis increases with tumor thickness and poor differentiation. Spindle cell SCC infiltrate deeply and show aggressive behavior. Verrucous lesions are well differentiated, but locally aggressive.

In a small proportion of cases (2.5%) skin carcinomas may spread into the perineural space of the trigeminal and facial nerves. While this is usually an incidental finding, in more advanced cases pain, lumps along the nerve, paresthesia or cranial nerve palsies may be seen.[1] Outcome is correlated with the extent of involvement.

Incomplete excision is associated with high recurrence rates, 30% in BCC and 50% in SCC.[1] Deep margin involvement is associated with a higher relapse rate than lateral margins. Reexcision or postoperative radiotherapy reduces the risk of recurrence.[1] The risk of recurrence with a positive margin will increase if the lesion has previously failed. Recurrence rates are higher for lesions of the facial region, those around the nose, eyes, and ears warranting particular care.[1] Recurrence rates are higher in younger patients,[10] especially women. Lesions on the lower limb, especially in the elderly, are associated with poorer outcomes. Tumors associated with chronic inflammation or scars and those occurring on the lower extremities are more likely to recur.[1] There may be a long latent period between the initial event and the development of the SCC. Immunosuppression, predicts for adverse outcome,[1] the ratio of SCC to BCC in immunosuppressed patients is the reverse of the general population.[11]

Surgery is the gold standard. Most studies suggest that both surgery and radiation therapy can achieve 5-year local control rates of 85–95%. One randomised trial[12] of surgery versus radiation therapy in BCC <4 cm of the face showed surgery to be superior. The study concludes that surgery is superior to radiation therapy both in terms of local control and cosmesis. The relative risks of failure with surgery is 0.7% and with radiation therapy is 7.5% (p = 0.001). The failure rate with surgery is lower than that commonly quoted in the literature and radiation therapy is given by three different techniques, none of which involved megavoltage therapy. The type of surgery may also influence the prospects for cure with 7.9% recurrence for non-Mohs modalities versus 3.1% for Mohs surgery.[13] The biological effective dose of radiation affects the probability of local control.[14]

Access to the full range of treatment modalities is desirable particularly in the management of advanced cases that may involve bone, cartilage, or nerves or recurrent lesions that are better managed in a multidisciplinary setting. The role of synchronous chemo–radiation therapy is being evaluated for locally advanced SCC.

■■■■■ **SUMMARY TABLE**

Prognostic Factors in Skin Cancer

Prognostic Factors	Tumor Related	Host Related	Environment Related
Essential	TNM category Recurrence[1] Histologic type[1] Perineural infiltration[14] Site[1]	Chronic inflammation, burns, radiation scars[1] Immunosuppression[11]	Surgical margins[1]
Additional	Grade Thickness	Age Gender Genetic factors Gorlin's syndrome	Radiation dose[14] Multidisciplinary care
New and promising			Chemo–radiotherapy

Sources:
• National Health and Medical Research Council. Clinical practice guidelines non melanoma skin cancer: Guidelines for the treatment and management in Australia 2002.
http://www.nhmrc.gov.au/publications/pdf/cp87.pdf.
• NCCN Clinical Practice Guidelines in Oncology: Basal Cell and Squamous Cell Carcinoma.
http://www. nccn.org/professionals/physician_gls/PDF/nmsc.pdf.
• National Cancer Institute: Skin Cancer (PDQ®): Treatment Guidelines 2005.
http://www.cancer.gov/cancertopics/pdq/treatment/skin/healthprofessional/.

REFERENCES

1. National Health and Medical Research Council, Clinical practice guidelines non melanoma skin cancer: Guidelines for the treatment and management in Australia. http://www.nhmrc.gov.au/publications/pdf/cp87.pdf, 2002.
2. Veness M, Richards S: Role of radiotherapy in treating skin cancer. *Aust J Dermatol* 44:159–156, 2003.
3. Marks R: Skin cancer — a practical guide to management. *Aust J Dermatol* 45:80, 2004.
4. Sobin LH, Wittekind Ch (eds.), UICC: *TNM Classification of malignant tumors*. 6th ed. New York, Wiley-Liss, 2002.
5. Silva JJ et al.: Results of radiotherapy for epithelial skin cancer of the pinna: the. *Int J Radiat Oncol Biol Phys* 47:451–459, 2000.
6. Poulsen M: Merkel cell carcinoma of the skin. *Lancet Oncol* 5:593–599, 2004.

7. Veness MJ et al.: Cutaneous head and neck squamous cell carcinoma metastatic to cervical lymph nodes (non parotid). *Laryngoscope* 113:1827–1833, 2003.

8. Palme CE et al.: Extent of parotid disease influences outcome in patients with metastatic cutaneous squamous cell carcinoma. *Arch Otolaryngol Head Neck Surg* 129:750–753, 2003.

9. Dellon AL et al.: Prediction of recurrence in incompletely excised basal cell carcinoma. *Plast Reconstr Surg* 75:860–871, 1985.

10. Leffell DJ: The scientific basis of skin cancer. *J Am Acad Dermatol* 42:18–22, 2000.

11. Ong CS et al.: Skin cancer in Australian heart transplant recipients. *J Am Acad Dermatol* 40:27–34, 1999.

12. Avril M, Auperin A: Basal cell carcinoma of the face: surgery or radiation therapy? Results of a randomised study. *Br J Cancer* 76:100–106, 1997.

13. Rowe DE, Carroll R, Day C: Prognostic factors for local recurrence, metastasis, and survival in squamous cell carcinoma of the skin, ear and lip. *J Am Acad Dermatol* 26:976–990, 1992.

14. Silva JJ et al.: Results of radiotherapy for epithelial skin cancer of the pinna: the Princess Margaret Hospital experience, 1982–1993. *Int J Radiat Oncol Biol Phys* 47:451–459, 2000.

CHAPTER 26

Cutaneous Malignant Melanoma

TREVOR W. BEER and PETER J. HEENAN

The incidence of cutaneous melanoma continues to rise in many parts of the world and remains a significant cause of morbidity and mortality. Prognosis has improved in many areas, largely due to a decrease in tumor thickness associated with earlier diagnosis.

Clinical stage is the most important determinant of prognosis. Patients with thin, early stage melanomas have an excellent outlook in general, but even in these patients there is no certainty of cure. Prognosis becomes poorer with increasing stage, but some patients may survive for extended periods with known metastatic disease. The American Joint Committee on Cancer (AJCC), validated in a series of 17,600 patients with melanoma, uses TNM categories to determine survival probability.[1,2]

Despite the large number of established and putative prognostic factors in melanoma, accurate prediction of prognosis in an individual patient remains difficult. Since the second edition of this publication,[3] the importance of mitotic rate and ulceration have been more clearly established. Many additional prognostic factors have been suggested, mainly from the use of histological, immunohistochemical, and molecular studies, but few have been widely tested in large studies.

The key determinants of prognosis in localized melanoma (stages I and II) are Breslow thickness and ulceration.[4] Clark's level of invasion may have some value in thin melanomas, but this is controversial.[5] Numerous other factors may be of prognostic relevance, particularly mitotic rate.[6,7] Most other suggested factors, including lymphocytic infiltration, regression, and cell type are of lesser importance in most studies, or findings are controversial and conflicting. Pregnancy does not significantly affect prognosis.[8]

Tumor growth phase has been shown to be poorly reproducible and of limited value, although it may assist in stratifying thin melanomas.[9] Histologic subtype provides little prognostic information when Breslow thickness is considered, although pure desmoplastic melanomas may have a slightly better prognosis.[10]

Prognostic Factors in Cancer, Third Edition, edited by Mary K. Gospodarowicz, Brian O'Sullivan, and Leslie H. Sobin.
Copyright © 2006 John Wiley & Sons, Inc.

In stage III disease (regional metastases), the key determinant of prognosis is the number of lymph nodes affected. Tumor burden (size of metastases) is important, with clinically detected disease faring worse than that only identified microscopically. Clinical or microscopic satellite & in-transit metastases dictate a prognosis similar to that of multiple nodal metastases. Ulceration of the primary tumor confers an adverse prognosis and tumors in older patients, those sited on the trunk, head, and neck may have a worse prognosis.

In stage IV (distant metastases), prognosis is worse with increasing number of metastatic sites and with metastasis to viscera.[11] High serum lactate dehydrogenase (a marker of liver involvement) and poor performance status are associated with reduced survival.[12]

Approximately 5% of patients present with metastatic melanoma for which a primary cannot be identified. In these patients, the outlook is much the same as that of patients with similar disease distribution associated with a known primary.[4]

Although many molecular and immunohistochemical studies have identified possible prognostic markers, multivariate analyses show that, in general, these are no better than standard morphologic criteria.[13] In the future, gene expression profiling using cDNA-microarray analysis may be of value.[14] Serum markers, such as S100β and melanoma inhibiting activity protein, can provide some prognostic information, but this is mostly relevant in monitoring treatment effects in advanced stage melanoma.[15]

A number of prognostic models have been derived combining a variety of clinical and pathological features. Some are complex and although they may show promise in whole populations, all suffer from the problem of limited predictive value for an individual patient.[4]

The site of primary melanoma has been shown to have prognostic relevance in some studies, but not others, even when controlled for tumor depth. In some series, tumors sited on the palms, soles, and subungual regions have a worse prognosis. Females have been shown to have slightly improved survival rates in only a proportion of studies. When controlled for thickness, race has been shown to be of relevance in some populations, with African Americans having a somewhat worse outcome.

The treatment of primary melanoma is complete excision. Most recommendations suggest a minimum margin of 10 mm for invasive melanoma, although histologically confirmed complete clearance may be all that is required.[16]

Clinical guidelines for melanoma management have been issued by a number of authorities across the world, with some available free on the internet.*

The therapeutic value of sentinel lymph node biopsy and elective lymph node dissection are controversial and appear to offer no consistent survival benefit.[17,18] Surgical removal of involved lymph nodes and limited extranodal metastatic disease may be advantageous.[4]

Vaccine and interferon therapies remain of unproven benefit, but interferon alpha 2-b has shown some encouraging results in certain circumstances.[19] Although disease-free survival may be improved, overall survival is not and the benefits need

Clinical Guidelines On The Internet
*NCCN Clinical Practice Guidelines in Oncology: Melanoma 2005. http://www.nccn.org

■■■■■■■■ **SUMMARY TABLE**

Prognostic Factors in Cutaneous Malignant Melanoma

Prognostic Factors	Tumor Related	Host Related	Environment Related
Essential	Stage T category N category M category		Completeness of excision

Additional	Ulceration
	Mitotic rate
	Regression
	Clark's level[a]
	Tumor infiltrating
	    lymphocytes
	Growth phase
	Desmoplastic type
	Vascular invasion
		Age
		Gender
		Site
		LDH[b]
		Performance
		    status[b]
			Lymph-node dissection
			Excision of metastases
			Chemotherapy
			Immunotherapy
			Radiotherapy

New and promising	Tumor suppressor genes Proliferation markers Angiogenesis Adhesion molecules Growth factors Serum S100β protein RT-PCR for circulating melanoma cells Telomerase MitF		Vaccine therapy Gene therapy

[a] Principally applies to thin melanomas.

[b] In stage IV disease.

• Scottish Intercollegiate Guidelines Network (SIGN). Cutaneous Melanoma 2003.
http://www.guideline. gov/summary/summary.aspx?doc_id=3877
• ESMO Minimum Clinical Recommendations for diagnosis, treatment and follow-up of cutaneous malignant melanoma 2005.
http://annonc.oupjournals.org/cgi/reprint/16/suppl_1/i66
• Australia: National Health and Medical Research Council 1999.
http://www.nhmrc.gov.au/publications

to be considered in the context of possible side effects. Radiotherapy may be of use palliatively, or in certain clinical situations, such as where complete surgical excision is not feasible.[4] Chemotherapy is largely confined to advanced metastatic disease or isolated limb perfusion for acrally sited lesions. Proof of a consistent or significant increase in survival is lacking.[20]

REFERENCES

1. AJCC (American Joint Committee on Cancer) Cancer Staging Handbook: TNM Classification of Malignant Tumors, 6th ed. New York, Springer-Verlag, 2002.
2. Balch CM, Soong SJ, Gershenwald JE, et al.: Prognostic factors analysis of 17,600 melanoma patients: validation of the American Joint Committee on Cancer melanoma staging system. *J Clin Oncol* 19:3622–3634, 2001.
3. Heenan PJ, Yu LL, English DR: Cutaneous malignant melanoma (Chapter 29), in Gospodarowicz MK, Henson DE, Hutter RVP, et al. (eds.): *Prognostic Factors in Cancer UICC*, 2nd ed. New York, Wiley-Liss, 2001.
4. Gershenwald JE, Balch CM, Soong S-J, et al.: Prognostic factors and natural history, in Balch CM, Houghton AN, Sober AJ, Song S-J (eds.): *Cutaneous Melanoma*, 4th ed. St Louis Quality Medical Publishing, 2003, pp. 25–54.
5. Leitner U, Buettner PG, Eigentler TK, Garbe C: Prognostic factors of thin cutaneous melanoma: An analysis of the Central Malignant Melanoma Registry of the German Dermatological Society. *J Clin Oncol* 22:3660–3667, 2004.
6. Azzola MF, Shaw HM, Thompson JF, et al.: Tumor mitotic rate is a more powerful prognostic indicator than ulceration in patients with primary cutaneous melanoma: an analysis of 3661 patients from a single center. *Cancer* 97:1488–1498, 2003.
7. Barnhill RL, Katzen J, Spatz A, et al.: The importance of mitotic rate as a prognostic factor for localized cutaneous melanoma. *J Cutan Pathol* 32:268–273, 2005.
8. O'Meara AT, Cress R, Xing G, et al.: Malignant melanoma in pregnancy. A population-based evaluation. *Cancer* 103:1217–1226, 2005.
9. Gimotty PA, Guerry DP, Ming ME, et al.: Thin primary cutaneous malignant melanoma: A prognostic tree for 10-year metastasis is more accurate than American Joint Committee on Cancer Staging. *J Clin Oncol* 22:3668–3676, 2004.
10. Busam KJ, Mujumdar U, Hummer A, et al.: Cutaneous desmoplastic melanoma: Reappraisal of morphologic heterogeneity and prognostic factors. *Am J Surg Pathol* 28:1518–1525, 2004.
11. Unger JM, Flaherty LE, Liu PY, et al.: Gender and other survival predictors in patients with metastatic melanoma on Southwest Oncology Group trials. *Cancer* 91:1148–1155, 2001.
12. Manola J, Atkins M, Ibrahim J, et al.: Prognostic factors in metastatic melanoma: a pooled analysis of Eastern Cooperative Oncology Group trials. *J Clin Oncol* 18:3782–3793, 2000.
13. Carlson JA, Ross JS, Slominski A, et al.: Molecular diagnostics in melanoma. *J Am Acad Dermatol* 52:743–775, 2005.
14. Nambiar S, Mirmohammadsadegh A, Bar A, et al.: Application of array technology: melanoma research and diagnosis. *Expert Rev Mol Diagn* 4:549–557, 2004.

15. Li N, Mangini J, Bhawan J: New prognostic factors of cutaneous melanoma: a review of the literature. *J Cutan Pathol* 29:324–340, 2002.

16. Heenan PJ: Local recurrence of melanoma. *Pathology* 36:1–5, 2004.

17. Medalie N, Ackerman AB: Controversies in Dermatology. Sentinel nody biopsy has no benefit for patients whose primary cutaneous melanoma has metastasized to a lymph node and therefore should be abandoned now. *Br J Dermatol* 151:298–307, 2004.

18. Morton DL, Cochran AJ: Controversies in Dermatology. The case for lymphatic mapping and sentinel lymphadenectomy in the management of primary melanoma. *Br J Dermatol* 151:308–319, 2004.

19. Kirkwood JM, Ibrahaim JG, Sosman JA, et al.: High-dose interferon alpha-2b significantly prolongs relapse-free and overall survival compared with the GM2-KLH/QS-21 vaccine in patients with resected stage IIB-III melanoma: results of intergroup trial E1694/S9512/C509801. *J Clin Oncol* 19:2370–2380, 2001.

20. Tsao H, Atkins MB, Sober AJ: Management of Cutaneous Melanoma. *N Engl J Med* 351:998–1012, 2004.

BREAST CANCER

CHAPTER 27

Breast Cancer

DANIEL F. HAYES

Breast cancer is a common disease in the developed world, causing considerable morbidity and mortality. However, much progress has been made in the areas of risk assessment, prevention, screening, primary care, and adjuvant systemic therapy of breast cancer, with recent statistics showing a dramatic reduction in annual overall mortality accompanied by decreasing ill effects of therapy.[1]

Risk is associated with gender, of course, and age, with 75% of all breast cancers occurring in women >50 years. Other risk factors include family history, early menarche, late first full-term pregnancy, moderate to excessive alcohol use, long-term combined estrogen and progesterone replacement therapy, and the presence of a deleterious mutation in one of two known breast cancer suppressor genes, BRCA1 and 2.[2] Risk can be reduced by prophylactic mastectomy, although this radical approach is rarely chosen by women of average-to-moderate risk.[3] Endocrine manipulation also reduces risk by ~50%. Although oophorectomy is effective in premenopausal women, like prophylactic mastectomy it is rarely an acceptable option.[4] Selective estrogen receptor modulators, such as tamoxifen and raloxifene, reduce risk by 50% in both young and older women.[5] Mammographic screening reduces mortality by ~20–30% over 10–15 years, presumably by virtue of early application of local and perhaps systemic therapy.[6] Breast preservation is associated with equal or superior outcomes to mastectomy, and prophylactic radiation, either to the breast or chest wall after mastectomy, clearly reduces local-regional recurrence and, perhaps surprisingly, distant recurrence and mortality.[6] Adjuvant systemic therapy clearly reduces distant metastases and recurrence,[7] and numerous systemic therapies are available that improve quality of life and modestly improve overall survival for patients with metastatic disease.[8]

Tumor-related features that predict outcomes in breast cancer must be divided between prognostic and predictive factors.[9] Prognostic factors are those that are associated with metastatic potential, such as the presence of a clinical T4 finding (fixation

Prognostic Factors in Cancer, Third Edition, edited by Mary K. Gospodarowicz, Brian O'Sullivan, and Leslie H. Sobin.
Copyright © 2006 John Wiley & Sons, Inc.

to the chest wall, peau d'orange, inflammation, skin ulceration, and nodules), pathologic lymph node involvement, tumor size, and grade. Predictive factors are associated with the likelihood that a specific treatment will work against the cancer in question. For breast cancer, these include estrogen and progesterone receptor (ER, PgR) content, which are very strong predictors of endocrine treatments, and expression of the HER2/erbB2 gene, which is required for activity of trastuzumab, a humanized monoclonal antibody directed against the HER2 protein.[10] Many factors can be both prognostic and predictive. For example, ER is a weak favorable prognostic factor in the absence of any systemic therapy and a strong predictive factor for benefit from endocrine treatment, while HER2 is a weak unfavorable prognostic factor, appears to be a weak-to-moderate negative predictive factor for SERM therapy and for nonanthracycline-based chemotherapy, an apparent neutral predictive factor for anthracyclines, and a powerful positive predictive factor for response to trastuzumab.[11]

Several endocrine manipulations are effective against ER positive breast cancer, and in the metastatic setting they can often be used in sequence, using one until it is no longer effective and then following with a second, to provide effective and often toxicity-free palliation.[8] These manipulations include additive hormonal treatments, such as SERMs and a progestational agent like megestrol acetate or medroxyprogesterone. These additive hormonal therapies are equally effective regardless of menopausal status. In contrast, ablative therapies elimate the production of estrogen, and are therefore specific to a woman's menstrual status. For premenopausal women, surgical oophorectomy or use of a luteinizing hormone releasing hormone agonist/ antagonist, such as goserelin or leuprolide, are equally effective. Recently, inhibition of the aromatization step of estrogen precursors (dihydroepiadrostenedione and testosterone) to estradiol and estrone has been shown to be very effective, even in patients who have progressed on a SERM. In the adjuvant setting, SERM therapy reduces the odds of recurrence and death by ~40 and 25%, respectively, in patients with ER positive cancers, and the aromatase inhibitors (AIs) appear to further reduce these events by an additional 20 and 15%, respectively.[7,12–14] Regardless of prognostic factors, all women with ER positive and/or PgR positive breast invasive breast cancer should receive some sort of adjuvant endocrine therapy, although the precise regimen is not currently established.

Currently, no clinically useful predictive factors for chemotherapy have been identified. In the metastatic setting, combination or serial single agent therapy is usually applied empirically until the patient appears to be refractory to available treatments and is resigned to best supportive care.[8] However, adjuvant chemotherapy reduces the annual odds of mortality in women with invasive breast cancer by ~40 and 20% in patients younger or older than 50 years, respectively.[7] Careful and thoughtful calculation of a woman's risk of recurrence in the absence of any therapy, based on prognostic factors, coupled with the relative reduction in risk provided by hormone therapy and chemotherapy, depending on her ER and PgR status, permit the clinician to provide a relatively concrete estimate of the absolute odds of a patient's benefiting from each therapy individually or in sequence, allowing her to judge if this benefit outweighs the potential toxicity from her perspective.[15–17]

In the metastatic setting, several clinical trials have demonstrated the benefits of trastuzumab for patients with HER2 positive breast cancer.[8] HER2 protein expression can be evaluated by immunohistochemistry. Since 95% or more of overexpression is due to amplification, HER2 status can also be determined by fluorescent *in situ* hybridization (FISH). The relative merit of each is controversial. Recently, exciting results from three prospective randomized clinical trials comparing adjuvant chemotherapy with or followed by trastuzumab vs. chemotherapy alone suggest a 50% reduction in distant recurrence and even a 30% reduction in mortality, with very short follow-up (1–2 years).[18–20] Long-term results of these trials, as well as those from a fourth trial, will determine the precise role of this agent in the early setting. Unfortunately, nearly 5% of patients receiving trastuzumab suffered some degree of heart dysfunction, although it was often reversible. Nonetheless, this disturbing complication further emphasizes the importance of careful selection of those patients most likely to benefit.

New prognostic factors include measures of tumor invasion and metastasis. In particular, enzyme-linked immunosorbent assays (ELISA) for urinary plasminogen activator (UPA) and plasminogen activator inhibitor 1 (PAI-1) have been shown to be moderate-to-strong poor prognostic factors, and these assays are in common use in certain countries in Europe.[21] More recently, simultaneous evaluation of expression of several genes has engendered considerable excitement. These assays can be performed by gene microarray analysis or by multiplex reverse transcription polymerase chain reaction (RT-PCR).[22,23] The latter is a particularly exciting technique, since it permits evaluation of formalin-fixed, paraffin-embedded tissues, which are more common in archived banks than are frozen tissues. The precise role of these newer assays is unclear, although the National Surgical Adjuvant Bowel and Breast Project (NSABP) has reported that one particular multiplex RT-PCR may be particularly accurate in distinguishing node negative, ER positive patients who will do well with tamoxifen alone versus those with a sufficiently high risk of relapse to justify chemotherapy.[24]

Several circulating assays have been reported for evaluation and monitoring of patients with breast cancer. In particular, assays for the MUC-1 protein, such as CA15-3 and CA27.29, and assays for carcinoembryonic antigen, can be helpful to guide metastatic therapy.[10,25] Likewise, the extracellular domain of HER-2 is shed and appears to track clinical course of patients with HER-2 positive breast cancer, although its clinical role has not been defined.[26] None of these assays is of value in evaluating patients with newly diagnosed, nonmetastatic breast cancer. Although a rising circulating marker in a patient who is otherwise free of disease after primary and adjuvant therapy has a relatively high positive predictive value for subsequent recurrence in the succeeding 3–6 months, the clinical utility of this information is unclear.[10,25] Recently, results of a prospective clinical trial of the relative worth of baseline and serial monitoring of circulating tumor cells (CTC) has suggested that elevated CTC levels are associated with a poorer prognosis and suggests a failure to benefit from systemic therapy in patients with metastatic breast cancer.[27] Further studies are underway to determine how best to apply this assay in routine clinical practice.

Finally, the field of pharmacogenomics is emerging, with the promise of further individualizing systemic therapy by prospective determination of inherited single nucleotide polymorphisms (SNPs) in genes associated either with drug metabolism and/or drug activity.[28] For example, recently reported preliminary studies have determined that the cytochrome p450 gene 2D6 is responsible for metabolism of the relatively inactive parent drug tamoxifen to the much more potent and high abundance product, 4-hydroxy N-desmethyl tamoxifen (endoxifen).[29] Further studies have suggested that deleterious SNPs in, or administration of drugs that inhibit, CYP2D6 reduce circulating levels of endoxifen and may have clinical implications.[30] Clearly, more work in this field, regarding not just tamoxifen, but all of the available systemic therapies for breast cancer, is needed.

■■■■■■■ **SUMMARY TABLE**

Prognostic Factors in Breast Cancer

Prognostic Factor	Tumor Related	Host Related	Environment Related
Essential	cTNM pTNM Grade ER PgR HER2		
Additional	UPA/PAI-1	Age Performance Status	
New and promising	Multi-gene expression analysis	SNPs in genes associated with drug metabolism and/or action	

Sources:
• National Cancer Institute: Breast Cancer (PDQ®): Treatment Guidelines 2005.
http://www.cancer.gov/cancertopics/pdq/treatment/breast/healthprofessional/.
• NCCN Clinical Practice Guidelines in Oncology: Breast Cancer 2005.
http://www.nccn.org/professionals/physician_gls/PDF/breast.pdf.
• ESMO Minimum Clinical Recommendations for diagnosis, treatment and follow-up of primary breast cancer 2005.
http://annonc.oupjournals.org/cgi/reprint/16/suppl_1/i7.
• Singapore Ministry of Health Clinical Practice Guidelines: Breast Cancer 2005.
http://www.moh.gov.sg/cmaweb/attachments/publication/cpg_Breast_Cancer-Mar_2004.pdf.

REFERENCES

1. Peto R, Borcham J, Clarke M, et al.: UK and USA breast cancer deaths down 25% in year 2000 at ages 20–69 years. *Lancet* 355:1822, 2000.

2. Domchek SM, Eisen A, Calzone K, et al.: Application of breast cancer risk prediction models in clinical practice. *J Clin Oncol* 21:593–601, 2003.

3. Meijers-Heijboer H, van Geel B, van Putten WL, et al.: Breast cancer after prophylactic bilateral mastectomy in women with a BRCA1 or BRCA2 mutation. *N Engl J Med* 345:159–164, 2001.

4. Rebbeck TR, Lynch HT, Neuhausen S, et al.: Prophylactic ooporectomy in carriers of BRCA1 and BRCA2 mutations. *N Eng J Med* 346:1616–1622, 2002.

5. Cuzick J, Powles T, Veronesi U, et al.: Overview of the main outcomes in breast-cancer prevention trials. *Lancet* 361:296–300, 2003.

6. Veronesi U, Boyle P, Goldhirsch A, et al.: Breast cancer. *Lancet* 365:1727–1741, 2005.

7. Early Breast Cancer Trialists' Collaborative Group T. Effects of chemotherapy and hormonal therapy for early breast cancer on recurrence and 15-year survival: an overview of the randomised trials. *Lancet* 365:1687–1717, 2005.

8. Ellis M, Hayes DF, Lippman ME: Treatment of Metastatic Breast Cancer, in Harris J, Lippman M, Morrow M, Osborne CK (eds.): *Diseases of the Breast,* 3rd ed. Philadelphia, Lippincott Williams & Wilkins, 2004, pp. 1101–1162.

9. Hayes DF: Clinical importance of prognostic factors: Moving from scientifically interesting to clinically useful, in Bronchud MH, Foote M, Giaccone G et al. (eds.): *Principles of Molecular Oncology*, 2nd ed. Totowa, NJ, Humana Press, Inc, 2004, pp. 51–72.

10. Bast RC Jr, Ravdin P, Hayes DF et al.: 2000 Update of recommendations for the use of tumor markers in breast and colorectal cancer: clinical practice guidelines of the American Society of Clinical Oncology. *J Clin Oncol* 19:1865–1878, 2001.

11. Yamauchi H, Stearns V, Hayes DF: When is a tumor marker ready for prime time? A case study of c-erbB-2 as a predictive factor in breast cancer. *J Clin Oncol* 19:2334–2356, 2001.

12. Coombes RC, Hall E, Gibson LJ, et al.: A randomized trial of exemestane after two to three years of tamoxifen therapy in postmenopausal women with primary breast cancer. *N Engl J Med* 350:1081–1092, 2004.

13. Goss PE, Ingle JN, Martino S, et al.: A randomized trial of letrozole in postmenopausal women after five years of tamoxifen therapy for early-stage breast cancer. *N Engl J Med* 349:1793–1802, 2003.

14. Howell A, Cuzick J, Baum M, et al.: Results of the ATAC (Arimidex, Tamoxifen, Alone or in Combination) trial after completion of 5 years' adjuvant treatment for breast cancer. *Lancet* 365:60–62, 2005.

15. Olivotto IA, Bajdik CD, Ravdin PM, et al.: Population-based validation of the prognostic model ADJUVANT! for early breast cancer. *J Clin Oncol* 23:2716–2725, 2005.

16. Ravdin PM, Siminoff LA, Davis GJ, et al.: Computer program to assist in making decisions about adjuvant therapy for women with early breast cancer. *J Clin Oncol* 19:980–991, 2001.

17. Whelan TJ, Loprinzi C: Physician/patient decision aids for adjuvant therapy. *J Clin Oncol* 23:1627–1630, 2005.

18. Perez EA, Suman VJ, Davidson N, et al.: Interim cardiac safety analysis of NCCTG N9831 intergroup adjuvant trastuzumab trial. *Proc Am Soc Clin Oncol* 23: 17s (abst 556), 2005.

19. Piccart-Gebhart MJ, Procter M, Leyland-Jones B, et al; Herceptin adjuvant (HERA) Trial Study Team: Trastuzmab after adjuvant chemotherapy in HER2-positive breast cancer. *N Engl J Med* 353:1659–1672, 2005.

20. Raymond E: NSABP. Doxorubicin and cyclophosphamide followed by paclitaxel with or without trastuzumab as adjuvant therapy for patients with HER-2 positive operable breast cancer: Combined analysis of NSABP B31/NCCTG-N9831. *Proc Am Soc Clin Oncol* 23: late breaking abstract; no page number, 2005.

21. Duffy MJ, Duggan C: The urokinase plasminogen activator system: a rich source of tumour markers for the individualised management of patients with cancer. *Clin Biochem* 37:541–548, 2004.

22. van de Vijver MJ, He YD, van't Veer LJ, et al.: A gene-expression signature as a predictor of survival in breast cancer. *N Engl J Med* 347:1999–2009, 2002.

23. Van't Veer LJ, Paik S, Hayes DF: Gene expression profiling of breast cancer: a new tumor marker. *J Clin Oncol* 23:1631–1635, 2005.

24. Paik S, Shak S, Tang G, et al.: A multi-gene RT-PCR assay using fixed, paraffin-embedded tumor tissue to predict the likelihood of breast cancer recurrence in node negative, estrogen receptor positive, tamoxifen-treated patients. *N Eng J Med* 351:2817–2826, 2004.

25. Bast RC Jr, Ravdin P, Hayes DF, et al.: Errata: 2000 Update of recommendations for the use of tumor markers in breast and colorectal cancer: clinical practice guidelines of the American Society of Clinical Oncology. *J Clin Oncol* 19:4185–4188, 2001.

26. Nunes RA, Harris LN: The HER2 extracellular domain as a prognostic and predictive factor in breast cancer. *Clin Breast Cancer* 3:125–135; discussion 136–137, 2002.

27. Cristofanilli M, Budd GT, Ellis MJ, et al.: Circulating tumor cells, disease progression, and survival in metastatic breast cancer. *N Engl J Med* 351:781–791, 2004.

28. Stearns V, Davidson NE, Flockhart DA: Pharmacogenetics in the treatment of breast cancer. *Pharmacogenomics J* 4:143–153, 2004.

29. Stearns V, Johnson MD, Rae JM, et al.: Active tamoxifen metabolite plasma concentrations after coadministration of tamoxifen and the selective serotonin reuptake inhibitor paroxetine. *J Natl Cancer Inst* 95:1758–1764, 2003.

30. Jin Y, Desta Z, Stearns V, et al.: CYP2D6 genotype, antidepressant use, and tamoxifen metabolism during adjuvant breast cancer treatment. *J Natl Cancer Inst* 97:30–39, 2005.

GYNECOLOGIC CANCERS

CHAPTER 28

Vulvar Cancer

DONALD E. MARSDEN and NEVILLE F. HACKER

Vulvar cancer accounts for ~4% of malignancies of the female genital tract. In the United States in 2004 there were an estimated 3970 new cases with 850 deaths.[1] Squamous cell carcinoma accounts for ~85% of cases, with malignant melanoma the next most common type while adenocarcinoma and basal cell carcinoma (BCC) are rare.

In recent years, there has been increasing emphasis on individualization of treatment for vulvar cancer, with emphasis on individualized, less radical surgery for early stage disease, with decreased surgical morbidity and excellent cure rates.[2]

The single most important prognostic factor in vulvar cancer is the number of positive groin nodes. Patients with three or more positive nodes have a significantly poorer prognosis. Where groin nodes are negative, 5-year survival rates of ~90% have been reported, whereas where nodes are positive the figure is ~50%. Extracapsular spread of tumor in nodes also portends a poor prognosis, and the size of the metastatic focus is also of prognostic significance, micrometastases <5 mm in diameter carrying a significantly better prognosis than macrometastases >15 mm in diameter.[3] Micrometastases, detected by immunohistochemistry in apparently negative nodes, confer a 20-fold increase in the risk of recurrence of the disease.[4]

Depth of tumor invasion, and the overall size of the tumor also correlate with prognosis.[5] The T1 tumors with <1 mm of invasion rarely metastasise to lymph nodes.[3]

For women with advanced vulvar cancer, Lataifeh et al.[6] reported that the disease-free survival of patients with negative groin nodes and those with only one micrometastasis was very similar, while the prognosis of patients with two or more positive groin nodes, whether unilateral or bilateral, was poor. Distant failure was more common in the group with two or more positive nodes.

Van der Velden et al.[7] reported that the risk of local recurrence correlated with tumor-free margins and residual lichen sclerosis or vulvar intraepithelial neoplasia. Rouzier et al.[8] reported that there were two types of local recurrence, namely, relapse

Prognostic Factors in Cancer, Third Edition, edited by Mary K. Gospodarowicz, Brian O'Sullivan, and Leslie H. Sobin.
Copyright © 2006 John Wiley & Sons, Inc.

at the site of the primary tumor or in the skin bridge, and relapse at a remote site on the vulva. The former was a strong predictor for cancer related death, whereas the latter was not. Primary site recurrence was associated with tumor size, depth of invasion, and margin status, whereas remote site relapse was associated with the presence of adjacent dermatosis.

The commonest histologic type of vulvar cancer is squamous cell carcinoma. Verrucous carcinoma and basal cell carcinoma have significantly better prognoses, while the prognosis for vulvar melanoma is more guarded. Adenocarcinoma may arise in Bartholin's glands, vestibular glands or sweat glands, and has a prognosis similar to that of squamous carcinomas of similar size and nodal status.

A multicenter study of patients with surgically staged vulvar cancer indicated that overexpression of CD44v6 was associated with an impaired prognosis with respect to disease-free survival and overall survival. CD 44 is a cell adhesion molecule that binds the extracellular matrix: certain isoforms have been implicated in tumor metastasis. This prognostic information was thought to add to that provided by the conventional prognostic indicators.[9] A recent study of 224 squamous carcinomas of the vulva at the Norwegian Radium Hospital indicated that low levels of p16ink4a protein and high levels of p21Waf1/Cip1 protein were associated with a shorter disease-related survival.[10]

Smoking is one of the predisposing factors to the development of the precursors of invasive carcinoma of the vulva, through the concentration of known carcinogens in the mucous of the female genital tract,[11] and is also associated with an increased incidence of anal and vulvar cancer.[12]

Immune deficiency due to human immunodeficiency virus (HIV) infection appears to be associated with an increased incidence of vulvar neoplasia and carcinoma in younger women, with a poorer prognosis, though there are only a few cases reported.[13]

A Dutch study of 75 women aged 80 years or older found that the ECOG performance status was the only independent prognostic variable of outcome.[14]

Two European studies highlighted the importance of treating vulvar cancer in tertiary referral centers. In a British study of 411 patients treated at 35 different hospitals, 16 of which treated one case or less per year, survival rates were dramatically lower than those from tertiary referral units in the United States, and similar findings emerged from a Dutch study. Failure to perform appropriate groin dissection was a common feature associated with poor outcome in both studies.[3]

As reflected above, the main current issues in vulvar cancer revolve around the management of locally extensive primary tumor and lymph nodes. Combined modality management is being investigated to both improve local control and decrease treatment morbidity.

███████ **SUMMARY TABLE**

Prognostic Factors for Vulvar Cancer

Prognostic Factors	Tumor Related	Host Related	Environment Related
Essential	T category N category M category	Age	Experience of treating centre
Additional	Extranodal spread Number of involved nodes Size of metastatic deposits in nodes Grade Pattern of invasion Depth of invasion	Smoking Immune status	Surgical margins Residual lichen sclerosis or VIN
New and promising	CD 44 p16INK4a p21Waf1/Cip 1		

Sources:
• National Cancer Institute: Vulva Cancer (PDQ®): Treatment Guidelines 2005.
http://www.cancer.gov/cancertopics/pdq/treatment/vulvar/healthprofessional/.
• Staging classifications and clinical practice guidelines of gynaecologic cancers 2003.
http://www.igcs.org/ guidelines/guideline_staging-booklet.pdf.

REFERENCES

1. Jemal A, Tiwari RC, Murray T et al.: Cancer Statistics 2004. *CA Cancer J Clin* 54:8–29, 2004.

2. de Hullu JA, Oonk MHM, van der Zee AGJ: Modern management of vulvar cancer. *Curr Opin Obstet Gynecol* 16:65–72, 2004.

3. Hacker NF: "Vulvar Cancer," in Berek JS, Hacker NF (eds.): Practical Gynecologic Oncology, 4th ed. Philadelphia, Lippincott, Williams and Wilkins, 2005.

4. Naryansingh GV, Miller ID, Sharma M, et al.: The prognostic significance of micrometastases in node-negative squamous cell carcinoma of the vulva. *Br J Cancer* 92:222–224, 2005.

5. Benedet JL, Ehlen TG: Vulvar Cancer, in Gospodarowicz MK, Henson DE, Hutter RVP, et al. (eds.): *Prognostic Factors in Cancer*. 2nd ed. New York, Wiley-Liss, 2001.

6. Lataifeh I, Nascimento MC, Nicklin JL, et al.: Patterns of recurrence and disease free survival in advanced squamous cell carcinoma of the vulva. *Gynecol Oncol* 95:701–705, 2004.

7. van der Velden J, Schilthuis MS, Hyde SE, et al.: Squamous cell cancer of the vulva with occult lymph node metastases in the groin: the impact of surgical technique on recurrence pattern and survival. *Int J Gynecol Cancer* 14:633–638, 2004.

8. Rouzier R, Haddad B, Plantier F, et al.: Local relapse in patients treated for squamous cell vulvar carcinoma: incidence and prognostic value. *Obstet Gynecol* 100:1159–1167, 2002.

9. Hefler LA, Concin N, Mincham D, et al.: The prognostic value of immunohistochemically detected CD44v3 and CD44v6 expression in patients with surgically staged vulvar carcinoma: a multicenter study. *Cancer* 94:125–130, 2002.

10. Knopp S, Bjorge T, Nesland JM, et al.: p16ink4a and p21Waf1/Cip 1 expression correlates with clinical outcome in vulvar carcinomas. *Gynecol Oncol* 95:37–45, 2004.

11. Jones RW: Vulval intraepithelial neoplasia: current perspectives. *Eur J Gynaecol Oncol* 26:393–402, 2001.

12. Chen C, Cook LS, Li XY, et al.: CYP2D6 genotype and the incidence of anal and vulval cancer. *Cancer Epidemiol, Biomarkers Prevention* 8:317–321, 1999.

13. Elit L, Voruganti S, Simunovic M: Invasive vulvar cancer in a woman with human immunodeficiency virus: case report and review of the literature. *Gynecol Oncol* 98:151–154, 2005.

14. Hyde SE, Ansink AC, Burger MPM, et al.: The impact of performance status on survival in patients 80 years and older with vulvar cancer. *Gynecol Oncol* 84:388–393, 2002.

CHAPTER 29

Uterine Cervix Cancer

JAN HAUSPY, IAN HARLEY, and ANTHONY W. FYLES

An estimated 493,000 women are diagnosed worldwide with invasive cervix carcinoma each year and 274,000 die (World Health Organization, WHO data). Cervical cancer is among the most common female cancers in the developing world. Response to therapy is excellent when diagnosed early; advanced disease remains a therapeutic challenge. The vast majority of cervical cancers can be detected in a very early stage with cervical pap smears. Women in the United States have a lifetime risk of 1/130 of developing cervical cancer.[1] Countries that have adapted a comprehensive screening program have seen a dramatic drop in deaths from cervical cancer due to early diagnosis.

Treatment guidelines relate to the stage of the disease. In stage IA1, a simple hysterectomy and in stage IA2 a radical hysterectomy with or without pelvic lymph node dissection (PLND) are standard. For stage IB1-IIA, <4-cm tumors, a radical hysterectomy with PLND or a radical pelvic radiotherapy with or without concurrent platinum-containing chemotherapy is performed. For stage IB2-IIA, >4-cm tumors, radiotherapy with external beam, and brachytherapy with concurrent platinum-containing chemotherapy is standard. In more advanced disease, stage IIB-IVA, radiotherapy with concurrent platinum-containing chemotherapy and in stage IVB platinum-containing chemotherapy and/or local radiotherapy for symptom relief are standard. Recurrence after radical surgery is usually addressed with chemoradiation, while for recurrence after radiotherapy surgical exenteration can be considered if the disease is confined to the pelvis. Fertility sparing treatment in young patients has been widely accepted. For stage IA1 lesions, conisation of the cervix is proposed with strict follow-up afterward, whereas for stage IA2 to IIA radical trachelectomy with laparoscopic pelvic lymph node dissection is accepted in selected cases for tumors up to 2 cm.[2] Neoadjuvant chemotherapy for locally advanced carcinoma of the cervix is still controversial and requires further investigation.[3]

Early stage cervical cancer is very often diagnosed by routine Pap smear, whereas more advanced lesions can reveal symptoms, such as PV bleeding, vaginal discharge,

Prognostic Factors in Cancer, Third Edition, edited by Mary K. Gospodarowicz, Brian O'Sullivan, and Leslie H. Sobin.

pain, and symptoms due to invasion of neighboring organs (i.e., bladder and large intestine) or regional lymph nodes.

Tumor category (T) has long been recognized as the most important determinant of outcome. The division of stage IB1 and IB2 based on tumor size stratifies prognosis with respect to survival and pelvic control. Tumor size has an independent effect on prognosis. The tumor size is studied by clinical measurement, but magnetic resonance imaging (MRI) has shown to be of prognostic value.[4] Pelvic and paraaortic lymph-node metastasis are the most significant independent prognostic indicators for survival.[5,6] Apart from the rare small-cell neuroendocrine carcinoma, histologic subtype does not appear to have prognostic significance. Some studies have shown an independent effect of histology, however, a population-based study did not show any survival difference between squamous-cell and non-squamous-cell carcinoma.[7]

In randomized controlled trials, concurrent radiation and cisplatin-based chemotherapy for advanced cervical carcinoma (IIb2, III, IVa without lymph-node involvement), positive nodes or margins at radical hysterectomy, provides a survival benefit over radiation therapy alone.[8,9]

Additional factors include depth of stromal invasion (DSI) and capillary/lymphatic space invasion (LVSI). The presence of deep stromal invasion (outer 1/3) and LVSI is associated with an increased risk of lymph node metastasis and DSI and LVSI have been regarded as independent prognostic factors. A recent review of the literature by Creasman[10] did not find LVSI to be a statistically significant factor for overall survival. Few studies have identified DSI as an independent factor for overall survival. A recent study from Japan of 115 patients with FIGO stage Ib-IIb cervical cancer found that DSI was not present on multivariate analysis.[11]

Anemia is associated with a poorer response and reduced survival. A recent GOG study indicated that hemoglobin levels during the last third of treatment are predictive of progression-free survival.[12] A German study identified midtherapy hemoglobin levels as a factor for overall survival. Hemoglobin levels $>13 \, g/L$, $11–13 \, g/L$ and $<11 \, g/L$ showed a significant difference in 3-year overall survival, 79, 63, and 32%, respectively (p = 0.0003).[13] Increased treatment duration is known to adversely affect local control, as are inadequate doses of radiation and omission of brachytherapy.[8,9]

Several biomarkers have been identified recently as predictors of poor prognosis. Hypoxia may directly induce resistance to radiation therapy and chemotherapy and indirectly lead to treatment resistance by modulating gene expression and effects of molecules, such as VEGF and HIF-1α.[14,15] HIF-1α overexpression has been associated with an adverse effect on survival,[16,17] but not consistently.[18] In a study by Dunst, patients with hypoxic readings at 19.8 Gy had a significantly reduced 3-year survival (53 vs. 68%, p = 0.04).[13] Membranous EGFR staining also had a significant effect on survival (HR 2.50, p = 0.011).[15] Hazelbag found that strong staining of PAI-1 in 108 patients with FIGO stage IA-II cervical carcinoma was a significant predictor for worse overall survival (HR 8.9, p = 0.04).[19] COX-2 expression was associated with poor survival,[20,21] but not always confirmed as an independent factor.[15]

Hypermethylation of gene promoter sequences is a frequent epigenetic event in many cancers, including cervical cancer. A study of 93 patients with invasive cervical cancer found promoter hypermethylation of the MYOD1 gene to be of significant prognostic value. Median survival was 1.9 and 6.1 years for MYOD1 methylation-positive and negative patients, respectively (p = 0.02).[22]

The association of human papilloma virus (HPV) with the pathogenesis of cervical cancer is well established. A study from Japan, of 97 patients with HPV-positive cervical cancers treated with primary radiotherapy, found that persistence of HPV after treatment was a powerful independent predictor for overall survival after multivariate analysis (HR 4.53, p = 0.0028).[23]

▦ SUMMARY TABLE

Prognostic Factors in Uterine Cervix Cancer

Prognostic Factor	Tumor Related	Host Related	Environment Related
Essential[8,9]	Stage T category N category Histologic type	Performance status	
Additional	Capillary–lymphatic-space invasion	Anemia during treatment	
New and promising	Tumor hypoxia VEGF, mEGFR, HIF-1α, COX-2 PAI-1 expression	Serum MYOD1 hypermethylation Persistence of HPV following treatment	

Sources:
• NCCN Clinical Practice Guidelines in Oncology: Cervix Cancer 2005.
http://www.nccn.org/professionals/physician_gls/PDF/cervical.pdf.
• Benedet JL, et al.: FIGO staging classifications and clinical practice guidelines in the management of gynecologic cancers. FIGO Committee on Gynecologic Oncology. *Int J Gynaecol Obstet* 70(2):209–262, 2000.

REFERENCES

1. Jemal A, et al.: Cancer statistics, 2005. *CA Cancer J Clin* 55:10–30, 2005.
2. Plante M, et al.: Vaginal radical trachelectomy: A valuable fertility-preserving option in the management of early-stage cervical cancer. A series of 50 pregnancies and review of the literature. *Gynecol Oncol* 98:3–10, 2005.
3. Neoadjuvant chemotherapy for locally advanced cervix cancer. *Cochrane Database Syst Rev*: CD001774, 2004.
4. Kodaira T, et al.: Comparison of prognostic value of MRI and FIGO stage among patients with cervical carcinoma treated with radiotherapy. *Int J Radiat Oncol Biol Phys* 56:769–777, 2003.
5. Ho CM, et al.: Multivariate analysis of the prognostic factors and outcomes in early cervical cancer patients undergoing radical hysterectomy. *Gynecol Oncol* 93:458–464, 2004.

6. Takeda N, et al.: Multivariate analysis of histopathologic prognostic factors for invasive cervical cancer treated with radical hysterectomy and systematic retroperitoneal lymphadenectomy. *Acta Obstet Gynecol Scand* 81:1144–1151, 2002.

7. Alfsen GC, et al.: Histologic subtype has minor importance for overall survival in patients with adenocarcinoma of the uterine cervix: a population-based study of prognostic factors in 505 patients with nonsquamous cell carcinomas of the cervix. *Cancer* 92:2471–2483, 2001.

8. Teng N: National Comprehensive Cancer Network Clinical Practice Guidelines in Oncology—v.1.2004. 2004, http://www.nccn.org/professionals/physician_gls/PDF/cervical.pdf

9. Benedet JL, et al.: FIGO staging classifications and clinical practice guidelines in the management of gynecologic cancers. FIGO Committee on Gynecologic Oncology. *Int J Gynaecol Obstet* 70:209–262, 2000.

10. Creasman WT, Kohler MF: Is lymph vascular space involvement an independent prognostic factor in early cervical cancer? *Gynecol Oncol* 92:525–529, 2004.

11. Shimada M, et al.: Stromal invasion of the cervix can be excluded from the criteria for using adjuvant radiotherapy following radical surgery for patients with cervical cancer. *Gynecol Oncol* 93:628–631, 2004.

12. Winter WE 3rd, et al.: Association of hemoglobin level with survival in cervical carcinoma patients treated with concurrent cisplatin and radiotherapy: a Gynecologic Oncology Group Study. *Gynecol Oncol* 94:495–501, 2004.

13. Dunst J, et al.: Anemia in cervical cancers: impact on survival, patterns of relapse, and association with hypoxia and angiogenesis. *Int J Radiat Oncol Biol Phys* 56:778–787, 2003.

14. Loncaster JA, et al.: Vascular endothelial growth factor (VEGF) expression is a prognostic factor for radiotherapy outcome in advanced carcinoma of the cervix. *Br J Cancer* 83:620–625, 2000.

15. Gaffney DK, et al.: Epidermal growth factor receptor (EGFR) and vascular endothelial growth factor (VEGF) negatively affect overall survival in carcinoma of the cervix treated with radiotherapy. *Int J Radiat Oncol Biol Phys* 56:922–928, 2003.

16. Bachtiary B, et al.: Overexpression of hypoxia-inducible factor 1alpha indicates diminished response to radiotherapy and unfavorable prognosis in patients receiving radical radiotherapy for cervical cancer. *Clin Cancer Res* 9:2234–2240, 2003.

17. Birner P, et al.: Overexpression of hypoxia-inducible factor 1alpha is a marker for an unfavorable prognosis in early-stage invasive cervical cancer. *Cancer Res* 60:4693–4696, 2000.

18. Haugland HK, et al.: Expression of hypoxia-inducible factor-1alpha in cervical carcinomas: correlation with tumor oxygenation. *Int J Radiat Oncol Biol Phys* 53:854–861, 2002.

19. Hazelbag S, et al.: Prognostic relevance of TGF-beta1 and PAI-1 in cervical cancer. *Int J Cancer* 112:1020–1028, 2004.

20. Ferrandina G, et al.: Prognostic role of the ratio between cyclooxygenase-2 in tumor and stroma compartments in cervical cancer. *Clin Cancer Res* 10:3117–3123, 2004.

21. Kim YB, et al.: Overexpression of cyclooxygenase-2 is associated with a poor prognosis in patients with squamous cell carcinoma of the uterine cervix treated with radiation and concurrent chemotherapy. *Cancer* 95:531–539, 2002.

22. Widschwendter A, et al.: DNA methylation in serum and tumors of cervical cancer patients. *Clin Cancer Res* 10:565–571, 2004.

23. Nagai Y, et al.: Persistence of human papillomavirus infection as a predictor for recurrence in carcinoma of the cervix after radiotherapy. *Am J Obstet Gynecol* 191:1907–1913, 2004.

CHAPTER 30

Ovarian and Fallopian Tube Cancer

SERGIO PECORELLI, BRUNELLA PASINETTI, GIANCARLO TISI,
LUCIA ZIGLIANI, and FRANCO E. ODICINO

Five-year survival rates for epithelial ovarian cancer are still unsatisfactory at ~45–50%[1] even though this represents a one-third improvement over the past 20 years. Ovarian cancers (borderline and frankly malignant) are staged following the definitions of the International Federation of Gynecology and Obstetrics (FIGO)[1] and the UICC[2]–AJCC[3] TNM classifications. The majority of patients are diagnosed with advanced stage disease and no screening procedures are currently recommended.[4]

The typical clinical presentation is with a suspicious pelvic mass, and/or abdominal distention with ascites. Staging investigations should include a complete blood count, chemistry profile with liver and renal function, serum CA 125 level, chest X-ray, and an abdominal-pelvic ultrasound or computerized tomography (CT). Surgical staging requires a laparotomy with a thorough examination of the abdominal cavity.[1] For early stage disease, FIGO I and IIA, surgery should involve total abdominal hysterectomy, bilateral salpingo-oophorectomy with omentectomy, staging biopsies, and at least sampling of the para-aortic and pelvic nodes. In younger patients with clinical Ia or Ic tumors wishing to conserve fertility, a unilateral salpingo-oophorectomy should be considered. In clinical stage II, III, and IV patients, management options include either cytoreductive surgery or alternatively neoadjuvant chemotherapy with interval cytoreduction in bulky stage III/IV disease particularly in nonsurgical candidates.[5]

OVARIAN CANCER

The stage and histologic type differentiating between malignant and borderline (low malignant potential) epithelial ovarian tumors are essential prognostic factors. Borderline tumors represent 5–10% of ovarian neoplasms and are mainly diagnosed in an

Prognostic Factors in Cancer, Third Edition, edited by Mary K. Gospodarowicz,
Brian O'Sullivan, and Leslie H. Sobin.

early stage with overall 5-year survival ranging from 85 to 95%. Prognosis for border-line tumors depends on disease extent as well as the histological subtype (primary tumor and extraovarian implants). Subgroups of borderline tumors with poor prognosis include advanced-stage mucinous tumors and micropapillary serous carcinoma (MPSC). Endocervical mucinous borderline tumor (EMBT) fare better compared with the intestinal mucinous borderline tumor (IMBT) and rare mixed epithelial borderline tumor (MEBT).[6]

Older age and poor performance status may impair the ability to undergo more aggressive treatment and are therefore associated with poorer outcome.[7] Patients treated by a trained gynecologic oncologist live better and longer than those treated by a general obstetrician–gynecologist or general surgeon.[1]

Histological grade is an additional prognostic factor, although a universal grading system has not been agreed upon.[1,3] DNA ploidy of frankly malignant ovarian carcinomas is prognostic, with aneuploid tumors conferring a worse prognosis compared with diploid tumors. Lymph-node involvement *per se* has a lesser impact on prognosis than intra-abdominal spread. In response to chemotherapy, both the half-life and absolute serum CA125 level correlates significantly with survival and with tumor regression.[8] The role of BRCA1 in nonfamilial ovarian cancers, which represent the vast majority of these diseases, is not yet clear.[9]

Ultraradical surgery typically entailing partial bowel resection is beneficial only if the patient can be rendered free of any gross residual disease. The role of pelvic and para-aortic lymphadenectomy remains controversial, although survival appears superior with FIGO stage IIIC with positive lymph-node disease compared to intra-abdominal spread.[10] For FIGO stage IIB–IIIC disease, upfront maximal surgical effort at cytoreduction with the goal of no residual disease affords improved survival. If initial maximal cytoreduction was not performed, interval debulking surgery (IDS) should be considered in patients responding to combined taxane plus platinum chemotherapy. This approach has demonstrated survival benefits for patients with suboptimally as well as optimally debulked disease, however, long-term follow-up is required for this approach to be considered standard. In addition, achieving a pathological complete remission after first-line chemotherapy is considered favorable.[11,12]

Cellular proliferative activity, reflected by mitotic counts, flow cytometric determination of the S-phase fraction, proliferation antigens, such as proliferating cell nuclear antigen—PCNA, and MIB-1 for detection of Ki-67 antigen, hold promise as future prognostic factors. Steroid receptor status, tumor angiogenesis markers, macrophage colony stimulating factors (CSF-1), and interleukin-6 (IL-6) have shown some promise.[13] Mutation of p53 and overexpression of mutant p53 products are much more common in advanced-stage (40–60%) than in early-stage disease (15%). Some studies have suggested that p53 overexpression in stage III–IV disease is associated with a 10–20% decrease in 5-year survival. Overexpression of c-erbB-2, ras, and myc oncogenes have been observed in a high number of ovarian cancer cases. LOH of the exons 21–23 on the long arm of the X chromosome independently correlates with reduced overall survival.[14–17] High levels of bikunin (an endogenous inhibitor of plasmin and other proteolytic enzymes) messenger ribonucleic acid (mRNA) in tumor tissue (mainly in tumor infiltrating macrophages) has been associated with improved prognosis regardless of stage, tumor size, histology and degree of differentiation.[18] The expression of human kallikrein (hK) gene family, hKs 6-10-11 has emerged as potential new serum biomarkers for ovarian cancer.[19]

FALLOPIAN TUBE CANCER

Carcinoma of the fallopian tube is a very rare neoplasm representing 0.3–1.1% of gynecologic malignancies. Its prevalence is 2.9–3.6 cases/1,000,000 women/year, thus limiting the possibility of a thorough analysis of potential prognostic factors. In 1991, the FIGO Committee on Gynecologic Oncology designed a specific staging classification for carcinoma of the fallopian tube, which was previously staged according to the ovarian cancer staging system.[1]

Stage represents the most important prognostic factor, with stage I patients demonstrating an 80% 5-year survival, with stage II, III, and IV 5-year survival rates of 50, 35, and 0%, respectively. Most fallopian tube carcinomas are serous adenocarcinomas, although histology *per se* has never been shown to be prognostic. The degree of differentiation and nuclear atypia as well as lymphatic spread are weakly prognostic. Pelvic, para-aortic, and groin lymph-node involvement is considered to represent regional metastases and are reported in 30–50% of cases undergoing primary surgery. Distant disease relapses, especially in the lymph nodes, is common.[20]

Surgical-pathological factors correlated with prognosis in early-stage patients include muscularis mucosa invasion compared to those limited to the mucosa. Improved prognosis was observed in patients with advanced disease who were administered chemotherapy. Among potential biological prognosis factors, ploidy and p53 overexpression have shown some promise, the latter particularly in stage 0 (carcinoma *in situ*).[20]

██████ **SUMMARY TABLES**

Prognostic Factors in Ovarian Cancer

Prognostic Factors	Tumor Related	Host Related	Environment Related
Essential	Stage Histology T category Grade Residual disease	Age Performance status	Quality of care— gynecologic oncologist
Additional	DNA ploidy (frankly malignant) N category CA125 Borderline tumors— residual disease	BRCA1 pCR at second look Resectability of recurrences/ metastases	Ultraradical surgery Lymphadenectomy (early stages) DDP + taxane based first-line chemotherapy
New and promising	Quantitative morphometric analyses Cellular proliferative activity Tumor angiogenesis Cytokines, chemokines, growth factors LOH p53 hK6-hK10-hK11	Bikunin derived from tumor-infiltrating macrophages	Interval debulking surgery (IDS) Intraperitoneal CT (low residual disease) Neoadjuvant chemotherapy

Sources:
• Staging classifications and clinical practise guidelines of gynaecological cancers by the FIGO Committee on Gynecologic Oncology and the International Gynecologic Cancer Society (IGCS) Guidelines Committee 2003.
http://www.figo.org/.
• NCCN Clinical Practice Guidelines in Oncology: Ovarian Cancer.
http://www.nccn.org/professionals/ physician_gls/PDF/ovarian.pdf.
• ESMO Minimum Clinical Recommendations for diagnosis, treatment and follow-up of epithelial ovarian carcinoma.
http://annonc.oupjournals.org/cgi/reprint/16/suppl_1/i13.

Prognostic Factors in Fallopian Tube Cancer

Prognostic Factors	Tumor Related	Host Related	Environment Related

Essential	Stage
	Residual disease
			Quality of care
			  gynecologic oncologist/
			  pathologist
			  obstetrician/
			  gynecologist
			  general surgeon
			Adjuvant Chemotherapy
			  (advanced stage)

Additional	Grade + degree of
	  nuclear atypia
	Histological type
	Lymph-node status
	Ploidy
	p53
	Depth of invasion
	  Closure of
	  fimbriated end
		Age (initial
		  stage)	

New and promising		p53 alterations	

REFERENCES

1. Heintz AP, Odicino F, Maisonneuve P, et al.: Carcinoma of the ovary. *Int J Gynaecol Obstet* 83:135–166, 2003.

2. Sobin L, Wittekind C, et al.: TNM classification of malignant tumors. 6th. ed. New York: Wiley-Liss; 2002.

3. *AJCC Cancer Staging Manual*. 6th ed. New York, Springer-Verlag, 2002.

4. du Bois A, Quinn M, Thigpen T, et al.: 2004 consensus statements on the management of ovarian cancer: final document of the 3rd International Gynecologic Cancer Intergroup Ovarian Cancer Consensus Conference (GCIG OCCC 2004). *Ann Oncol* 16:viii7–viii12, 2005.

5. Rose PG, Nerenstone S, Brady MF, et al.: Secondary surgical cytoreduction for advanced ovarian carcinoma. *N Engl J Med* 351:2489–2497, 2004.

6. Morice P, Camatte S, Rey A, et al.: Prognostic factors for patients with advanced stage serous borderline tumours of the ovary. *Ann Oncol* 14:592–598, 2003.

7. Chan JK, Loizzi V, Lin YG, et al.: Stages III and IV invasive epithelial ovarian carcinoma in younger versus older women: what prognostic factors are important? *Obstet Gynecol* 102:156–161, 2003.

8. Tate S, Hirai Y, Takeshima N, et al.: CA125 regression during neoadjuvant chemotherapy as an independent prognostic factor for survival in patients with advanced ovarian serous adenocarcinoma. *Gynecol Oncol* 96:143–149, 2005.

9. Nelson HD, Huffman LH, Fu R, et al.: Genetic risk assessment and BRCA mutation testing for breast and ovarian cancer susceptibility: systematic evidence review for the U.S. Preventive Services Task Force. *Ann Intern Med* 143:362–379, 2005.

10. Panici PB, Maggioni A, Hacker N, et al.: Systematic aortic and pelvic lymphadenectomy versus resection of bulky nodes only in optimally debulked advanced ovarian cancer: a randomized clinical trial. *J Natl Cancer Inst* 97:560–566, 2005.

11. Trimbos JB, Vergote I, Bolis G, et al.: Impact of adjuvant chemotherapy and surgical staging in early-stage ovarian carcinoma: European Organisation for Research and Treatment of Cancer-Adjuvant ChemoTherapy in Ovarian Neoplasm trial. *J Natl Cancer Inst* 95:113–125, 2003.

12. Shibata K, Kikkawa F, Mika M, et al.: Neoadjuvant chemotherapy for FIGO stage III or IV ovarian cancer: Survival benefit and prognostic factors. *Int J Gynecol Cancer* 13:587–592, 2003.

13. Ferrandina G, Lauriola L, Zannoni GF, et al.: Increased cyclooxygenase-2 (COX-2) expression is associated with chemotherapy resistance and outcome in ovarian cancer patients. *Ann Oncol* 13:1205–1211, 2002.

14. Nielsen JS, Jakobsen E, Holund B, et al.: Prognostic significance of p53, Her-2, and EGFR overexpression in borderline and epithelial ovarian cancer. *Int J Gynecol Cancer* 14:1086–1096, 2004.

15. Camilleri-Broet S, Hardy-Bessard AC, Le Tourneau A, et al.: HER-2 overexpression is an independent marker of poor prognosis of advanced primary ovarian carcinoma: a multicenter study of the GINECO group. *Ann Oncol* 15:104–112, 2004.

16. Skirnisdottir I, Seidal T, Sorbe B: A new prognostic model comprising p53, EGFR, and tumor grade in early stage epithelial ovarian carcinoma and avoiding the problem of inaccurate surgical staging. *Int J Gynecol Cancer* 14:259–270, 2004.

17. Hogdall EV, Ryan A, Kjaer SK, et al.: Loss of heterozygosity on the X chromosome is an independent prognostic factor in ovarian carcinoma: from the Danish "MALOVA" Ovarian Carcinoma Study. *Cancer* 100:2387–2395, 2004.

18. Matsuzaki H, Kobayashi H, Yagyu T, et al.: Plasma bikunin as a favorable prognostic factor in ovarian cancer. *J Clin Oncol* 23:1463–1472, 2005.

19. Borgono CA, Fracchioli S, Yousef GM, et al.: Favorable prognostic value of tissue human kallikrein 11 (hK11) in patients with ovarian carcinoma. *Int J Cancer* 106:605–610, 2003.

20. Baekelandt M, Jorunn Nesbakken A, Kristensen GB, et al.: Carcinoma of the fallopian tube. *Cancer* 89:2076–2084, 2000.

CHAPTER 31

Endometrial Cancer

FERNANDA G. HERRERA and MICHAEL F. MILOSEVIC

Endometrial cancer is diagnosed in ~142,000 women worldwide each year, and 42,000 associated deaths. There are at least two broad types of endometrial cancer based on differences in pathogenesis.[1] Type I endometrial cancer, comprising 90% of cases, is associated with prolonged estrogen stimulation and a favorable prognosis. In contrast, Type II endometrial cancer is estrogen independent and associated with a greater risk of recurrence and death. Overall, the 5-year survival of patients with endometrial cancer is ~80%.[2] The standard surgical treatment for early stage endometrial cancer is a total abdominal hysterectomy (TAH), bilateral salpingo-oophorectomy (BSO), with or without pelvic lymphadenectomy. Radiotherapy and chemotherapy may be used postoperatively to reduce the risk of recurrence.

Advanced age, beyond 70 or 80 years, is a strong independent predictor of poor prognosis.[2–5] High-body mass index (BMI) has been associated with an increased risk of death,[6] with diabetes mellitus and hypertension additional risk factors for type I endometrial cancer, at least in part because of their association with obesity. The effects of insulin resistance and insulin-like growth factors are under investigation.[7] The survival of African-American women with endometrial cancer is 25% lower than white women living in the United States (61.8 vs. 86.2%).[8]

The TNM 2002 classification for endometrial cancer parallels the International Federation of Gynecology and Obstetrics (FIGO) classification, and mandates surgical staging of all operable patients. Seventy to eighty percent are surgical stage I tumors at diagnosis. The 5-year overall survival rates for surgical stage I, II, III, and IV disease are 88, 75, 55, and 16%, respectively.[2] Endometrioid adenocarcinoma accounts for ~80% of cases. Serous and clear cell histologies are less common, but more likely to be associated with peritoneal or distant metastases and poor prognosis.[1,2] High histologic grade and deep myometrial invasion are independent adverse prognostic factors, particularly in endometrioid tumors. High grade or deeply invasive

Prognostic Factors in Cancer, Third Edition, edited by Mary K. Gospodarowicz, Brian O'Sullivan, and Leslie H. Sobin.

tumors are associated with a higher risk of pelvic lymph node involvement, disease recurrence, and reduced survival.[2,9,10] In stage I disease, 5-year overall survival ranges from 66% in high-grade disease involving the outer one-half of the myometrium, to 93% in grade I disease confined to the endometrium.[2] Histologic evidence of tumor invading vascular and lymphatic spaces is often seen in association with other adverse prognostic factors, including high-grade, deep invasion, and pelvis lymph node metastases, but is also an independent adverse prognostic factor.[9,11]

Metastases to pelvic and para-aortic lymph nodes are associated with a poor prognosis. The risk of nodal involvement increases with increasing histologic grade and depth of myometrial invasion (3% for grade 1 disease confined to the endometrium, 28% for grade 3 tumors that extend to the outer one-third of the myometrium[2]). Paraaortic metastases are seen in ~50% of patients with pelvic nodal involvement.[2] The presence of extrauterine disease is associated with a high risk of recurrence and lower survival. Positive peritoneal cytology has been linked to poor outcome, but largely due to its association with other adverse surgico-pathologic factors.[12] Positive cytology as the only manifestation of extra-uterine disease is clinically inconsequential.[13] Distant metastases carry a uniformly poor prognosis.

PTEN is a tumor suppressor gene that is overexpressed in the setting of high-estrogen levels. Loss of PTEN function is an early event in the carcinogenesis of type I endometrial cancer, and has been associated with more advanced disease at presentation.[14] Abnormalities of the KRAS2 oncogene and defects in DNA mismatched repair are also seen in type I cancers.[1] Mutations of the p53 tumor suppressor gene occur late in the development of type I tumors, but early in type II tumors, and have been associated with aggressive clinical behavior and poor survival.[14] Overexpression of HER-2/neu may be an important step in the hormone-independent growth of type II disease and carries a poor prognosis.[15] Hypoxia-inducible factor 1α (HIF-1α) expression has been identified in ~50% of patients with stage I endometrial cancer and has independent adverse prognostic significance.[16] High levels of the angiogenic protein vascular endothelial growth factor (VEGF-D) and its receptor (VEGFR-3) may both be independent adverse prognostic factors.[17]

It is not known whether all patients with endometrial cancer should undergo lymphadenectomy, or alternatively whether the procedure should be confined to those at greatest risk of harboring occult nodal metastases. Lymphadenectomy may or may not have a direct therapeutic effect on patient survival. The role of postoperative radiotherapy in the management of endometrial cancer is currently evolving. There have been two recent phase III trials of postoperative radiotherapy in patients with[5] and without[4] lymph node dissection at the time of surgery. Both showed ~60% reduction in the risk of pelvic recurrence with radiotherapy relative to surgery alone, but no difference in overall survival. Many of the recurrences in the surgery only arms were confined to the upper vagina and might have been prevented with postoperative vaginal brachytherapy.[5,18] Isolated vaginal recurrences can be salvaged with radiotherapy at the time of recurrence.[19] Overall postoperative radiotherapy is important in minimizing the morbidity associated with uncontrolled pelvic disease.[4] Hormonal treatment with progestational agents may be beneficial in patients with recurrent disease. Cytotoxic chemotherapy is being investigated both as adjuvant treatment for patients with advanced disease at presentation, and for recurrence.[1,2]

■■■■■■ **SUMMARY TABLE**

Prognostic Factors in Endometrial Cancer

Prognostic Factors	Tumor Related	Host Related	Environment Related
Essential	pT category cN category M category Histologic type Grade		
Additional	pN category Lymphovascular space invasion	Age Race Comorbidities	Adjuvant radiation in intermediate and high-risk patients
New and promising	KRAS2, HER-2/neu PTEN, p53 HIF-1α, VEGF		

Source:
• Clinical Practice Guidelines for Endometrial Carcinoma. National Comprehensive Cancer Network NCCN, 2005.
http://www.nccn.org/proffesionals/physicians_gls/PDF/uterine.pdf.

REFERENCES

1. Amant F, Moerman P, Neven P, et al.: Endometrial cancer. *Lancet* 366:491–505, 2005.
2. Creasman WT, Odicino F, Maisonneuve P, et al.: Carcinoma of the corpus uteri. *Int J Gynaecol Obstet* 83:79–118, 2003.
3. Alektiar KM, Venkatraman E, Abu-Rustum N, et al.: Is endometrial carcinoma intrinsically more aggressive in elderly patients? *Cancer* 98:2368–2377, 2003.
4. Creutzberg CL, van Putten WL, Koper PC, et al.: Surgery and postoperative radiotherapy versus surgery alone for patients with stage-1 endometrial carcinoma: multicentre randomised trial. PORTEC Study Group. Post Operative Radiation Therapy in Endometrial Carcinoma. *Lancet* 355:1404–1411, 2000.
5. Keys HM, Roberts JA, Brunetto VL, et al.: A phase III trial of surgery with or without adjunctive external pelvic radiation therapy in intermediate risk endometrial adenocarcinoma: a Gynecologic Oncology Group study. *Gynecol Oncol* 92:744–751, 2004.
6. Calle EE, Rodriguez C, Walker-Thurmond K, et al.: Overweight, obesity, and mortality from cancer in a prospectively studied cohort of U.S. adults. *N Engl J Med* 348:1625–1638, 2003.

7. Berstein LM, Kvatchevskaya JO, Poroshina TE, et al.: Insulin resistance, its consequences for the clinical course of the disease, and possibilities of correction in endometrial cancer. *J Cancer Res Clin Oncol* 130:687–693, 2004.

8. SEER Cancer Statistics Review, 1975–2002. National Cancer, Institute, 2002.

9. Benedet JL, Miller AM: Endometrial Cancer, in Gospodarowicz MK, Henson DE, Hutter RVP, et al. (eds.): *Prognostic Factors in Cancer*. 2nd ed. New York, Wiley-Liss, 2001.

10. Mariani A, Webb MJ, Keeney GL, et al.: Surgical stage I endometrial cancer: predictors of distant failure and death. *Gynecol Oncol* 87:274–280, 2002.

11. Briet JM, Hollema H, Reesink N, et al.: Lymphvascular space involvement: an independent prognostic factor in endometrial cancer. *Gynecol Oncol* 96:799–804, 2005.

12. Mariani A, Webb MJ, Keeney GL, et al.: Endometrial cancer: predictors of peritoneal failure. *Gynecol Oncol* 89:236–242, 2003.

13. Tebeu PM, Popowski Y, Verkooijen HM, et al.: Positive peritoneal cytology in early-stage endometrial cancer does not influence prognosis. *Br J Cancer* 91:720–724, 2004.

14. Salvesen HB, Akslen LA: Molecular pathogenesis and prognostic factors in endometrial carcinoma. *APMIS* 110:673–689 2002.

15. Mariani A, Sebo TJ, Katzmann JA, et al.: HER-2/neu overexpression and hormone dependency in endometrial cancer: analysis of cohort and review of literature. *Anticancer Res* 25:2921–2007, 2005.

16. Sivridis E, Giatromanolaki A, Gatter KC, et al.: Association of hypoxia-inducible factors 1alpha and 2alpha with activated angiogenic pathways and prognosis in patients with endometrial carcinoma. *Cancer* 95:1055–1063, 2002.

17. Yokoyama Y, Charnock-Jones DS, Licence D, et al.: Expression of vascular endothelial growth factor (VEGF)-D and its receptor, VEGF receptor 3, as a prognostic factor in endometrial carcinoma. *Clin Cancer Res* 9:1361–1369, 2003.

18. Solhjem MC, Petersen IA, Haddock MG: Vaginal brachytherapy alone is sufficient adjuvant treatment of surgical stage I endometrial cancer. *Int J Radiat Oncol Biol Phys* 62:1379–1384, 2005.

19. Creutzberg CL, van Putten WL, Koper PC, et al.: Survival after relapse in patients with endometrial cancer: results from a randomized trial. *Gynecol Oncol* 89:201–209, 2003.

CHAPTER 32

Gestational Trophoblastic Disease

HEXTAN Y.S. NGAN, KAREN K.L. CHAN, and KEVIN F. TAM

Gestational trophoblastic disease (GTD) is a disease of the proliferative trophoblastic allografts and includes partial mole (PM), complete hydatidiform mole (CM), invasive mole, metastatic mole, choriocarcinoma (CC), placental site trophoblastic tumor (PSTT), and epithelioid trophoblastic tumor (ETT). While CC, PSTT, and ETT are definitely neoplastic, the various types of molar pregnancies are basically benign, but with a potential to behave like a malignant disease. This potential malignant behavior is identified by the failure of regression of the human chorionic gonadotrophin (hCG) in the absence of a normal pregnancy and is termed gestational trophoblastic neoplasia (GTN). GTN may be diagnosed when the plateau of HCG lasts for four measurements over a period of 3 weeks or longer (days 1, 7, 14, 21); or when there is a rise in HCG of 3 weekly consecutive measurements or longer, over at least a period of 2 weeks (days 1, 7, 14); or when the HCG level remains elevated for 6 months or more; or if there is a histological diagnosis of CC.[1] In GTN, unlike other solid malignancies, metastasis does not always mean poor prognosis. If the metastatic lesion is a mole rather than CC, the prognosis is much better. Histological confirmation, however, is uncommon because most cases of GTN are treated with chemotherapy. Thus other prognostic factors in addition to metastasis have to be taken into consideration in assessing the prognosis in GTN.

The prognostic factors of GTN are age, serum human chorionic gonadotrophin level (hCG), interval from treatment to antecedent pregnancy, size, number, and site (liver and brain) of metastatic lesions, type of antecedent pregnancies and previous treatment with chemotherapy. These are included and weighted in the FIGO 2000 staging and classification system.[1] Choriocarcinoma tends to be aggressive and should be treated aggressively. New prognostic factors include Doppler ultrasonography of the uterine artery, apoptotic activities, and Mcl-1 expression.[2–4] PSTT arises from the intermediate trophoblasts and behaves quite differently from that of GTN.

Prognostic Factors in Cancer, Third Edition, edited by Mary K. Gospodarowicz, Brian O'Sullivan, and Leslie H. Sobin.
Copyright © 2006 John Wiley & Sons, Inc.

The main prognostic factors are the presence of lung metastasis and the last known pregnancy >4 years prior to presentation with PSTT.[5] Epithelial trophoblastic tumor is a rare GTD and has a similar behavior to that of PSTT.

GTN is treated by chemotherapy. Appropriate treatment includes early prompt treatment, as well as the use of effective regimens. It is essential to monitor the serum hCG of patients with molar pregnancy, since ≈6–36% of moles progress to GTN. Since early diagnosis and treatment is most difficult in GTN following normal pregnancy, a high index of suspicion is important and pregnancy tests should be performed for unexplained irregular bleeding and a solitary lung nodule or unusual cerebral signs in a young woman.

Using the FIGO 2000 scoring system,[1] GTN is categorized into low- and high-risk groups. The UICC[6] has adopted the FIGO staging and scoring system and in addition to a score, a staging system based on tumor extension outside the uterus and the presence of metastasis outside the lung was adopted.[1] Treatment of low-risk GTN stage I-III: score <7 is by single agent chemotherapy.[7–9] Methotrexate is most widely used and actinomycin-D can be considered if there is liver impairment. Other drugs include 5-FU and etoposide. High-risk GTN, stage II-IV: score >6, should be treated by multiple-agent chemotherapy.[7] Various studies have shown poor outcome with the use of only single agent therapy in high-risk disease. Inadequate chemotherapy also allows for the emergence of drug-resistant tumor refractory to subsequent treatment. EMA-CO (etoposide + methotrexate + dactinomycin and vincristine + cyclophosphamide) is a widely used regimen. Alternative regimens have included MAC: methotrexate, actinomycin-D, cyclophosphamide; and CHAMOC: cyclophosphamide, hydroxyurea, actinomycin-D, methotrexate, vincristine. For a resistant tumor or in the setting of relapsed disease, the EMA-CE regimen in which etoposide and cisplatin are substituted for vincristine and cyclophosphamide in the EMA-CO regimen; APE (dactinomycin, cisplatin, etoposide); PVB (cisplatin, vinblastine, bleomycin); PEBA (cisplatin, etoposide, bleomycin, adriamycin); MBE: (methotrexate, bleomycin, etoposide), and carboplatin/taxol can be considered. Ifosfamide, carboplatin, etoposide with autologous bone marrow transplant have been used, but are associated with significant toxicity and should be used cautiously.

In order to achieve the best outcomes, high-risk patients should ideally be treated in centers specialized in treating GTN. Surgery plays a role in the removal of solitary tumor in drug resistant cases or in the emergency setting with hemorrhage from brain, liver, or uterine sites. In suitable cases, embolization of feeding vessels, such as the uterine arteries can spare a definitive operation and thus retain a patient's reproductive potential. Although radiotherapy has a limited role, it may be indicated to prevent or decrease hemorrhage from brain or liver metastases.

There is increasing evidence that the spectrum of gestational trophoblastic disease is characterized by altered expression of several growth regulatory factors and oncogenes.[10] These include factors involved in the antigenic relationships between normal placenta, molar pregnancy, and gestational choriocarcinoma. In addition, the expression of proto-oncogenes (e.g., MDM2, EGFR, c-erb-2,3,4 and bcl-2), tumor suppressor genes (e.g., TP53, p21, RB and DOC-2/hDab2), and other growth factors have been implicated in trophoblast cellular proliferation. Cell adhesion molecules including matrix-degrading proteases (e.g., serine proteases and matrix metalloproteinases, MMPs), which are thought to influence the implantation and invasion of normal and abnormal trophoblastic cells, have also been implicated.[10] These new and promising factors may, in the future, have both prognostic and therapeutic consequences.

TABLE 32.1   FIGO Scoring System for Gestational Trophoblastic Neoplasia (Ref. 1)[a]

FIGO Scoring	0	1	2	4
Age	<40	$\geqslant40$		
Antecedent pregnancy	Mole	Abortion	Term	
Interval months from index pregnancy	<4	$4-<7$	$7-<13$	$\geqslant13$
Pre-treatment serum hCG (IU/L)	$<10^3$	$10^3-<10^4$	$10^4-<10^5$	$\geqslant10^5$
Largest tumor size (including uterus) cm	<3	$3-<5$	$\geqslant5$	
Site of metastases	Lung	Spleen, kidney	Gastrointestinal	Liver, brain
Number of metastases		1–4	5–8	>8
Previous failed chemotherapy			Single drug	2 or more drugs

[a]Low-risk score <7.
High-risk score $\geqslant7$.

■■■■■■ **SUMMARY TABLE**

Prognostic Factors in Gestational Trophoblastic Disease

Prognostic Factors	Tumor Related	Host Related	Environment Related
Essential	HCG Site of metastasis Number of metastatic sites	Antecedent pregnancy Time interval	Prior chemotherapy
Additional	Tumor size Number of metastasis	Age	
New and promising	Uterine pulsatility index		

Sources:
• Society of Obstetricians and Gynecologists of Canada. Gestational Trophoblastic Disease Clinical Practice Guidelines 2002.
http://www.sogc.org/sogcnet/sogc_docs/common/guide/pdfs/ps114.pdf.
• Staging classifications and clinical practice guidelines of gynaecologic cancers
http://www.igcs.org/guidelines/guideline_staging-booklet.pdf.p119–142, 2003.
• National Cancer Institute: Gestational Trophoblastic Disease (PDQ®): 2005.
http://www.cancer.gov/cancertopics/pdq/treatment/gestationaltrophoblastic/healthprofessional/.
• British Columbia Cancer Agency Cancer Management Guidelines.
http://www.bccancer.bc.ca/HPI/CancerManagementGuidelines/Gynecology/GestationalTrophoblastic Neoplasia/default.htm.

REFERENCES

1. FIGO Oncology Committee: FIGO staging for gestational trophoblastic neoplasia 2000. FIGO Oncology Committee. *Int J Gynaecol Obstet* 77:285–287, 2002.

2. Agarwal R, Strickland S, McNeish IA, et al: Doppler ultrasonography of the uterine artery and the response to chemotherapy in patients with gestational trophoblastic tumors. *Clin Cancer Res* 8:1142–1147, 2002.

3. Fong PY, Xue WC, Ngan HY, et al.: Mcl-1 expression in gestational trophoblastic disease correlates with clinical outcome: a differential expression study. *Cancer* 103:268–276, 2005.

4. Chiu PM, Ngan YS, Khoo US, et al.: Apoptotic activity in gestational trophoblastic disease correlates with clinical outcome: assessment by the caspase-related M30 CytoDeath anti-body. *Histopathology* 38:243–249, 2001.

5. Papadopoulos AJ, Foskett M, Seckl MJ, et al.: Twenty-five years' clinical experience with placental site trophoblastic tumors. *J Reprod Med* 47:460–464, 2002.

6. Sobin LH, Wittekind C: TNM classification of malignant tumors (6th ed.), New York, Wiley-Liss, 2002.

7. Gestational Trophoblastic Disease (PDQ®): Treatment Guidelines. National Cancer Institute, U.S., 2003. http://www.cancer.gov/cancertopics/pdq/treatment/gestationaltrophoblastic/healthprofessional/.

8. Staging classifications and clinical practice guidelines of gynaecological cancers by the FIGO Committee on Gynecologic Oncology and the International Gynecologic Cancer Society (IGCS) Guidelines Committee, 2003. http://www.figo.org/.

9. British Columbia Cancer Agency Cancer Management Guidelines: British Columbia Cancer Agency, Canada, 2001. http://www.bccancer.bc.ca/HPI/CancerManagementGuidelines/Gynecology/GestationalTrophoblasticNeoplasia/default.htm.

10. Fulop V, Mok SC, Berkowitz RS: Molecular biology of gestational trophoblastic neoplasia: a review. *J Reprod Med* 49:415–422, 2004.

UROLOGICAL TUMORS

CHAPTER 33

Penile Cancer

SIMON HORENBLAS and JUANITA M. CROOK

Carcinoma of the penis is a rare malignancy, accounting for <1% of urological cancers in males. The vast majority (95%) are squamous cell carcinomas (SCC). Rare disorders like melanoma and soft tissue sarcomas will not be considered. Most information regarding the clinical course and prognostic factors is based on relatively few retrospective series; there are no known prospective clinical trials for penile cancer. The TNM system is the most widely used staging classification.[1]

Size of the tumor has been replaced by depth of infiltration as a classification criterion of the primary tumor. Despite prognostic significance of size alone, infiltration is considered more important with respect to local and regional recurrence.[2,3] In the clinic, it is not always easy to judge the depth of infiltration. On average, a 25% difference is seen between clinical and pathological classification.[3] Application of newer imaging modalities, such as magnetic resonance imaging (MRI) may improve staging accuracy.[4] Regional lymph-node involvement is the most important prognostic factor for survival. Five-year survival for patients without lymph node involvement is >90%. Cure can be achieved in patients with single nodal metastasis in 75%, decreasing to 20% in patients with multiple lymph-node metastases.[5]

The sentinel node biopsy in clinically node-negative patients with penile cancer is useful.[6,7] Five-year disease-specific survival is 96% and 66% for patients with a tumor negative versus positive sentinel node (p = 0.001).[8] The early resection of occult inguinal metastases detected on dynamic sentinel node biopsy is an independent prognostic factor for disease specific survival (p = 0.006).[9] Disease specific 3-year survival of patients with positive lymph nodes detected during surveillance was only 35% as compared to 84% for those who underwent early resection (log rank p = 0.0017).[8]

The solid and cord pattern of histologic growth have been abandoned in favor of superficial spreading, vertical, multicentric, and verrucous patterns. These have been added to the WHO histological classification of tumors of the penis.[10] Growth pattern is

Prognostic Factors in Cancer, *Third Edition*, edited by Mary K. Gospodarowicz, Brian O'Sullivan, and Leslie H. Sobin.
Copyright © 2006 John Wiley & Sons, Inc.

related to regional metastatic involvement. The metastatic rate is 82% in vertical-growth carcinoma in contrast to no evidence of metastasis in verrucous carcinoma. The most common pattern is the superficial spreading type (42%), followed by vertical growth (32%). In combination with pathologic tumor stage, and presence of >50% poorly differentiated cancer, vascular invasion is the strongest predictor of nodal metastasis.[11,12] Paradoxically, despite easy access to the bloodstream through invasion into the spongiosus–cavernous tissue, hematogenous dissemination is uncommon, and is always preceded by lymphatic spread.

Grade has predictive value for the presence of regional metastasis. Elective lymph-node dissection has been justified on the basis of high probability of occult metastasis in poorly differentiated SCC-tumors.[5,13,14] Grade and lymphatic involvement are independent prognostic factors for survival.[15] The 5-year survival for poorly differentiated tumors is 47%, in contrast to 79 and 68% in well- and moderately differentiated tumors, respectively. Solsona et al. assessed the predictive value of grade for lymph-node involvement. While grade by itself was not predictive, the combination of corpus cavernosum invasion and poor differentiation was associated with an 80% incidence of lymphatic invasion.

The exact depth of penetration has been proposed as a classification criterion. The threshold for penile metastasis is ~4–6 mm invasion into the corpus spongiosum.[16] Currently, infiltration into the various structures of the penis is considered to be a classification criterion in the TNM classification.[2] Hematogenous spread is a late event in the natural history of SCC of the penis and is always preceded by lymphatic spread.

An association of overexpression of p53, Ki-67, and COX-2 with poor prognosis has been documented.[17–19] Ploidy does not add significant prognostic information.[20]

Based on the International Agency for Research on Cancer data, the incidence rates vary from 0.4 to 0.9/100,000 in developed countries to as high as 7.9/100,000 in less developing nations. Possible explanations include: access to healthcare, difference in hygiene related to water supply, difference in sexual attitude, and difference in smoking habits. The infrequency of penile cancer after neonatal circumcision is well documented.[21] Neonatal circumcision is associated with a three-fold decrease in risk of penile carcinoma, although in some series up to 20% of cases had been circumcised neonatally.[22] Circumcision at infancy prevents the most prominent finding associated with penile cancer: an unretractable foreskin and the associated irritation and infection. Reported incidence of phimosis in men with penile cancer range from 42 to 92%. A Swedish case-control study of 244 men with penile cancer estimated that 45% suffered at least one episode of balanitis in contrast to 8% in the control group.[23] In this study, phimosis and balanitis were significant independent risk factors. Studies in China and India, using multivariate analyses, corroborate these findings.

Recent findings on the oncogenic potential of the sexually transmittable human papilloma viruses (HPV) have renewed interest and research in its role in penile carcinoma. The overall incidence of HPV in penile carcinoma is 40–45% as detected by PCR (polymerase chain reaction) amplification of DNA HPV 16 and 18.[24,25]

There is epidemiological evidence to support an association between smoking and anogenital SCC.[26,27] The majority of studies indicate that smoking close to the time of diagnosis is associated with an increase in risk, which supports the hypothesis that smoking has a late-stage or promotional role.

For patients treated with primary radiation therapy, interstitial brachytherapy results in a higher rate of penile preservation. For external radiation, fraction sizes <2 Gy, treatment interruptions, and total doses <60 Gy are to be avoided.[28]

There is optimism that new prognostic factors will emerge. Analysis of microarray data and proteomics should yield new insight into the genetic make up of various types of tumors.

▮▮▮ SUMMARY TABLE

Prognostic Factors in Penile Cancer

Prognostic Factors	Tumor Related	Host Related	Environment Related
Essential	Depth of invasion T category N category M category Grade		
Additional	Lymphovascular invasion Histology p53 Ki67	Phimosis	Presence of HPV Smoking Radiation dose/ fractionation
New and promising	Microarray Proteomics		

Sources:
• National Cancer Institute: Penile Cancer (PDQ®): Treatment Guidelines 2005.
http://www. cancer. gov/cancertopics/pdq/treatment/penile/healthprofessional/.
• The Management of Penile Cancer 2000.
http://www.sua.org.sg/whatsnew/whatsnew_penis.htm.

REFERENCES

1. Sobin LH, Wittekind Ch (eds.), UICC: *TNM Classification of malignant tumors.* 6th ed. New York, Wiley-Liss, 2002.
2. Solsona E, Iborra I, Rubio J, et al.: Prospective validation of the association of local tumor stage and grade as a predictive factor for occult lymph node micrometastasis in patients with penile carcinoma and clinically negative inguinal lymph nodes. *J Urol* 165: 1506, 2001.
3. Horenblas S, van Tinteren H, Delemarre J F, et al.: Squamous cell carcinoma of the penis: accuracy of tumor, nodes and metastasis classification system, and role of lymphangiography, computerized tomography scan and fine needle aspiration cytology. *J Urol* 146: 1279, 1991.

4. Lont A P, Besnard A P, Gallee M P, et al.: A comparison of physical examination and imaging in determining the extent of primary penile carcinoma. *BJU Int* 91: 493, 2003.

5. Horenblas S, van Tinteren H: Squamous cell carcinoma of the penis. IV. Prognostic factors of survival: analysis of tumor, nodes and metastasis classification system. *J Urol* 151: 1239, 1994.

6. Tanis P J, Lont A P, Meinhardt W, et al.: Dynamic sentinel node biopsy for penile cancer: reliability of a staging technique. *J Urol* 168: 76, 2002.

7. Valdes Olmos R A, Tanis P J, Hoefnagel C A, et al.: Penile lymphoscintigraphy for sentinel node identification. *Eur J Nucl Med* 28: 581, 2001.

8. Kroon B K, Horenblas S, Meinhardt W, et al.: Dynamic sentinel node biopsy in penile carcinoma: evaluation of 10 years experience. *Eur Urol* 47: 601, 2005.

9. Kroon B K, Horenblas S, Lont A P, et al.: Patients with penile carcinoma benefit from immediate resection of clinically occult lymph node metastases. *J Urol* 173: 816, 2005.

10. Cubilla A L, Dillner J, Schellhammer F, et al.: Tumours of the penis. In: Pathology and genetics of tumours of the urinary system and male genital organs. Eble J N, Sauter G, Epstein J I, et al. (eds.): Lyon, IARC Press, Chapt. 5, 2004, p. 279.

11. Slaton J W, Morgenstern N, Levy D A, et al.: Tumor stage, vascular invasion and the percentage of poorly differentiated cancer: independent prognosticators for inguinal lymph node metastasis in penile squamous cancer. *J Urol* 165: 1138, 2001.

12. Ficarra V, Zattoni F, Cunico S C, et al.: Lymphatic and vascular embolizations are independent predictive variables of inguinal lymph node involvement in patients with squamous cell carcinoma of the penis: Gruppo Uro-Oncologico del Nord Est (Northeast Uro-Oncological Group) Penile Cancer data base data. *Cancer* 103: 2507, 2005.

13. Solsona E, Algaba F, Horenblas S, et al.: EAU Guidelines on Penile Cancer. *Eur Urol* 46: 1, 2004.

14. Crook J M, Jezioranski J, Grimard L, et al.: Penile brachytherapy: results for 49 patients. *Int J Radiat Oncol Biol Phys* 62: 460, 2005.

15. Horenblas S, van Tinteren H, Delemarre J F, et al.: Squamous cell carcinoma of the penis. III. Treatment of regional lymph nodes. *J Urol* 149: 492, 1993.

16. Cubilla A L, Piris A, Pfannl R, et al.: Anatomic levels: important landmarks in penectomy specimens: a detailed anatomic and histologic study based on examination of 44 cases. *Am J Surg Pathol* 25: 1091, 2001.

17. Berdjis N, Meye A, Nippgen J, et al.: Expression of Ki-67 in squamous cell carcinoma of the penis. *BJU Inter* 96: 146, 2005.

18. Golijanin D, Tan J Y, Kazior A, et al.: Cyclooxygenase-2 and microsomal prostaglandin E synthase-1 are overexpressed in squamous cell carcinoma of the penis. *Clin Cancer Res* 10: 1024, 2004.

19. Lopes A, Bezerra A L, Pinto C A, et al.: p53 as a new prognostic factor for lymph node metastasis in penile carcinoma: analysis of 82 patients treated with amputation and bilateral lymphadenectomy. *J Urol* 168: 81, 2002.

20. Gustafsson O, Tribukait B, Nyman C R, et al.: DNA pattern and histopathology in carcinoma of the penis. A prospective study. *Scand J Urol Nephrol Suppl* 110: 219, 1988.

21. Lerman S E, Liao J C: Neonatal circumcision. *Pediatr Clin North Am* 48: 1539, 2001.

22. Dillner J, von Krogh G, Horenblas S, et al.: Etiology of squamous cell carcinoma of the penis. *Scand J Urol Nephrol Suppl* 189: 189–193, 2000.

23. Hellberg D, Valentin J, Eklund T, et al.: Penile cancer: is there an epidemiological role for smoking and sexual behaviour? *Br Med J (Clin Res ed)* 295: 1306, 1987.

24. Gross G, Pfister H: Role of human papillomavirus in penile cancer, penile intraepithelial squamous cell neoplasias and in genital warts. *Med Microbiol Immunol (Berlin)* 193: 35, 2004.

25. Bezerra A L, Lopes A, Santiago G H, et al.: Human papillomavirus as a prognostic factor in carcinoma of the penis: analysis of 82 patients treated with amputation and bilateral lymphadenectomy. *Cancer* 91: 2315, 2001.

26. Daling J R, Sherman K J, Hislop T G, et al.: Cigarette smoking and the risk of anogenital cancer. *Am J Epidemiol* 135: 180, 1992.

27. Harish K, Ravi R: The role of tobacco in penile carcinoma. *Br J Urol* 75: 375, 1995.

28. Sarin R, Norman A R, Steel G G, et al.: Treatment results and prognostic factors in 101 men treated for squamous carcinoma of the penis. *Int J Radiat Oncol Biol Phys* 38: 713, 1997.

CHAPTER 34

Prostate Cancer

LOUIS J. DENIS and PADRAIG R. WARDE

Prostate cancer is an extremely common malignancy with estimated 679,000 new cases diagnosed worldwide in 2002 and 221,000 deaths.[1] The UICC TNM classification is the means by which prostate cancer is staged and prognosis defined at diagnosis.[2] The other main prognostic factors include prostate specific antigen (PSA) and Gleason score.[3] Patient assessment should include history including family history, comorbidity, urinary function, symptoms suggesting metastasis, and physical examination including digital rectal exam. Serum PSA level and the Gleason score should be ascertained and depending on their levels, bone scan or computerized tomography (CT) of the abdomen and pelvis may be indicated.

Treatment approaches include active monitoring, hormone therapy, radical prostatectomy (RP), brachytherapy, or external beam radiotherapy (EBRT), depending on tumor and patient characteristics. Estimated life expectancy is an important factor in determining local treatment choice. Randomized clinical trials have shown the efficacy of adjunctive hormonal therapy in patients with locally advanced disease (T3–T4) treated with radiation therapy. In metastatic disease (M1 or N1), hormonal therapy is the mainstay of treatment. Chemotherapy has recently been shown to prolong survival in patients with hormone refractory disease and its role as adjuvant therapy in localized disease is currently being assessed.[4]

The local disease extent has been demonstrated to be an independent marker of prognosis.[3] It is assessed by digital rectal examination and described by T category. Other methods of assessment of local extent including magnetic resonance imaging (MRI) with or without endorectal coil may be of value.[5] Histologic grade plays a key role in determining progression and overall survival.[6] The Gleason system is the preferred grading system.[6] Other histopathologic factors include DNA ploidy, presence of perineural invasion, and percent positive cores on needle biopsy.[7] The most promising is percent positive cores.[8] The PSA is useful in the

Prognostic Factors in Cancer, Third Edition, edited by Mary K. Gospodarowicz, Brian O'Sullivan, and Leslie H. Sobin.

diagnosis and monitoring of prostate cancer. A number of PSA variables have been proposed to increase the sensitivity including the "percent free PSA". The PSA velocity and doubling time are valuable predictors in recurrent and hormone refractory disease.[9–11]

The presence of pelvic lymph node involvement correlates clearly with outcome.[12] The number of involved lymph nodes and lymph node density (the number of positive lymph nodes divided by the total number of lymph nodes removed), are also important in determining prognosis. Surgical margin status after radical prostatectomy has also been demonstrated to be an independent predictor of patient outcome and tumor volume (extent) is currently being evaluated.[13] In androgen-independent prostate cancer (AIPC), time to PSA recurrence, nadir PSA on androgen deprivation therapy, and PSA doubling time have been identified as significant risk factors for cancer specific survival in a cohort of men who had never been treated with cytotoxic chemotherapy.[14] Other factors including lactate dehydrogenase, alkaline phosphatase, Gleason score, performance status, age, hemoglobin presence and extent of visceral disease, and extent of osseous involvement have also been suggested to have prognostic importance in AIPC.[15,16]

Age at diagnosis is not a prognostic factor in localized disease.[17] The presence of significant comorbid illnesses has a definite impact on outcome.[18]

There are major geographic variations in prostate cancer death rates and some studies have suggested that inferior access to healthcare by lower socioeconomic groups is the main contributor to this disparity in prostate cancer mortality.[19] Access to quality care clearly influences outcome and higher procedure volumes, both at the physician and institution level, have been associated with improved patient outcomes.[20] Other factors such as the ability to achieve clear surgical margins, or use of appropriate radiation dose have been shown to affect results.[21,22]

Genomic- and proteomic-based studies have led to the identification of a large number of candidate biomarkers in prostate cancer. The potential prognostic use of new markers (both in malignant and nonmalignant tissues and body fluids) has recently been reviewed and includes microvessel density, growth factors, markers of proliferation/apoptosis (e.g., Bcl-2), as well as genomic alterations (e.g., chromosome 7, 8 gains/losses).[23,24] The most promising factors currently in the assessment of malignant tissue are microvessel density and Ki-67.[7,24]

The essential prognostic factors in prostate cancer include the anatomic disease extent as defined by TNM category, PSA level, and Gleason score. With the introduction of widespread early detection with PSA, a major shift in the proportion of patients presenting with early stage disease has been observed.[25] The identification of prognostic factors for disease progression in low grade, low PSA, early stage disease is critical in treatment selection. In patients with a high risk of relapse, the role of adjuvant chemotherapy and bisphosphonates is the key clinical issue. In hormone refractory and metastatic disease, the development of more effective systemic agents is the most important therapeutic challenge.

████████ **SUMMARY TABLE**

Prognostic Factors in Prostate Cancer

Prognostic Factors	Tumor Related	Host Related	Environment Related
Essential	TNM categories PSA Gleason Score		
Additional	PSA velocity PSA doubling time % positive biopsy DNA ploidy Margin status	Age Comorbidity Performance status	Access to care Quality of care
New and promising	Ki-67 MIB1 Microvessel density		

Sources:
• NCCN Clinical Practice Guidelines in Oncology: Prostate Cancer 2005.
http://www.nccn.org/professionals/physician_gls/PDF/prostate.pdf.
• British Columbia Cancer Agency Cancer Management Guidelines:Prostate 2004.
http://www.bccancer. bc.ca/HPI/CancerManagementGuidelines/Genitourinary/Prostate/default.htm.
• European Association Urology: Guidelines on Prostate Cancer 2005.
http://www.uroweb.org/files/ uploaded_files/2003_Prostate_Cancer_update.pdf.
• American Society of Clinical Oncology Recommendations for the Initial Hormonal Management of Androgen-Sensitive Metastatic, Recurrent, or Progressive Prostate Cancer 2004.
http://www.asco.org/asco/ downloads/JCO.2004.04.579v1.pdf.

REFERENCES

1. http://www-depdb.iarc.fr/globocan/GLOBOframe.htm:
2. Sobin LH, Wittekind C: UICC TNM classification of malignant tumours, 6th ed., New York, John Wiley & Sons, Inc., 2002.
3. D'Amico AV, Moul J, Carroll PR, et al.: Cancer-specific mortality after surgery or radiation for patients with clinically localized prostate cancer managed during the prostate-specific antigen era. *J Clin Oncol* 21:2163–2172, 2003.
4. Denis L, Bartsch G, Khoury S, et al.: Prostate Cancer. Paris, Health Publications, 2003.
5. Brassell SA, Rosner IL, McLeod DG: Update on magnetic resonance imaging, ProstaScint, and novel imaging in prostate cancer. *Curr Opin Urol* 15:163–166, 2005.

6. Amin M, Boccon-Gibod L, Egevad L, et al.: Prognostic and predictive factors and reporting of prostate carcinoma in prostate needle biopsy specimens. *Scand J Urol Nephrol* 39:20–33, 2005.

7. Ross JS, Sheehan CE, Dolen EM, et al.: Morphologic and molecular prognostic markers in prostate cancer. *Adv Anat Pathol* 9:115–128, 2002.

8. Cooperberg MR, Pasta DJ, Elkin EP, et al.: The University of California, San Francisco Cancer of the Prostate Risk Assessment score: a straightforward and reliable preoperative predictor of disease recurrence after radical prostatectomy. *J Urol* 173:1938–1942, 2005.

9. Cavanaugh SX, Kupelian PA, Fuller CD, et al.: Early prostate-specific antigen (PSA) kinetics following prostate carcinoma radiotherapy: prognostic value of a time-and-PSA threshold model. *Cancer* 101:96–105, 2004.

10. D'Amico AV, Chen MH, Roehl KA, et al.: Preoperative PSA velocity and the risk of death from prostate cancer after radical prostatectomy. *N Engl J Med* 351:125–135, 2004.

11. D'Amico AV, Moul J, Carroll PR, et al.: Surrogate end point for prostate cancer specific mortality in patients with nonmetastatic hormone refractory prostate cancer. *J Urol* 173:1572–1576, 2005.

12. Daneshmand S, Quek ML, Stein JP, et al.: Prognosis of patients with lymph node positive prostate cancer following radical prostatectomy: long-term results. *J Urol* 172:2252–2255, 2004.

13. Srigley JR, Amin M, Boccon-Gibod L, et al.: Prognostic and predictive factors in prostate cancer: historical perspectives and recent international consensus initiatives. *Scand J Urol Nephrol Suppl*:8–19, 2005.

14. Shulman MJ, Benaim EA: The natural history of androgen independent prostate cancer. *J Urol* 172:141–145, 2004.

15. Wyatt RB, Sanchez-Ortiz RF, Wood CG, et al.: Prognostic factors for survival among Caucasian, African-American and Hispanic men with androgen-independent prostate cancer. *J Natl Med Assoc* 96:1587–1593, 2004.

16. Halabi S, Small EJ, Kantoff PW, et al.: Prognostic model for predicting survival in men with hormone-refractory metastatic prostate cancer. *J Clin Oncol* 21:1232–1237, 2003.

17. Parker CC, Gospodarowicz M, Warde P: Does age influence the behaviour of localized prostate cancer? *BJU Int* 87:629–637, 2001.

18. Hall WH, Jani AB, Ryu JK, et al.: The impact of age and comorbidity on survival outcomes and treatment patterns in prostate cancer. *Prostate Cancer Prostatic Dis* 8:22–30, 2005.

19. Jemal A, Ward E, Wu X, et al.: Geographic patterns of prostate cancer mortality and variations in access to medical care in the United States. *Cancer Epidemiol Biomarkers Prev* 14:590–595, 2005.

20. Edwards BK, Brown ML, Wingo PA, et al.: Annual report to the nation on the status of cancer, 1975–2002, featuring population-based trends in cancer treatment. *J Natl Cancer Inst* 97:1407–1427, 2005.

21. Zietman AL, DeSilvio ML, Slater JD, et al.: Comparison of conventional-dose vs high-dose conformal radiation therapy in clinically localized adenocarcinoma of the prostate: a randomized controlled trial. *JAMA* 294:1233–1239, 2005.

22. Eastham JA, Kattan MW, Riedel E, et al.: Variations among individual surgeons in the rate of positive surgical margins in radical prostatectomy specimens. *J Urol* 170:2292–2295, 2003.

23. Schalken JA, Bergh A, Bono A, et al.: Molecular prostate cancer pathology: current issues and achievements. *Scand J Urol Nephrol Suppl*:82–93, 2005.

24. Verhagen PC, Tilanus MG, de Weger RA, et al.: Prognostic factors in localised prostate cancer with emphasis on the application of molecular techniques. *Eur Urol* 41:363–371, 2002.

25. Cooperberg MR, Lubeck DP, Mehta SS, et al.: Time trends in clinical risk stratification for prostate cancer: implications for outcomes (data from CaPSURE). *J Urol* 170:S21–S25; discussion S26–S27, 2003.

CHAPTER 35

Germ Cell Testis Tumors

PETER W. CHUNG and HANS-JOACHIM SCHMOLL

Testicular germ cell tumors are uncommon, but increasing incidence has been observed.[1] The main pathologic categories are seminoma and non-seminomatous germ cell tumors (NSCGTs), which occur in approximately equal proportions.

Patient assessment includes a full history, physical examination, imaging [computerized tomography (CT) abdomen/pelvis, chest radiograph/CT] and serum levels of tumor markers alpha-fetoprotein (AFP), human chorionic gonadotropin (HCG), and lactate dehydrogenase (LDH). Radical orchidectomy is both a diagnostic and a therapeutic procedure but not in routine clinical use anymore. Pathology assessment and treatment in centers experienced in management of these tumors is crucial.[2]

The overall prognosis is very favorable, and even in cases of relapsed disease, salvage treatment is curative. Practice guidelines for the management of testis tumors according to stage and prognostic factors are widely available.[3,4] Treatment decision should be based on prognostic factors. For stage I disease, a surveillance strategy is used in both seminoma and NSGCT. Alternative management in stage I seminoma includes adjuvant radiotherapy or adjuvant carboplatin (one cycle AUC 7). For patients with stage I non-seminoma, alternatives to surveillance, which is in particular indicated for low-risk patients, are adjuvant BEP chemotherapy, in particular for high risk stage I with vascular or lymphatic invasion in the pathologic specimen, or nerve-sparing retroperitoneal node dissection (NS-RPLND). For patients with seminoma and small volume retroperitoneal lymph node metastases (stage IIA/B), radiotherapy is the standard treatment. In stage IIA marker negative nonseminoma, NS-RPNLD or chemotherapy are used. For patients with marker positive stage IIA or more extensive disease (stage IIB), chemotherapy is the mainstay of treatment with surgery playing an important role in the management of residual disease after chemotherapy.

With excellent survival, prognostic factors in early disease reflect mainly the risk of relapse. In clinical stage I seminoma, age, lymphovascular invasion, tumor size, and rete

Prognostic Factors in Cancer, Third Edition, edited by Mary K. Gospodarowicz, Brian O'Sullivan, and Leslie H. Sobin.
Copyright © 2006 John Wiley & Sons, Inc.

testis invasion have been identified as predictors of relapse. In a pooled analysis of 638 patients' data, tumor size ($\geq$4 cm) and rete testis involvement independently predicted for increased risk of relapse.[5] In stage I NSGCT vascular invasion predicts for a 50% risk of relapse.[6-9] Extent of involvement with embryonal carcinoma and percent MIB1 staining within the primary tumor are also of value,[8-10] but not mandatory prognostic factors for treatment decision. In stage II seminoma, the size of the retroperitoneal lymph nodes is the most important predictor for relapse and survival, and in bulky retroperitoneal tumors ($\geq$5 cm), chemotherapy is the treatment of choice.[11,12] In stage II NSGCT the size and number of nodes involved at RPLND indicate the likelihood of relapse. Patients who have nodal size 2–5 cm and/or more than five nodes involved, have an increased likelihood of relapse and receive adjuvant chemotherapy or primary chemotherapy.[13,14] Elevated serum tumor markers prior to RPLND predict for subsequent relapse in the absence of adjuvant chemotherapy patients with low-volume disease can be observed since chemotherapy is effective at relapse.[15]

Serum tumor markers have been incorporated into the TNM classification.[4] The classification was based on data from >5800 patients treated with cisplatin-based chemotherapy studied by the International Germ Cell Cancer Collaborative Group (IGCCCG). The majority of patients had NSGCT.[16] In general, the prognosis for metastatic seminoma is better than that of NSGCT. Standard treatment in good prognosis patients is three cycles of BEP chemotherapy with four cycles in intermediate/poor prognosis patients.[2] High-dose chemotherapy is being investigated as first-line treatment in poor prognosis patients. The rate of tumor marker decline and normalization also has prognostic significance. Patients with unsatisfactory decline or prolonged time to marker normalization had worse outcomes, even taking into account prognostic groupings.[17,18] Prognostic factors in salvage therapy are complete response to first-line therapy, prolonged duration of disease-free interval (>3–6 months), and lower marker levels of AFP/HCG.[12] These factors have been used to select patients for intensive salvage, such as high-dose chemotherapy.

Considerable efforts were undertaken to understand the molecular alterations in testicular germ cell tumors and the relationship to treatment outcomes. In particular, the number of copies of the isochromosome of the short arm of chromosome 12 has been studied.[19] In patients with predominant embryonal carcinoma histology, cluster analysis of p53, apoptotic index, and expression of Ki67 have been studied.[20] Patients with high Ki67, low apoptosis, and low p53 had better survival than predicted according to IGCCC groupings. Further studies will be required to understand the role these molecular alterations play in clinical practice.

Although the majority of patients with testicular germ cell tumors are cured with modern therapy, there remains controversy in management in both early stage and advanced disease. In stage I disease, debate still surrounds the choice of surveillance versus adjuvant treatment and the application of specific treatment to minimize morbidity while maintaining the cure rate. This risk-adapted approach has much to do with the more recent recognition of treatment-associated late toxicity together with excellent salvage therapy in early disease, but suffers from the relative weakness of risk models in predicting disease relapse. In stage IIA/B, controversy exists regarding the optimal role of radiotherapy versus chemotherapy in seminoma, and surgery versus chemotherapy in NSGCT. Although testicular germ cell tumors may be the model of the curable neoplasm, in advanced disease, there are a proportion of patients who succumb to disease despite aggressive therapy. For these patients, the role of early dose-intensification and the role and timing of high-dose chemotherapy is yet to be clarified. Ongoing randomized studies employing high-dose chemotherapy as first line treatment in poor prognosis patients will determine the balance between efficacy and toxicity. Finally, as a single cycle of high dose chemotherapy may be inadequate to cure patients who have primary chemo-refractory disease, the role of multiple cycles of high-dose therapy is under study.

▆▆▆▆▆ SUMMARY TABLE

Prognostic Factors in Germ Cell Testis Tumors

Prognostic Factors	Tumor Related	Host Related	Environment Related
Essential	Histologic type T category N category M category AFP, HCG, LDH Site of metastases		
Additional	Rate of marker decline	Delay in diagnosis	Physician expertise
New and promising	Copy number of i(12p) p53 Ki67 Apoptotic index		

Source:
• NCCN Clinical Practice Guidelines in Oncology:Testicular Cancer 2005.
http://www.nccn.org/ professionals/physician_gls/PDF/testicular.pdf.

REFERENCES

1. Huyghe E, Matsuda T, Thonneau P: Increasing incidence of testicular cancer worldwide: a review. *J Urol* 170: 5–11, 2003.
2. Schmoll HJ, et al.: European consensus on diagnosis and treatment of germ cell cancer: a report of the European Germ Cell Cancer Consensus Group (EGCCCG). *Ann Oncol* 15: 1377–1399, 2004.
3. Motzer R, et al.: Testicular Cancer, in Clinical Practice Guidelines in Oncology. 2005, National Comprehensive Cancer Network, http://www.nccn.org/professionals/physician_gls/PDF/testicular.pdf

4. Sobin LH, Wittekind C: *International Union against Cancer: TNM classification of malignant tumors*. 6th ed., New York: Wiley-Liss. xxiii, 2002, p. 266.

5. Warde P, et al.: Prognostic factors for relapse in stage I seminoma managed by surveillance: a pooled analysis. *J Clin Oncol* 20: 4448–4452, 2002.

6. Alexandre J, et al.: Stage I non-seminomatous germ-cell tumors of the testis: identification of a subgroup of patients with a very low risk of relapse. *Eur J Cancer* 37: 576–582, 2001.

7. Roeleveld TA, et al.: Surveillance can be the standard of care for stage I nonseminomatous testicular tumors and even high risk patients. *J Urol* 166: 2166–2170, 2001.

8. Albers P, et al.: Risk factors for relapse in clinical stage I nonseminomatous testicular germ cell tumors: results of the German Testicular Cancer Study Group Trial. *J Clin Oncol* 21: 1505–1512, 2003.

9. Vergouwe Y, et al.: Predictors of occult metastasis in clinical stage I nonseminoma: a systematic review. *J Clin Oncol* 21: 4092–4099, 2003.

10. Atsu N, et al.: A novel surveillance protocol for stage I nonseminomatous germ cell testicular tumors. *BJU Intern* 92: 32–35, 2003.

11. Chung PW, et al.: Stage II testicular seminoma: patterns of recurrence and outcome of treatment. *Eur Urol* 45: 754–759 2004, discussion 759–760.

12. Bosl GJ, et al.: Cancer of the testis, *in* DeVita VT, Hellman S, Rosenberg SA, (eds.), *Cancer: Principles and Practice of Oncology*, Philadelphia, Lippincott Williams & Wilkins; p. 1269–1293, 2005.

13. Kondagunta GV, et al.: Relapse-free and overall survival in patients with pathologic stage II nonseminomatous germ cell cancer treated with etoposide and cisplatin adjuvant chemotherapy. *J Clin Oncol* 22: 464–467, 2004.

14. Beck SD, et al.: Impact of the number of positive lymph nodes on disease-free survival in patients with pathological stage B1 nonseminomatous germ cell tumor. *J Urol* 174: 143–145, 2005.

15. Rabbani F, et al.: Low-volume nodal metastases detected at retroperitoneal lymphadenectomy for testicular cancer: pattern and prognostic factors for relapse. *J Clin Oncol* 19: 2020–2025, 2001.

16. van Dijk MR, et al.: Survival of patients with nonseminomatous germ cell cancer: a review of the IGCC classification by Cox regression and recursive partitioning. *Br J Cancer* 90: 1176–1183, 2004.

17. Mazumdar M, et al.: Predicting outcome to chemotherapy in patients with germ cell tumors: the value of the rate of decline of human chorionic gonadotrophin and alpha-fetoprotein during therapy. *J Clin Oncol* 19: 2534–2541, 2001.

18. Fizazi K, et al.: Early predicted time to normalization of tumor markers predicts outcome in poor-prognosis nonseminomatous germ cell tumors. *J Clin Oncol* 22: 3868–3876, 2004.

19. George DW, et al.: Update on late relapse of germ cell tumor: a clinical and molecular analysis. *J Clin Oncol* 21: 113–122, 2003.

20. Mazumdar M, et al.: Cluster analysis of p53 and Ki67 expression, apoptosis, alpha-fetoprotein, and human chorionic gonadotrophin indicates a favorable prognostic subgroup within the embryonal carcinoma germ cell tumor. *J Clin Oncol* 21: 2679–2688, 2003.

CHAPTER 36

Renal Cell Cancer

CHRISTOPHE GHYSEL, STEVEN JONIAU, and HENDRIK VAN POPPEL

Renal cell carcinoma (RCC) accounts for 2–3% of all adult malignancies with the highest incidence in the fifth to seventh decades of life. It is the most lethal of all urological cancers.[1] Approximately 30% of patients present with metastatic disease and another 30% of patients who undergo nephrectomy for localized disease will subsequently develop metastases.[2,3] RCC has the reputation of having an individual unpredictable outcome. Rare cases of spontaneous tumor regression and extended survival despite the presence of metastases have been described. Approximately 90% of renal tumors are RCC, and 85% of these are clear cell tumors. Other less common cell types include papillary, chromophobe, and Bellini duct (collecting duct) tumors. A number of RCC are hereditary types, including von Hippel–Lindau syndrome, and are associated with different cell types.[2,4]

Over the past decade, the rate of incidental findings of renal mass on imaging studies for evaluation of unrelated symptoms has increased to >60%. Less than 10% now present with the typical triad of flank mass, flank pain, and hematuria or symptoms resulting from metastatic disease.[5] Patient assessment includes history and physical examination, with special attention for supraclavicular adenopathy, an abdominal mass, lower extremity edema, varicocele, or subcutaneous nodules. Laboratory evaluation should include a complete blood cell count, calcium, liver function studies, lactate dehydrogenase (LDH) and serum creatinin, erythrocyte sedimentation rate (ESR) and urinalysis. Computerized tomography (CT) of the chest, abdomen, and pelvis are essential imaging studies. Magnetic resonance imaging (MRI) is used in evaluating the inferior vena cava or as a substitute for CT in case of contrast allergy or renal insufficiency. A bone scan is performed when elevated serum alkaline phosphatase or bone pain is present. Computerized tomography or MRI of the brain is performed for symptoms suspicious of brain metastases.

Prognostic Factors in Cancer, Third Edition, edited by Mary K. Gospodarowicz, Brian O'Sullivan, and Leslie H. Sobin.
Copyright © 2006 John Wiley & Sons, Inc.

Radical nephrectomy remains the gold standard. A partial nephrectomy is accepted for tumors <5 cm. Resection of the adrenal is controversial. Seven percent of tumors >5 cm have micrometastatic adrenal involvement.[6] The role of lymphadenectomy also remains a subject of debate. Regional lymph-node extension is an important prognostic factor, usually associated with poor survival. Nevertheless, there may be a subset of patients with micrometastatic lymph-node involvement who could benefit from lymphadenectomy.[7]

In metastatic RCC, prognosis is dependent on the number of metastatic sites, location of metastasis, time between diagnosis and metastatic disease, neutrophil count, LDH, and C-reactive protein levels.[8] Current strategies advocate debulking nephrectomy in the context of modern immunotherapies. Two randomized trials, SWOG 8949 and EORTC 30947, have confirmed a survival benefit of 5.8 months over immunotherapy alone.[8] Resection of solitary metastases can achieve prolonged survival. Factors that positively influence prognosis in metastatectomy are a time interval of >2 years between nephrectomy and metastasis, location of metastasis in the lung, and T category.[9]

Treatment with interferon-α, IL-2, or combinations leads to responses in 10–20%. Favorable prognostic factors include good performance status, long disease-free interval, and disease predominantly confined to the lung. Several tumor and dendritic cell based vaccines are currently under evaluation.[10] Since RCC is a highly vascular tumor, the study of angiogenesis inhibitors appears particularly relevant and promising. Thalidomide is a potent *in vivo* angiogenesis inhibitor and is currently under investigation in an ECOG randomized phase III trial.[11]

The T category, grade, and performance status are prognostic indicators,[5,12] the most important being anatomic tumor extent at diagnosis. An elevated ESR, hypercalcemia, gender-specific anaemia, and an elevated alkaline phosphatase level are laboratory values that are well supported as prognostic factors for RCC. Histologic grade correlates most strongly with prognosis in every T category. The most commonly used grading system is that of Fuhrman,[13] based on nuclear and nucleolar size, shape, and content. Controversy exists concerning the interobserver reproducibility of grading, which has prompted the development of quantitative nuclear morphometric parameters and DNA ploidy, which have shown to be independent prognostic factors. The presence and extent of histological necrosis in tumor specimens was found to be independent predictors of survival in localised but not in metastatic disease.[14]

During the last several years, new outcome-prediction models for RCC, such as UISS and SSIGN scoring systems, have been developed.[12] Motzer et al[15] developed a prognostic factor model for survival with previously untreated metastatic RCC, which incorporates performance status, time from diagnosis to treatment with interferon alpha, hemoglobin, LDH, and serum calcium. This model has now been validated[16] with prior radiotherapy and sites of metastasis being additional prognosticators.

Loss of chromosomes 3p, 14q, 8p, and 9p have been shown to be the most frequent mutations in clear cell carcinoma. Loss of heterozygosity on chromosome 8p and 9p is a potentially more powerful predictor of recurrence than is tumor grade.[17] Microvascular invasion is a strong independent prognostic factor.[13,18] Other molecular markers including CA 9, vimentin, and p53, have been tested, but none has demonstrated independent prognostic significance. In recent years many studies have focused on investigating proliferation markers, such as PCNA, and Ki-S5.[11] Primary apoptosis evaluated with apoptotic indices and CD 95 expression was an independent prognostic factor for overall survival.[19]

Kidney cancer is now known to consist of several different types of tumors caused by different genes. Although at present, therapy is still largely based on surgical resection, understanding the molecular pathways should provide the foundation for the development of disease specific molecular therapeutic strategies.[4]

▰▰▰ SUMMARY TABLE

Prognostic Factors in Renal Cell Cancer

Prognostic Factors	Tumor Related	Host Related	Environment Related
Essential	Stage T category		

Additional	Grade
	Histologic type
	Microvascular
	  involvement
	Nuclear
	  morphometry
	Symptoms
	ESR
		Performance status
		Hereditary diseases
			Adrenalectomy
			Lymph-node
			  dissection
			Resection of
			  metastases

New and promising	DNA ploidy
	Genetic alterations
	Molecular markers
	Apoptosis
	Proliferation
	  markers
	Histologic necrosis
			Immunotherapy
			Angiogenesis
			  inhibition

Sources:
• Clinical Practice Guidelines in Oncology: National Comprehensive Cancer Network. Kidney Cancer 2005. http://www.nccn.org/professionals/physician_gls/PDF/kidney.pdf.
• National Cancer Institute: Kidney Cancer (PDQ®): Treatment Guidelines 2005. http://www.cancer.gov/ cancertopics/pdq/treatment/renalcell/healthprofessional/.

REFERENCES

1. Jemal A, Tiwari RC, Murray T, et al.: Cancer statistics, 2004. *CA Cancer J Clin* 54:8–29, 2004.
2. Novick AC CS: Renal Tumors, in Walsh PC RA, Vaughan ED, et al. (eds.): *Campbell's Urology* 8th ed., Philadelphia, Saunders, 2002.

3. Kirkali Z, Tuzel E, Mungan MU: Recent advances in kidney cancer and metastatic disease. *BJU Int* 88:818–824, 2001.

4. Linehan WM, Vasselli J, Srinivasan R, et al.: Genetic basis of cancer of the kidney: disease-specific approaches to therapy. *Clin Cancer Res* 10:6282S–6289S, 2004.

5. Pantuck AJ, Zisman A, Belldegrun AS: The changing natural history of renal cell carcinoma. *J Urol* 166:1611–1623, 2001.

6. De Sio M, Autorino R, Di Lorenzo G, et al.: Adrenalectomy: defining its role in the surgical treatment of renal cell carcinoma. *Urol Int* 71:361–367, 2003.

7. Joslyn SA, Sirintrapun SJ, Konety BR: Impact of lymphadenectomy and nodal burden in renal cell carcinoma: retrospective analysis of the National Surveillance, Epidemiology, and End Results database. *Urology* 65:675–680, 2005.

8. Flanigan RC, Mickisch G, Sylvester R, et al.: Cytoreductive nephrectomy in patients with metastatic renal cancer: a combined analysis. *J Urol* 171:1071–1076, 2004.

9. Swanson DA: Surgery for metastases of renal cell carcinoma. *Scand J Surg* 93:150–155, 2004.

10. Lam JS, Belldegrun AS, Figlin RA: Advances in immune-based therapies of renal cell carcinoma. *Expert Rev Anticancer Ther* 4:1081–1096, 2004.

11. Lam JS, Shvarts O, Leppert JT, et al.: Renal cell carcinoma 2005: new frontiers in staging, prognostication and targeted molecular therapy. *J Urol* 173:1853–1862, 2005.

12. Kirkali Z, Lekili M: Renal cell carcinoma: new prognostic factors? *Curr Opin Urol* 13:433–438, 2003.

13. Lang H, Lindner V, Letourneux H, et al.: Prognostic value of microscopic venous invasion in renal cell carcinoma: long-term follow-up. *Eur Urol* 46:331–335, 2004.

14. Lam JS, Shvarts O, Said JW, et al.: Clinicopathologic and molecular correlations of necrosis in the primary tumor of patients with renal cell carcinoma. *Cancer* 103:2517–2525, 2005.

15. Motzer RJ, Bacik J, Mazumdar M: Prognostic factors for survival of patients with stage IV renal cell carcinoma: memorial sloan-kettering cancer center experience. *Clin Cancer Res* 10:6302S–6303S, 2004.

16. Mekhail TM, Abou-Jawde RM, Boumerhi G, et al.: Validation and extension of the Memorial Sloan-Kettering prognostic factors model for survival in patients with previously untreated metastatic renal cell carcinoma. *J Clin Oncol* 23:832–841, 2005.

17. Presti JC Jr, Wilhelm M, Reuter V, et al.: Allelic loss on chromosomes 8 and 9 correlates with clinical outcome in locally advanced clear cell carcinoma of the kidney. *J Urol* 167:1464–1468, 2002.

18. Goncalves PD, Srougi M, Dall'lio MF, et al.: Low clinical stage renal cell carcinoma: relevance of microvascular tumor invasion as a prognostic parameter. *J Urol* 172:470–474, 2004.

19. Richter EN, Oevermann K, Buentig N, et al.: Primary apoptosis as a prognostic index for the classification of metastatic renal cell carcinoma. *J Urol* 168:460–464, 2002.

CHAPTER 37

Bladder Cancer

RICHARD J. SYLVESTER and ADRIAN P. M. VAN DER MEIJDEN

In the United States, bladder cancer is the fourth most frequent cancer in men and the ninth most frequent cancer in women, accounting for 4.6% of all malignancies.[1] Among patients with bladder cancer, three-quarters are male, and at the initial diagnosis, three-quarters present with superficial bladder cancer as opposed to muscle invasive or metastatic disease.[1] Two-thirds of cases are observed in developed countries where, due to its recurrent nature and the need for long-term follow up, it is an important disease from an economic point of view.[2] Environmental risk factors include cigarette smoking, exposure to chemicals, and infection with schistosomiasis.[2]

The most frequent symptom of bladder cancer is painless, gross hematuria. Key investigations include urine analysis, cytology, intravenous pyelogram or computerized tomography (CT) scan, cystoscopy, and bladder biopsy. Tumor markers in the urine have been shown to be more sensitive than urine cytology, especially for low-grade/stage disease, but none of them have been able to replace the combination of cystoscopy and urine cytology.[3]

As there are important differences in the prognosis and treatment of superficial bladder cancer, muscle invasive (locally advanced) disease, and metastatic bladder cancer, these three entities are discussed separately.[1,4]

The diagnosis of superficial tumors (Ta, T1, and Tis) is made by transurethral resection (TUR) of the Ta T1 papillary tumors and in carcinoma *in situ* (Tis) by multiple bladder biopsies. A meta-analysis has shown that after TUR of all visible tumor, patients should receive one immediate postoperative intravesical instillation using a chemotherapeutic drug.[5] According to the prognostic factors, this may be sufficient treatment in low-risk tumors; otherwise it is followed by more adjuvant intravesical chemotherapy or immunotherapy in intermediate and high-risk patients.

Prognostic Factors in Cancer, Third Edition, edited by Mary K. Gospodarowicz,
Brian O'Sullivan, and Leslie H. Sobin.
Copyright © 2006 John Wiley & Sons, Inc.

Prognostic factors in superficial bladder cancer have been determined by the analysis of various databases, some of which include data from multiple, randomized clinical trials.[6] While the primary endpoint in clinical trials is generally overall survival, this is not a good endpoint in superficial bladder cancer. The natural course of the disease is such that many patients survive >10–15 years and a large percentage may die from other causes.[1,6] Therefore two other endpoints have been used in practice: recurrence of superficial tumors and progression to muscle invasive disease. According to their prognostic factors, patients are categorized into risk groups: good, intermediate, and poor prognosis.[7]

For tumor recurrence, the most important prognostic factors are the number of tumors prior to TUR, the previous recurrence rate, and the maximum tumor diameter. For progression to muscle invasive disease, the G grade, the T category and the presence of Tis are the most important prognostic factors.[6] Patients with a small, single primary tumor are at the lowest risk of recurrence while patients with Tis and/or T1G3 lesions have the highest risk of progression. The result of the first cystoscopy 3 months after TUR is also a very important risk factor for both further tumor recurrence and progression.[8] It has been shown that after TUR, intravesical chemotherapy is able to prevent recurrence, but not progression.[9] Meta-analyses have shown that intravesical immunotherapy using BCG is not only superior to chemotherapy in reducing recurrence, but is also more effective in delaying or preventing progression.[10,11] Adjuvant therapy after TUR is determined by the risk group to which the patient belongs. In patients at low risk of progression, the urologist might predominantly aim to prevent recurrences using intravesical chemotherapy. However, when the risk of progression is high, intravesical BCG, which has more side effects than chemotherapy, might be selected.[12]

Many molecular tumor markers have been investigated to determine whether they might be used to predict the prognosis of the patient. The p53 tumor suppressor gene has especially been studied, often in small series. Conclusions on its potential use have not been reached.[13,14]

In contrast to superficial tumors, muscle invasive cancers cannot be eradicated by TUR alone. After staging the tumor by CT scan or magnetic resonance imaging (MRI) (and in selected cases, bone scintigraphy), the gold standard consists of radical cystoprostatectomy plus urinary diversion. Alternatively, patients can be offered external beam irradiation or in selected cases interstitial radiotherapy. Before applying definitive therapy, neoadjuvant chemotherapy might be considered and after cystectomy, adjuvant systemic chemotherapy is an option.[15,16]

In a meta-analysis of 3000 patients, neo-adjuvant chemotherapy showed a 14% reduction in the relative risk of death and an absolute improvement of 5% in the 5-year survival, from 45 to 50%.[17] Previous trials investigating the role of adjuvant combination therapy after cystectomy have methodological flaws and are underpowered.[15,18] A recent meta-analysis concluded that more data are needed to determine the role of adjuvant chemotherapy.[18] The most important prognostic factors are the lymph node status and T category.[19]

Systemic combination chemotherapy is the treatment of choice for metastatic bladder cancer. For many years the gold standard has been MVAC. However, its use is often limited by adverse effects, especially in frail patients. As compared to MVAC, gemcitabine/cisplatin-based regimens have been shown to have an apparently similar median survival of slightly >1 year, but less toxicity.[16] Prognostic factors for survival in metastatic bladder cancer include performance status, presence of visceral metastases, and alkaline phosphatase level.[20] Molecular markers, such as p53, p21, Ki 67, and the Rb gene have prognostic importance but their exact significance has not yet been established.[14]

◼◼◼◼ SUMMARY TABLES

Prognostic Factors in Superficial Bladder Cancer (Ta, T1, Tis)

Prognostic Factors	Tumor Related	Host Related	Environment Related
Essential	Grade T category Carcinoma *in situ* Number of tumors Prior recurrence rate		Quality of TUR One immediate instillation after TUR Intravesical treatment

Additional	Tumor size
	Recurrence at
	   3 months
		Age
		Gender
		Cigarette
		   smoking	

New and promising	p53 NMP22 COX-2 Lymphovascular invasion		

Prognostic Factors in Locally Advanced and Metastatic Bladder Cancer (T2–T4, M0-1)

Prognostic Factors	Tumor Related	Host Related	Environment Related
Essential	T category[a] N category[a] Sites of metastases[b]	Performance status[b] Alkaline phosphatase[b]	
Additional	Grade[a] Histologic cell type[a] Lymphatic/vascular invasion[a] Concomitant Cis[a] Tumor size[a] Hydronephrosis[a]	Age[a,b] Performance status[a] Hemoglobin[a,b] Response to chemotherapy[a,b]	Extent of lymphadenectomy[a]
New and promising	p53[a,b] p21[a,b] Rb[a,b] Ki 67[b] EGF receptor[a] E-cadherin[a] Microvessel density[a]		Lymph node density[a]

[a]Locally advanced bladder cancer.
[b]Metastatic bladder cancer.

Sources:
• National Cancer Institute: Bladder Cancer (PDQ®): Treatment Guidelines 2005.
http://www.cancer.gov/cancertopics/pdq/treatment/bladder/healthprofessional/.
• NCCN Clinical Practice Guidelines in Oncology: Bladder Cancer 2005.
http://www.nccn.org/professionals/ physician_gls/PDF/bladder.pdf.
• ESMO Minimum Clinical Recommendations for diagnosis, treatment and follow-up of invasive bladder cancer 2005.
http://annonc.oupjournals.org/cgi/reprint/16/suppl_1/i43.
• American Urological Association Clinical Guidelines Bladder Cancer 1999.
http://www.auanet.org/timssnet/ products/clinical_guidelines/bladdercancer.pdf.

REFERENCES

1. Jemal A, Murray T, Ward E, et al.: Cancer statistics, 2005. *CA Cancer J Clin* 55: 10–30, 2005.
2. Bassi P, Pagano F: Bladder cancer, in Gospodarowicz MK, Henson DE, Hutter RVP, et al. (eds.): *Prognostic Factors in Cancer*. 2nd ed. New York, Wiley-Liss, 2001.

3. Lotan A, Roehrborn: Sensitivity and specificity of commonly available bladder tumor markers versus cytology: results of a comprehensive literature review and meta-analysis. *Urology* 61: 109–118, 2003.

4. International Union Against Cancer. *TNM classification of malignant tumors*, 6th ed., Sobin LH, Wittekind Ch (eds.): Wiley-Liss, New York, 2002.

5. Sylvester RJ, Oosterlinck W, van der Meijden APM: A single immediate postoperative instillation of chemotherapy decreases the risk of recurrence in patients with stage Ta T1 bladder cancer: a meta-analysis of published results of randomized trials. *J Urol* 171: 2186–2190, 2004.

6. Millan-Rodriguez F, Chechile-Toniolo G, Salvador-Bayarri J, et al.: Multivariate analysis of the prognostic factors of primary superficial bladder cancer. *J Urol* 163: 73–78, 2000.

7. Millan-Rodriguez F, Chechile-Toniolo G, Salvador-Bayarri J, et al.: Primary superficial bladder cancer risk groups according to progression, mortality and recurrence. *J Urol* 164: 680–684, 2000.

8. Holmang S, Johansson SL: Stage Ta-T1 bladder cancer: the relationship between findings at first followup cystoscopy and subsequent recurrence and progression. *J Urol* 167: 1634–1637, 2002.

9. van der Meijden AP, Sylvester RJ: BCG immunotherapy for superficial bladder cancer: an overview of the past, the present and the future. *EAU Update Series* 1: 80–86, 2003.

10. Boehle A, Jocham D, Bock PR: Intravesical bacillus Calmette-Guerin versus mitomycin C for superficial bladder cancer: a formal meta-analysis of comparative studies on recurrence and toxicity. *J Urol* 169: 90–95, 2003.

11. Sylvester RJ, van der Meijden APM, Lamm DL: Intravesical bacillus Calmette-Guerin reduces the risk of progression in patients with superficial bladder cancer: a meta-analysis of the published results of randomized trials. *J Urol* 168: 1964–1970, 2002.

12. van der Meijden AP, Sylvester RJ: BCG immunotherapy for superficial bladder cancer: an overview of the past, the present and the future. *EAU Update Series* 1: 80–86, 2003.

13. Schmitz-Drager BJ, Goebell PJ, Ebert T, et al.: p53 immunohistochemistry as a prognostic marker in bladder cancer. *Eur Urol* 38: 691–700, 2000.

14. Kausch I, Boehle A: Molecular aspects of bladder cancer III. Prognostic markers of bladder cancer. *Eur Urol* 41: 15–29, 2002.

15. Pectasides D, Pectasides M, Nikolaou M: Adjuvant and neoadjuvant chemotherapy in muscle invasive bladder cancer: literature review. *Eur Urol* 48: 60–68, 2005.

16. Rosenberg JE, Carroll PR, Small EJ: Update on chemotherapy for advanced bladder cancer. *J Urol* 174: 14–20, 2005.

17. Advanced Bladder Cancer (ABC) Meta-Analysis Collaboration. Neoadjuvant chemotherapy in invasive bladder cancer: update of a systematic review and meta-analysis of individual patient data. *Eur Urol* 48: 202–206, 2005.

18. Advanced Bladder Cancer (ABC) Meta-Analysis Collaboration. Adjuvant chemotherapy in invasive bladder cancer: a systematic review and meta-analysis of individual patient data. *Eur Urol* 48: 189–201, 2005.

19. Gschwend JE, Dahm P, Fair WR: Disease specific survival as endpoint of outcome for bladder cancer patients following radical cystectomy. *Eur Urol* 41: 440–448, 2002.

20. Sengelov L, Kamby C, von der Maase H: Metastatic urothelial cancer: evaluation of prognostic factors and change in prognosis during the last twenty years. *Eur Urol* 39: 634–642, 2001.

OPHTHALMIC TUMORS

CHAPTER 38

Uveal Melanoma

JERRY A. SHIELDS and CAROL L. SHIELDS

Uveal melanoma is the most common primary intraocular malignancy. It occurs in approximately six patients per million people per year in the United States. It is more common in Caucasians and is very uncommon in people of African or Asian heritage. Uveal melanoma poses clinical challenges because of its tendency to metastasize by hematogenous routes to distant sites, particularly the liver.[1,2] There have been many publications related to prognosis for uveal melanoma.[3–20] Mortality figures have varied somewhat from series to series, depending on many complex factors.[4,5] There is an ~15% tumor-related mortality at 5 years after treatment, 30% at 10 years, and 50% at 15 years. We indicate that the figures are lower for smaller melanomas with fewer risk factors and greater for large melanomas with more risk factors.

Most uveal melanomas occur in the choroid, followed by ciliary body and iris. The diagnosis is usually made by clinical evaluation using indirect ophthalmoscopy and slit lamp biomicroscopy, and supported by ancillary diagnostic methods including ultrasonography, fundus photography, slit lamp photography, fluorescein angiography, and transillumination.

Many years ago it was almost universally believed that enucleation was the only appropriate management for suspected uveal melanoma. Eventually, enucleation was challenged by some authorities who proposed that eye removal may not prevent metastasis and may even promote tumor dissemination.[13] That concept was challenged by others, who believed that prompt enucleation was in the patient's best interests.[14] Due to this controversy, several alternative approaches, designed to save the eye, became popular. These included observation for tumor growth before initiating treatment, and active treatment by methods of laser photocoagulation, local tumor removal without removing the entire eye, thermotherapy, charged particle irradiation, and plaque brachytherapy.[1,2] According to current knowledge, no method is superior with regard

Prognostic Factors in Cancer, Third Edition, edited by Mary K. Gospodarowicz,
Brian O'Sullivan, and Leslie H. Sobin.
Copyright © 2006 John Wiley & Sons, Inc.

to patient prognosis.[11] However, as with other neoplasms, the prognosis appears to be worse in older or immunosuppressed patients.[3,6]

The TNM classification has limitations in predicting prognosis for uveal melanoma and is not used by most clinicians who manage this neoplasm.[9] The main clinical factors predictive of prognosis include tumor size, location, and growth pattern.[1-3,6]

Studies have shown that tumors with greater basal diameter and greater thickness have an increased chance of metastasis.[1-3,6] Five-year mortality following enucleation is 16% for small melanoma (<3 mm thickness), 32% for medium melanoma (3–8 mm thickness), and 53% for large melanoma (>8 mm thickness).[11] Iris melanoma has a better prognosis than ciliary body or choroidal melanoma. This is possibly because it is discovered at an earlier stage than melanoma located in the posterior uvea. Tumors that arise in the ciliary body have a worse prognosis, perhaps because they usually attain a larger size before diagnosis. Tumors in the choroid tend to have an intermediate prognosis.[1-3,6] Uveal melanoma can occur as a solitary nodule or it can assume diffuse, relatively flat growth pattern. Diffuse uveal melanoma tends to be more invasive and has a greater tendency to extend extrasclerally than does nodular melanoma.[1-3,6] Despite its relatively flat appearance, metastasis occurs in 24% of patients by 5 years.[12] A particularly aggressive type of diffuse melanoma is the ring melanoma of the ciliary body, which also carries a worse prognosis.[1] Extrascleral extension is present in ~8% of all patients with uveal melanoma and is an important risk factor for metastasis. Patients with this finding have a worse prognosis regardless of the treatment employed.[1-3]

Some of the aforementioned clinical factors like tumor size, location, growth pattern, and extrascleral extension can also be ascertained histopathologically, and hence are both clinical and pathologic prognostic factors. Strict pathologic risk factors include cell type, mitotic activity, atypical microvasculature, and tumor infiltrating lymphocytes. It has been recognized that cell type of uveal melanoma is related to prognosis. Patients with tumors composed of pure spindle cells have a more favorable prognosis and those with a component of epithelioid cells (mixed or epithelioid cell types) have a worse prognosis.[1,3,8,10] Melanomas with a low mitotic activity are associated with a better prognosis while those with greater mitotic activity carry a worse prognosis.[1,3,8] In many cases, extrascleral extension is evident clinically. In some cases, however, extrascleral extension is microscopic and only detected in eyes that are enucleated. There is increased mortality in patients with extrascleral extension of the tumor.[1,3,8] More recently it has been found that the histopathological presence of networks of closed vascular loops and other abnormal vascular patterns are associated with a less favorable prognosis.[18,19] Some uveal melanomas have demonstrated evidence of infiltration of lymphocytes in the tumor. This is also believed to be associated with decreased survival.[6,10]

There are other new and promising cytologic and genetic factors that relate to prognosis for uveal melanoma.[3,6,10] Ploidy abnormalities represent abnormal amount of DNA in cells. Flow cytometry studies have suggested that DNA aneuploidy is associated with increased mortality. The aneuploidy pattern has been correlated with the presence of epithelioid cells.[3,6,10] Cytogenetic abnormalities have been associated with chromosomes 3, 6, and 8. It appears that monosomy of chromosome 3 is associated with a much worse prognosis.[19,20] Future clinical trials will hopefully be beneficial in clarifying their clinical relevance and applicability.

■■■■■■■ SUMMARY TABLE

Prognostic Factors in Uveal Melanoma

Prognostic Factors	Tumor Related	Host Related	Environment Related
Essential	Size Location (iris better prognosis) Growth pattern Cell type Extrascleral extension		
Additional	Lymphocytic infiltration Mitotic activity Microvasculature pattern		
New and promising	Aneuploidy Cytogenetic abnormalities (e.g., chromosome 3,6,8)		

Source:
• National Cancer Institute: Intraocular (Eye) Melanoma (PDQ®): Treatment Guidelines 2005.
http://www.cancer.gov/cancertopics/pdq/treatment/intraocularmelanoma/healthprofessional.

REFERENCES

1. Shields JA, Shields CL: Uveal melanoma, in Shields JA, Shields CL (eds.): *Intraocular Tumors. A Text and Atlas*. Philadelphia, Saunders, 1992, pp. 117–205.

2. Shields JA, Shields CL: Uveal melanoma, in Shields JA, Shields CL (eds.): *Atlas of Intraocular Tumors*. Philadelphia, Lippincott Williams and Wilkins. 1999, pp. 74–132.

3. Seddon JM, Moy CS: Choroidal melanoma: prognosis, in Ryan SJ. (ed.): *Retina* 3rd ed. St. Louis, CV Mosby, 2001, pp. 687–697.

4. Diener-West M, Earle JD, Fine SL, et al.: The COMS Randomized trial of iodine-125 brachytherapy for choroidal melanoma, III.: Initial mortality findings. COMS report 18. *Arch Ophthalmol* 119:967–982, 2001.

5. Kujala E, Makitie T, Kivela T: Very long-term prognosis of patients with malignant uveal melanoma. *Invest Ophthalmol Vis Sci* 44:4651–4659, 2003.

6. Singh AD, Shields CL, Shields JA: Prognostic factors in uveal melanoma. *Melanoma Res* 11:255–263, 2001.

7. Shields CL, Shields JA, Kiratli H, et al.: Risk factors for metastasis of small choroidal melanocytic lesions. *Ophthalmology* 102:1351–1361, 1995.

8. Isager P, Ehlers N, Overgaard J: Prognostic factors for survival after enucleation for choroidal and ciliary body melanomas. *Acta Ophthalmol Scand* 82:517–525, 2004.

9. Kujala E, Kivela T: Tumor, Node, Metastasis Classification of Malignant Ciliary Body and Choroidal Melanoma Evaluation of the 6th Edition and Future Directions. *Ophthalmology* 2005, in press.

10. Mooy CM, De Jong PT: Prognostic parameters in uveal melanoma: a review. *Surv Ophthalmol* 41:215–228, 1996.

11. Diener-West M, Hawkins BS, Markowitz JA, et al.: A review of mortality from choroidal melanoma. II. A meta-analysis of 5-year mortality rates following enucleation, 1966 through 1988. *Arch Ophthalmol* 110:245–250, 1992.

12. Shields CL, Shields JA, De Potter P, et al.: Diffuse choroidal melanoma. Clinical features predictive of metastasis. *Arch Ophthalmol* 114:956–963, 1996.

13. Zimmerman LE, McLean IW: An evaluation of enucleation in the management of uveal melanomas. *Am J Ophthalmol* 87:741–760, 1979.

14. Seigel D, Myers M, Ferris F, et al.: Survival rates after enucleation of eyes with malignant melanoma. *Am J Ophthalmol* 87:751–765, 1979.

15. Shields CL, Cater J, Shields JA, et al.: Combined plaque radiotherapy and transpupillary thermotherapy for choroidal melanoma: tumor control and treatment complications in 270 consecutive patients. *Arch Ophthalmol* 120:933–940, 2002.

16. Folberg R, Mehaffey M, Gardner LM, et al.: The microcirculation of choroidal and ciliary body melanomas. *Eye* 11:227–238, 1997.

17. Makitie T, Summanen P, Tarkkanen A, et al.: Microvascular loops and networks as prognostic indicators in choroidal and ciliary body melanomas. *J Natl Cancer Inst* 91:359–367, 1999.

18. Durie FH, Campbell AM, Lee WR, et al.: Analysis of lymphocytic infiltration in uveal melanoma. *Invest Ophthalmol Vis Sci* 31:2106–2110, 1990.

19. Prescher G, Bornfeld N, Hirche H, et al.: Prognostic implications of monosomy 3 in uveal melanoma. *Lancet* 347:1222–1225, 1996.

20. Sisley K, Rennie IG, Parsons MA, et al.: Abnormalities of chromosomes 3 and 8 in posterior uveal melanoma correlate with prognosis. *Genes Chromosomes Cancer* 19:22–28, 1997.

CHAPTER 39

Retinoblastoma

VIKAS KHETAN, HELEN S. L. CHAN, LISA WANG, and BRENDA L. GALLIE

Retinoblastoma is the commonest malignant eye tumor of childhood, affecting 15 per 100,000 live births.[1,2] Nonhereditary retinoblastoma is always unilateral. Children predisposed to hereditary retinoblastoma because they carry a mutant *RB1* allele usually develop bilateral disease, but may only have unilateral disease. However, only 10% of children have familial retinoblastoma, and most germline *RB1* alleles are novel, so the major factor negatively affecting outcome is timeliness of diagnosis. In regions where primary healthcare is readily available, retinoblastoma rarely extends outside the eye(s) and survival exceeds 96%. However, where access to healthcare is limited, extraocular disease is common with very poor survival rates.

Prognostic factors affecting risk will be described for retinoblastoma at three levels: risk to develop retinoblastoma; risk to lose the eye with intraocular disease despite current best therapies; and risk of death due to metastatic disease with current best therapies. No multicenter clinical trials have been performed to evaluate systematically therapy for intraocular or extraocular retinoblastoma. Such trials will require global collaboration.

RISK TO DEVELOP RETINOBLASTOMA

A germline mutant *RB1* allele increases the risk for retinoblastoma 40,000-fold. Without accurate identification of the *RB1* gene status, all probands who are bilaterally affected, or unilaterally affected with family history, definitely have germline mutations; 50% of offspring will inherit the mutant allele and have 95% risk of tumors.[3] Since there is a 10% chance of either parent being an unaffected carrier, each sib has a 9.5% chance of developing tumor. Of unilaterally affected probands without family history, 15% will have a germline mutation; 7.5% of their offspring, and 0.75% of their sibs will develop retinoblastoma.

Prognostic Factors in Cancer, Third Edition, edited by Mary K. Gospodarowicz,
Brian O'Sullivan, and Leslie H. Sobin.

With full molecular analysis 93% of *RB1* mutant alleles can be identified, supporting accurate identification of infants at risk, facilitating early diagnosis and intervention and vastly improving visual outcome and saving eyes.[4] A simple molecular test for the proband's mutation accurately distinguishes relatives at high risk from those at the normal population risk (0.0007%), who then avoid invasive clinical surveillance for tumor development. *RB1* "null" mutant alleles that result in nonfunctional protein carry a 99% risk of tumor; *RB1* alleles with partial function result in 30–70% risk of tumor.[5]

RISK FOR THE EYE WITH INTRAOCULAR RETINOBLASTOMA

Early diagnosis vastly improves the prognosis to cure retinoblastoma and keep the eye. The most common presenting sign is leukocoria, with parents noticing the white tumor directly visible through the pupil. Diagnosis is clinical, supported by the demonstration of calcification in the tumor on ultrasound and computerized tomography (CT) scan. CT/magnetic resonance imaging (MRI) scan also screens for the rare "trilateral retinoblastoma", an intracranial primitive neuroectodermal tumor. Intraocular biopsy is *not* indicated and risks tumor dissemination.

For the past 40 years, prognosis of intraocular retinoblastoma depended on the Reese–Ellsworth classification, designed to predict outcome of external beam radiation (EBRT). Since 1990, chemotherapy with focal (laser and cryo) therapy has replaced EBRT as primary therapy, to avoid the severe long-term side effect of EBRT, high risk for second primary tumors. EBRT remains a valuable tool to salvage eyes that fail chemotherapy/focal therapy. The new International Intraocular Retinoblastoma Classification (IIRC) more accurately specifies prognosis of eyes treated with chemotherapy and focal therapy[6] (Table 39.1). The TNM stage is not widely used for intraocular retinoblastoma (T1-3).[7] In a world survey of retinoblastoma classification,[8] the IIRC more accurately reflected prognosis for eyes treated with chemotherapy and focal therapy than the Reese–Ellsworth Classification.

Worldwide chemotherapy has included three drugs: carboplatin, etoposide, and vincristine (CEV). The Toronto protocol adds high-dose cyclosporine simultaneous with chemotherapy to countermultidrug resistance. Comparison of results without[8] and with[9] cyclosporine, supports a current open multicenter clinical trial in retinoblastoma.

RISK OF DEATH FROM METASTATIC RETINOBLASTOMA

Retinoblastoma can metastasize by direct extension into the orbit, into the brain and meninges via the optic nerve, regionally to lymph nodes and mandible,[10] and to distant sites through the blood stream from the choroid and anterior chamber, particularly localizing to bone and bone marrow. The cure rate and survival for extraocular retinoblastoma is extremely poor. The survival for patients with regional disease ranges from 63 to 84%.[12,13] The survival in patients with central nervous system (CNS) disease ranges from 0 to 20%.[12,14] With bone marrow metastasis only survival

TABLE 39.1   Prognosis for Eye by the International Intraocular Retinoblastoma Classification

Group	Tumor Feature	Recommended Therapy	Eye Salvage Chemotherapy and Focal Therapy n = 440,[8] %	Eye Salvage All Treatments[8] n = 1914,[8] %
A	≤3 mm confined to the retina >3 mm from fovea, >1.5 mm from optic disk	Focal – laser and cryotherapy	98	98
B	>3 mm confined to the retina Subretinal fluid ≤3 mm from tumor, No subretinal seeding	3–5 cycles CEV	95	86
C	Tumor(s) discrete Subretinal fluid, present or past, no seeding, >3 mm and <0.25 retina Local subretinal seeding, present or past, <3 mm from tumor Local fine vitreous seeding	6–8 cycles CEV	84	71
D	Tumor(s) massive or diffuse Subretinal fluid, present or past, no seeding, > 0.25 < total retinal detachment Diffuse subretinal seeding, present or past Diffuse or massive vitreous seeding	6–8 cycles CEV	57	17
E	Risk of extraocular extension Tumor touching the lens Neovascular glaucoma Tumor anterior to anterior vitreous face Diffuse infiltrating tumor Opaque media from hemorrhage Tumor necrosis with aseptic orbital cellulitis Phthisis bulbi	Enucleation	11	3

ranges between 0 to 100%.[13-17] The Toronto protocol is the only report of favorable survival in patients with CNS involvement.[18] The precipitous drop in survival between intraocular and extraocular disease justifies rapid initiation of treatment when retinoblastoma is first diagnosed. Current treatment of metastatic retinoblastoma offers hope. "Cure" with long-term follow-up is possible with chemotherapy, orbital and focal radiation, intrathecal chemotherapy, and bone marrow/stem cell transplant.

The 2002 TNM classification for metastatic retinoblastoma[7] does not reflect differences in outcome for disease affecting the CNS versus bone marrow. The newly proposed International Retinoblastoma Classification (IRC)[11] addresses these issues. Stage 0 is intraocular retinoblastoma without pathology; stage 1 includes enucleated patients with no residual disease; stage 2 is enucleated patients with microscopic residual disease; stage 3 is regional disease; stage 4a is metastatic disease non CNS; and stage 4b is CNS disease.

▬▬▬▬ **SUMMARY TABLE**

Prognostic Factors in Retinoblastoma

Prognostic Factors	Tumor Related	Host Related	Environment Related
Essential	International Intraocular RB Classification (Groups A–E)[6] International RB Classification (Stage 0–4)[11]	Germline mutant RB1 allele	Access to care
Additional	Multidrug resistance gene (s)		Cyclosporine therapy Multidisciplinary team with management expertise
New and promising			Global retinoblastoma collaboration[9]

REFERENCES

1. Cheng C Y, Hsu W M: Incidence of eye cancer in Taiwan: an 18-year review. *Eye* 18, 152–158, 2004.
2. Seregard S, Lundell G, Svedberg H, Kivela T: Incidence of retinoblastoma from 1958 to 1998 in Northern Europe: advantages of birth cohort analysis. *Ophthalmology* 111, 1228–1232, 2004.

3. Gallie B, Erraguntla V, Heon E, Chan H: Pediatric Ophthalmology and Strabismus. Taylor D, Hoyt C (eds.): Elsevier, 2004, pp. 486–504.

4. Richter S, et al.: Sensitive and Efficient Detection of RB1 Gene Mutations Enhances Care for Families with Retinoblastoma. *Am J Hum Genet* 72, 253–269, 2003.

5. Lohmann D R, Gallie B L, Retinoblastoma: Revisiting the model prototype of inherited cancer. *Am J Med Genet* 129C, 23–28, 2004.

6. Murphree A L: Intraocular retinoblastoma: the case for a new group classification. *Ophthalmol Clinics N Am* 18, 41–53, 2005.

7. *TNM Classification of Malignant Tumours.* Sobin L H, Wittekind C (eds.): Wiley-Liss New York, 2002.

8. Wang L, Panzarella T, Murphree A L, et al.: International Congress of Ocular Oncology Gallie B L, (ed.): Whistler, British Columbia, 2005, submitted to NEJM.

9. Chan H S L, Heon E, Gallie B L: Good long term results of multidrug resistance-reversal chemotherapy for advanced intraocular retinoblastoma without upfront elective consolidation radiation. *Proceedings of the American Association for Cancer Research* 46, Abstract 4732, 2005.

10. Pandya J, et al.: Predilection of retinoblastoma metastases for the mandible. *Med Pediatr Oncol* 38, 271–273, 2002.

11. Chantada G, et al.: in International Retinoblastoma Symposium and International Congress of Ocular Oncology, Gallie B L, Paton K (eds.): Whistler, British Columbia, Canada, 2005.

12. Antoneli C B, et al.: Extraocular retinoblastoma: a 13-year experience. *Cancer* 98, 1292–1298, 2003.

13. Chantada G, et al.: Treatment of overt extraocular retinoblastoma. *Med Pediatr Oncol* 40, 158–161, 2003.

14. Namouni F, et al.: High-dose chemotherapy with carboplatin, etoposide and cyclophosphamide followed by a haematopoietic stem cell rescue in patients with high-risk retinoblastoma: a SFOP and SFGM study. *Eur J Cancer* [A] 33A, 2368–2375, 1997.

15. Dunkel I J, et al.: Successful treatment of metastatic retinoblastoma. *Cancer* 89, 2117–2121, 2000.

16. Kremens B, et al.: High-dose chemotherapy with autologous stem cell rescue in children with retinoblastoma. *Bone Marrow Transplant* 31, 281–284, 2003.

17. Chantada G, et al.: Results of a prospective study for the treatment of retinoblastoma. *Cancer* 100, 834–842, 2004.

18. Chan H S L, et al.: 11th International Retinoblastoma Symposium and the 14th Meeting of the International Society for Genetic Eye Disease, Paris, France, 2003.

HEMATOLOGIC MALIGNANCIES

CHAPTER 40

Hodgkin Lymphoma

LENA SPECHT

Hodgkin lymphoma is uncommon, constituting 10–15% of all lymphomas. It contains two disease entities, nodular lymphocyte predominant (LP) Hodgkin lymphoma and classical Hodgkin lymphoma, the latter being subdivided into nodular sclerosis, mixed cellularity, lymphocyte rich classical, and lymphocyte depleted.[1]

LP Hodgkin lymphoma usually presents as localized peripheral lymphadenopathy and B-symptoms are rare. Treatment is local involved field radiotherapy except in rare disseminated cases. Classical Hodgkin lymphoma usually presents as central and peripheral lymphadenopathy, most commonly above the diaphragm, and B-symptoms occur in 40% of patients. Treatment of classical Hodgkin lymphoma has changed over the past few years. In early-stage disease combined treatment with two or four cycles of chemotherapy followed by involved field radiotherapy is now standard. In advanced disease, six-to-eight cycles of chemotherapy is standard with radiotherapy reserved for patients who do not reach complete remission. Dose-intensified chemotherapy regimens are being employed for patients with adverse prognostic factors.[2] With modern treatment, prognosis is excellent in early stage disease with cure rates well over 90%, and even for patients with advanced disease 5-year survival exceeds 80%.[3]

Patient assessment should include a careful history identifying risk factors for lymphoma (e.g., immune deficiency or autoimmune disease), duration and growth rate of lymph node enlargement, presence or absence of B-symptoms (unexplained fever, night sweats, and/or unexplained weight loss of >10% of the usual body weight in the 6 months prior to diagnosis), symptoms suggesting extralymphatic involvement, performance status, and comorbid illness.[4] Physical examination should include evaluation of all lymph-node regions, inspection of Waldeyer's ring, evaluation of the presence or absence of hepatosplenomegaly, inspection of the skin, and detection of palpable masses. Laboratory studies should include a complete blood count, erythrocyte sedimentation rate (ESR), albumin, evaluation of renal and liver function, and

Prognostic Factors in Cancer, Third Edition, edited by Mary K. Gospodarowicz, Brian O'Sullivan, and Leslie H. Sobin.
Copyright © 2006 John Wiley & Sons, Inc.

viral serologies [human immunodeficiency virus (HIV), Epstein–Barr virus (EBV)]. Radiological studies include standard posteroanterior and lateral chest radiographs and computerized tomography (CT) scans of the neck, chest, abdomen, and pelvis. Functional imaging with fluoro-deoxy-glucose positron emission tomography (FDG–PET) is now gaining widespread acceptance, and several studies suggest that it is more sensitive than CT scans.[5] Liver and bone marrow biopsies may be used for patients at particular risk of involvement. Laparotomy with splenectomy, which used to be part of the staging procedure, is no longer performed.

The anatomic extent of disease is the most important prognostic factor.[6] The TNM classification employed for other malignancies is not a workable staging system for the lymphomas, because the site of origin of the disease is often unclear, and there is no way to differentiate among T, N, and M. Since no other convincing and tested overall staging system is yet available, the Ann Arbor staging classification is still recommended.[7]

The Ann Arbor stage is not a sensitive indicator of prognosis. The extent of disease may vary considerably in stages other than stage I, and the volume of disease in individual regions is not taken into account at all. Consequently, numerous studies have investigated other prognostic factors in the lymphomas. The important prognostic factors have in the vast majority of studies proved to be surrogate measures of the total tumor burden (e.g., number of nodal and extranodal sites, size of tumor masses, hemoglobin, lymphocyte count, serum albumin, ESR, B-symptoms) or the physiologic reserve of the patient (e.g., age, performance status).[8] Direct measurement of the tumor burden using modern imaging seems promising for prognostic evaluation.[9]

Prognostic factors in early stage disease (CS I–II) include measures of the anatomic extent of disease, such as Ann Arbor stage, tumor bulk, number of involved regions, and the presence of extranodal disease.[2,6,8] B-symptoms and ESR are also essential tumor related factors. Based on combinations of these factors different groups divide patients into early favorable and early unfavourable (intermediate) groups.[2,4,10–14] Lymphocyte predominant histology is associated with a particularly indolent course.[2] Age and immune status are essential host related factors.[6] Additional tumor related factors are hemoglobin and albumin, and gender is an additional host related factor. An early PET-scan after 1–2 cycles of chemotherapy has recently been shown to be of great prognostic importance, and may well in the future become essential in the evaluation of patients.[5]

Prognostic factors in advanced disease (CS III–IV) also include measures of the anatomic extent of disease, such as Ann Arbor stage, tumor bulk, and number of involved nodal and extranodal regions. LP histology does not carry a better prognosis in advanced disease.[2] The extent and volume are more difficult to quantify in advanced disease, and B-symptoms and a large number of biologic parameters have been shown to influence prognosis and to be correlated with both tumor burden and possibly the proliferative potential of the tumor.[6] Age and immune status are essential host related factors. An International Prognostic Score (IPS) for advanced disease has been developed incorporating seven risk factors: Age $\geq$45 years, male sex, stage IV disease, hemoglobin <10.5 g/dL, serum albumin <4.0 g/dL, leukocytosis $\geq$15 $\times$ 10^9/L, and lymphocytopenia $<0.6 \times 10^9$/L or $<8\%$ of white blood cell count. Patients are divided according to the number of risk factors.[2,4,11,12,14,15] However, stratification of patients on the basis of the IPS score is still an experimental approach. As for early stage disease an early PET-scan after 1–2 cycles of chemotherapy is very promising as an indicator of prognosis.[5]

■■■■■ SUMMARY TABLE

Prognostic Factors in Hodgkin Lymphoma

Prognostic Factors	Tumor Related	Host Related	Environment Related

Essential	Stage[a]
	Tumor bulk
	Number of involved nodal
	    and extranodal regions
	B-symptoms
	Histologic type[b]
	ESR[b]
	IPS score[c] (based on factors
	    marked[a])
	Hemoglobin[a,c]
	Albumin[a,c]
	White cell count[a,c]
	Lymphocyte count[a,c]
		Age[a]
		Gender[a,c]
		Immune
		    status	

Additional	Hemoglobin[b] Albumin[b] ESR[c] Alkaline phosphatase[c]	Gender[b]	
New and promising	Early PET-scan		

[a] Essential prognostic factors in advanced stage only.
[b] Early stage disease only.
[c] Advanced disease only.

Sources:
• NCCN Clinical Practice Guidelines in Oncology:Hodgkin's Lymphoma 2005.
http:// www. nccn.org/professionals/physician_gls/PDF/hodgkins.pdf.
• ESMO Minimum Clinical Recommendations for diagnosis, treatment and follow-up of Hodgkin's Disease.
http://annonc.oupjournals.org/cgi/reprint/16/suppl_1/i54.

REFERENCES

1. Jaffe ES, Harris NL, Stein H, et al.: World Health Organization Classification of Tumours. *Pathology and Genetics of Tumours of Haematopoietic and Lymphoid Tissues.* Lyon, IARC Press, 2001.

2. Diehl V, Thomas RK, Re D: Part II: Hodgkin's lymphoma—diagnosis and treatment. *Lancet Oncol* 5:19–26, 2004.

3. Diehl V, Harris NL, Mauch PM: Hodgkin's lymphoma, in DeVita VT, Hellman S, Rosenberg SA (eds.): *Cancer. Principles and Practice of Oncology,* 7th ed. Philadelphia, Lippincott, Williams & Wilkins, 2005, pp. 2020–2075.

4. Specht L: Staging systems and staging investigations at presentation, in Magrath I (ed.): *The Lymphoid Malignancies,* (3rd ed.) London, Hodder Arnold, 2005, in press.

5. Hutchings M, Eigtved AI, Specht L: FDG-PET in the clinical management of Hodgkin lymphoma. *Crit Rev Oncol Hematol* 52:19–32, 2004.

6. Specht L: Hodgkin's Disease, in Gospodarowicz M, Henson DE, Hutter RVP, et al. (eds.): *Prognostic Factors in Cancer,* 2nd ed. New York, Wiley-Liss, 2001, pp, 673–687.

7. Sobin LH, Wittekind Ch (eds.), UICC: *TNM Classification of malignant tumors.* 6th ed. New York, Wiley-Liss, 2002.

8. Specht LK, Hasenclever D: Prognostic Factors, in Hoppe RT, Armitage JO, Diehl V, et al. (eds.): *Hodgkin's Disease,* 2nd Ed. Philadelphia, Lippincott Williams & Wilkins, 2006, in press.

9. Gobbi PG, Broglia C, Di Giulio G, et al.: The clinical value of tumor burden at diagnosis in Hodgkin lymphoma. *Cancer* 101:1824–1834, 2004.

10. Clinical practice guidelines for the diagnosis and management of Hodgkin lymphoma: The Cancer Council Australia, 2004. www.cancer.org.au.

11. Adult Hodgkin's lymphoma: treatment: National Cancer Institute, 2005. www.cancer.gov.

12. Hoppe RT: Hodgkin's disease, *Practice guidelines in oncology*: National Comprehensive Cancer Network, 2005. www.nccn.org.

13. Jost LM, Stahel RA: ESMO Minimum Clinical Recommendations for diagnosis, treatment and follow-up of Hodgkin's disease. *Ann Oncol* 16:i54–i55, 2005.

14. Sutcliffe S, De Lena M: Hodgkin's lymphoma, in Cancer management guidelines: British Columbia Cancer Agency, 2005. www.bccancer.bc.ca.

15. Hasenclever D, Diehl V: A prognostic score for advanced Hodgkin's disease. International Prognostic Factors Project on Advanced Hodgkin's Disease. *N Engl J Med* 339: 1506–1514, 1998.

CHAPTER 41

Non-Hodgkin Lymphomas

MARY K. GOSPODAROWICZ, MICHAEL CRUMP, and EMANUELE ZUCCA

Non-Hodgkin lymphomas are a diverse group of lymphoid malignancies with large variations in the genetics, molecular disease patterns, and course of disease. With current treatment, approximately 50% of patients diagnosed with lymphoma will succumb to their disease.[1] The exact etiology for most of lymphomas is unknown, but the association with immune dysregulation and infection is well documented. The infectious etiology has been confirmed in a number of MALT type marginal zone lymphomas.

In the last decade, molecular and genetic studies led to improved understanding of the pathobiology of lymphomas.[2–7] The current WHO Classification is based largely on histologic pattern and immunophenotype that characterizes lymphomas into B-cell malignancies and T/NK-cell malignancies. With the exceptions of mycosis fungoides and anaplastic large cell lymphoma, the T/NK phenotype carries a worse prognosis.[8] Gene expression profiling provided a molecular framework for the study of lymphoma and new classifications based on the gene expression patterns have been proposed.[1,9] For example, in diffuse large-cell lymphoma, three gene expression groups germinal center B-cell-like, activated B-cell-like, and primary mediastinal lymphoma represent distinct prognostic entities.[10] Diffuse large B-cell lymphoma and follicular lymphoma are the most common disease entities.[9] Most prognostic factor information is based on the study of these two diseases. Follicular lymphomas are generally associated with better prognosis than diffuse large-cell lymphomas and the number of nodal sites is a strong prognostic factor.

The anatomic extent of disease is also of major importance. The Ann Arbor staging classification is the accepted classification for non-Hodgkin's lymphoma and is included in the AJCC and UICC manuals.[11] Stage I and II presentations are frequently referred to as localized presentations, while stages III and IV are disseminated disease. In addition to histologic classification and extent of disease, tumor bulk or burden is found to be an important predictor of outcome in localized presentations.

Prognostic Factors in Cancer, Third Edition, edited by Mary K. Gospodarowicz, Brian O'Sullivan, and Leslie H. Sobin.
Copyright © 2006 John Wiley & Sons, Inc.

Tumor burden may manifest itself as degree of invasion and direct extension in the extranodal organs. Systemic symptoms including fever, night sweats, and weight loss, so-called B symptoms, are usually associated with more extensive disease, but their presence has an independent prognostic factor in any stage disease.[1,12] The presence of anemia, elevated LDH is usually associated with increased tumor burden and is an adverse factor. High beta-microglobulin level is also associated with an adverse prognosis in all patients with lymphomas.[12]

The International Prognostic Index (IPI) developed for diffuse large-cell lymphoma over 10 years ago stratifies patients according to the presence of adverse factors including older age, advanced stage, poor performance status, elevated lactate dehydrogenase (LDH), and a number of extranodal sites into prognostic groups. It is widely used to interpret the outcomes of treatment.[1,12] A modification of IPI was developed for follicular lymphoma, so-called FLIPI.[13] The adverse prognostic factors in FLIPI are age >60 years, stages III–IV, hemoglobin <120 g/L, >4 nodal areas involved, and abnormal LDH level. Patients in the low-risk group (0–1 adverse factor) had 70% 10-year survival, while those in a high-risk group (3 or more adverse factors) had 35% 10-year survival.[13] A prognostic model constructed using age, performance status, LDH level, and bone marrow has been proposed to predict the outcome of peripheral T-cell lymphomas.[14]

The presenting site of lymphoma is a prognostic factor; extranodal lymphomas presenting in brain and testis are associated with particularly adverse prognosis.[12] These differences are observed in the presence of a single histologic entity—diffuse large cell lymphoma. The presentation in skin is associated with excellent prognosis even in the face of diffuse cutaneous disease.[15] The histologic type does not exert the same prognostic influence in skin lymphomas as in other presentations. This may be explained by the different gene expression patterns present in different types of cutaneous lymphoma.[15]

In MALT type of marginal zone lymphoma, the presence of *Helicobacter pylori* infection usually indicates a favorable prognosis. Complete remissions are obtained with antibiotic therapy with excellent outcomes. Eradication of all the infections associated with MALT lymphomas at different anatomic sites, *Borellia burgdorferi*, *Campylobacter jejunum*, and *Chlamydia psittaci* has been associated with regression of MALT lymphomas.[16,17] The presence of t11;18 translocation is relatively common and is associated with adverse outcome following antibiotic therapy.[17] In the cutaneous lymphoma, generally associated with excellent prognosis, the site of involvement is an independent prognostic factor with patients presenting with diffuse large B-cell lymphoma in the leg having much worse outcome than those presenting in other body sites.[15] In contrast to cutaneous lymphoma, nasal T/NK type lymphoma is associated with poor prognosis.[16] In this and the other lymphomas involving head and neck, local disease extent is a powerful prognostic factor. A specific prognostic index has been proposed for CNS lymphoma taking into account older age, poor performance status, elevated LDH, high CSF protein concentration and involvement of deep regions of the brain.[18]

New prognostic factors include molecular factors, such as p53, CD44, proliferation indices are associated with adverse prognosis.[19] Furthermore, expression of CD5,

MMP9, Cyclin D2, has been associated with adverse outcomes while the expression of CD10, Bcl-6, has been associated with favorable prognosis in diffuse large-cell lymphoma.[19]

There is little doubt that access to care and quality of care affect the outcome in lymphomas. However, there is paucity of publications on this subject. Age was the factor identified in the NHS study of socioeconomic factors leading to delays in the diagnosis of lymphoma.[20]

The future approaches to the management of lymphomas will be based on genetic and molecular information. Currently, although gene expression analysis defines subtypes of non-Hodgkin's lymphoma on the basis of cell of origin with different outcomes after treatment, this technology is not widely available or practical for routine clinical use. The molecular profiling not only allows recognition of important gene signatures involved in the pathobiology of lymphoma, but also permits identification of potential new therapeutic targets.[1,7,10]

◼◼◼◼◼ **SUMMARY TABLE**

Prognostic Factors in Non-Hodgkin Lymphomas

Prognostic Factors	Tumor Related	Host Related	Environment Related
Essential	Histologic type Stage B-symptoms Extranodal site Tumor bulk LDH		
Additional	Number of nodal areas Number of extranodal sites	Age Comorbidity Performance status Hemoglobin $\beta2$ microglobulin	Access to care Quality of care
New and promising	Gene profile of lymphoma cells P53 CD44 CD10 Bcl-6 BCl-2 FOXP-1	Gene profiling of non-malignant tumor-infiltrating immune cells	

Sources:
• NCCN Clinical Practice Guidelines in Oncology:Non-Hodgkin's Lymphoma 2005.
http://www. nccn.org/professionals/physician_gls/PDF/nhl.pdf.
• ESMO Minimum Clinical Recommendations for diagnosis, treatment and follow-up of newly diagnosed large cell Non-Hodgkin's 2005.
• Lymphoma.
http://annonc.oupjournals.org/cgi/reprint/16/suppl_1/i58.
• National Cancer Institute: Non- Hodgkin's Lymphoma (PDQ®): Treatment Guidelines 2005.
http://www. cancer.gov/cancertopics/pdq/treatment/adult-non-hodgkins/healthprofessional/.

REFERENCES

1. Cheson BD: What is new in lymphoma? *CA Cancer J Clin* 54:260–272, 2004.

2. de Jong D: Molecular pathogenesis of follicular lymphoma: a cross talk of genetic and immunologic factors. *J Clin Oncol* 23:6358–6363, 2005.

3. Farinha P, Gascoyne RD: Molecular pathogenesis of mucosa-associated lymphoid tissue lymphoma. *J Clin Oncol* 23:6370–6378, 2005.

4. Glas AM, Kersten MJ, Delahaye LJ, et al.: Gene expression profiling in follicular lymphoma to assess clinical aggressiveness and to guide the choice of treatment. *Blood* 105:301–307, 2005.

5. Lossos IS: Molecular pathogenesis of diffuse large B-cell lymphoma. *J Clin Oncol* 23:6351–6357, 2005.

6. Savage KJ, Monti S, Kutok JL, et al.: The molecular signature of mediastinal large B-cell lymphoma differs from that of other diffuse large B-cell lymphomas and shares features with classical Hodgkin lymphoma. *Blood* 102:3871–3879, 2003.

7. Dave SS, Wright G, Tan B, et al.: Prediction of survival in follicular lymphoma based on molecular features of tumor-infiltrating immune cells. *N Engl J Med* 351:2159–2169, 2004.

8. Rudiger T, Weisenburger DD, Anderson JR, et al.: Peripheral T-cell lymphoma (excluding anaplastic large-cell lymphoma): results from the Non-Hodgkin's Lymphoma Classification Project. *Ann Oncol* 13:140–149, 2002.

9. Morton LM, Wang SS, Devesa SS, et al.: Lymphoma incidence patterns by WHO subtype in the United States, 1992–2001. *Blood* 107:265–276, 2006.

10. Staudt LM, Dave S: The biology of human lymphoid malignancies revealed by gene expression profiling. *Adv Immunol* 87:163–208, 2005.

11. Sobin LH, Wittekind C: UICC TNM, classification of malignant tumours (6th ed.). New York, John Wiley & Sons, Inc., 2002.

12. Evans LS, Hancock BW: Non-Hodgkin lymphoma. *Lancet* 362:139–146, 2003.

13. Solal-Celigny P, Roy P, Colombat P, et al.: Follicular lymphoma international prognostic index. *Blood* 104:1258–1265, 2004.

14. Gallamini A, Stelitano C, Calvi R, et al.: Peripheral T-cell lymphoma unspecified (PTCL-U): a new prognostic model from a retrospective multicentric clinical study. *Blood* 103: 2474–2479, 2004.

15. Hoefnagel JJ, Dijkman R, Basso K, et al.: Distinct types of primary cutaneous large B-cell lymphoma identified by gene expression profiling. *Blood* 105:3671–3678, 2005.

16. Coffey J, Hodgson DC, Gospodarowicz MK: Therapy of non-Hodgkin's lymphoma. *Eur J Nucl Med Mol Imaging* 30:S28–S36, 2003.

17. Bertoni F, Zucca E: State-of-the-art therapeutics: marginal-zone lymphoma. *J Clin Oncol* 23:6415–6420, 2005.

18. Ferreri AJ, Blay JY, Reni M, et al.: Prognostic scoring system for primary CNS lymphomas: the International Extranodal Lymphoma Study Group experience. *J Clin Oncol* 21:266–272, 2003.

19. Gascoyne RD: Emerging prognostic factors in diffuse large B cell lymphoma. *Curr Opin Oncol* 16:436–441, 2004.

20. Neal RD, Allgar VL: Sociodemographic factors and delays in the diagnosis of six cancers: analysis of data from the "National Survey of NHS Patients: Cancer". *Br J Cancer* 92:1971–1975, 2005.

CHAPTER 42

Leukemias

PATRICIA DISPERATI, FERNANDO SUAREZ-SAIZ, HAYTHAM KHOURY, and
MARK D. MINDEN

ACUTE LEUKEMIAS

The acute leukemias are a heterogeneous group of malignant diseases characterized by
their increased proliferation and lack of differentiation. In addition to the presence of
an abnormal clonal population, failure of normal blood cell production is also prominent in the acute leukemias. In the absence of any therapy, patients with acute leukemia
will die in days to a few months. With therapy some patients are cured while for others
treatment barely changes the natural history of the disease. In considering prognosis of
acute leukemias one should consider (1) the nature or type of the disease; (2) the specific therapy that is given; and (3) the time (historical) or location in which the therapy
is given. The acute leukemias can be divided into lymphoid or myeloid origin based
upon the cell of origin and the presence of markers characteristic of the lineage.

Acute Myeloid Leukemia

Acute myeloid leukemia (AML) is a collection of diseases arising in a myeloid bone
marrow stem cell, due to acquired genetic changes. In the past, AML has been classified according to FAB criteria, however, this is now being replaced by WHO criteria
that include cytogenetic and molecular aspects of the disease.[1] A variety of prognostic factors have been suggested for AML, such as age and presenting white count,
however, the importance of these can mostly be accounted for by specific genetic
changes present in the leukemia cells.[2] It is of note that the outcome of a AML with
a particular genetic change is modified by the precise therapy that is given. Patients
with t(15;17), t(8;21) and inv(16) have the best prognosis provided they are treated
with a regimen that includes all trans retinoic acid for the first instance and a regimen

Prognostic Factors in Cancer, Third Edition, edited by Mary K. Gospodarowicz,
Brian O'Sullivan, and Leslie H. Sobin.

that includes high dose cytarabine for the latter two.[3,4] Translocations of MLL and losses of chromosome 5 and 7 are associated with poor outcomes regardless of therapy.[5] Patients with normal cytogenetics are at intermediate risk. Patients with high white blood count disease tend to have mutations of FLT3, Kit, and ras genes.[5] Although these patients frequently achieve remission, there is a high relapse rate and eventual death. Allogeneic stem cell transplant can improve the outcome in intermediate and high risk patients, but is of little added value in the good risk patients.[6]

Acute Lymphoblastic Leukemia

Acute lymphoblastic leukemia (ALL) is a heterogeneous group of diseases traditionally divided into three broad subgroups: B-precursor ALL, T-precursor ALL, and B-mature (Burkitts) Leukemia.[16] Like AML, the morphologic classification is being replaced by cytogenetic/molecular descriptions.[1] Also, as in AML, age and white blood count have been noted as prognostic factors.[17] The effect of age may be twofold. First, the genetic changes associated with ALL vary across the span of age. For example t(9;22) is <5% in patients <18, but represents 25–30% of cases in patients >18. Prior to imatinib t(9;22) was associated with a high relapse rate and death.[18,19] The second manner that age contributes to outcome is that in the past, younger patients received more intensive therapy than older patients. This may be detrimental to the older patients, as patients of the same age treated with a pediatric protocol fare better than the same age group treated with an adult protocol.[20] Age may also affect how well a patient can tolerate a particular treatment.[21] The maximum age that can tolerate very intensive therapy is yet to be determined. In T-ALL the presence of the Hox11 gene portends a high response rate and long term remission while, long-term remission is less for patients expressing Lyl1 or Tal1.[22] Finally, the presence or absence of certain genes involved in drug metabolism provide increased risk or protection against the development of ALL. For example, the GSTM1 null genotype was significantly increased in children with ALL (OR 1.7; 95% CI, 1.0, 2.7).[23]

CHRONIC LEUKEMIAS

Unlike acute leukemias, chronic leukemias are characterized by increased numbers of mature cells, and in the early stages, preservation of bone marrow function. In contrast to the acute leukemias, patients with chronic leukemias can survive for years without any treatment. Here, we will comment on the most common chronic leukemias, specifically chronic lymphocytic leukemia (CLL) and chronic myelogenous leukemia (CML).

Chronic Lymphocytic Leukemia

Chronic lymphocytic leukemia is a lymphoproliferative disorder with expansion of mature, CD5 positive, long-lived nonfunctional B-lymphocytes. Aside from cases where allogeneic bone marrow transplant can be pursued, it is an indolent, incurable disease. The 5-year survival is ~51%.[27] Scales, such as the Rai and Binet, are of prognostic use. They take into account lymphadenopathy, organomegaly (spleen and liver), and cytopenias. Poor risk clinical prognostic factors include a doubling time of lymphocytes of <12 months, older age, male sex, high lymphocyte count, high lactic dehydrogenase levels, and comorbidities. The prognostic utility of these clinical parameters has been enhanced by measurement of CD38, and zeta associated protein 70 (ZAP-70); high expression of these predict for early progression of disease.[28;29]

Cytogenetic analysis, with the use of fluorescence *in situ* hybridization (FISH) has shown that deletions of 17p and −11q have worse survival, whereas deletion of 13q indicates better prognosis.[30] Somatic hypermutation in the variable regions of the heavy chain immunoglobulin (IgV$_H$) has also been associated with prognosis. The presence of mutation (>2% difference in nucleotide sequence of the IgV$_H$ when compared to germline) indicates longer survival, 24 years versus 8 years.[31]

Chronic Myelogenous Leukemia

Chronic myelogenous leukemia (CML) is a myeloproliferative stem-cell disorder characterized by the presence of the bcr-abl fusion gene, a result of the balanced translocation between the long arms of chromosomes 9 and 22, the t(9;22)(q34;q11), also known as the Philadelphia (Ph) chromosome.[36] The median age of presentation is 55–60 years, with a slight male predominance. The natural history of CML is progression from chronic phase (CP) to accelerated (AP) and/or blast crisis (BC) after 3–4 years.

Prognostic models, such as Sokal, Hasford,[37] and the European score, rely on clinical and pathological data at presentation, including age, liver and spleen size, number of blasts, basophils, and eosinophils in the peripheral blood, and platelet count. These models were developed and validated during a period in which the main forms of therapy were hydroxyurea or oral busulfan. Although these agents controlled blood counts they did not impact significantly on survival. The first agent to affect long-term survival was interferon. Patients who had a major response to interferon, that is a reduction in Ph+ve cells to <30% had improved survival.[36,38,39] Interferon has now been replaced by imatinib as the treatment of choice for CML.[40,41] Patients who have an early response to imatinib have a better long-term progression free survival than those who have a slow response. Patients with a deletion of chromosome 9 in the region of the abl gene, have a greater tendancy to progress, whether on interferon therapy or on imatinib.[42] Finally, patients on imatinib who develop point mutations of the abl gene show disease progression due to drug resistance.[43]

■■■■■■ **SUMMARY TABLES**

Prognostic Factors in Acute Myeloid Leukemia

Prognostic Factors	Tumor Related	Host Related	Environment Related
Essential	Cytogenetics[7] t(15;17), t(8;21), inv(16), t(16;16) −5q, −7q, −5, −7 inv(3), t(6;9), t(9;22) Mutations FLT3[5] MLL	Age[a]	Secondary leukemia treatment related[8]
Additional	LDH at presentation Extramedullary disease Multidrug resistance genes[9] Remission duration[10] Response to therapy/minimal residual disease[11]		
New and promising	Gene expression profile[12] Overexpression of WT1, PRAME and BAALC[13,14] Cellular localization of NPM[15]		

[a] Age alters both tumor-and host-related factors.[2]

Source:
• National Cancer Institute: Acute Myeloid Leukemia (PDQ®): Treatment Guidelines 2005.
http://www.cancer.gov/cancertopics/pdq/treatment/adultAML/healthprofessional.
• NCCN Clinical Practice Guidelines in Oncology: Acute Myeloid Leukemia 2005.
http://www.nccn.com/ professionals/physician_gls/PDF/aml.pdf.

Prognostic Factors in Acute Lymphoblastic Leukemia

Prognostic Factors	Tumor Related	Host Related	Environment Related
Essential	CNS disease t(9;22)	Age	
Additional	Cytogenetics[5] and molecular genetics Immunophenotype MRD[24] Genes mutations p53, Rb, P14, p15, p21, HOX11L2, Caspase 3 and Calcitonin Multidrug resistance (MDR1, MRP, LRP)	Gender	
New and promising	DNA microarray[25] Proteomics	Pharmacogenetics[26]	

Source:
• National Cancer Institute: Acute Lymphoblastic Leukemia (PDQ®): Treatment Guidelines 2005.
http://www.cancer.gov/cancertopics/pdq/treatment/adultALL/healthprofessional.

Prognostic Factors in Chronic Lymphocytic Leukemia

Prognostic Factors	Tumor Related	Host Related	Environment Related
Essential	Clinical staging: Hemoglobin, platelet count, spleen size		
Additional	Cytogenetics −13q, +12, −11q, −17p, CD38 IgV$_H$ mutations β2 microglobulin Lymphocyte doubling time p53 defects Serum thymidine kinase ZAP-70	Infection susceptibility profile	
New and promising	Gene expression profiling[32–34] VEGF, VEGFR Soluble CD23 mcl-1 protein expression and mcl-1 promoter insertion Telomere length and telomerase activity Minimal residual disease[35]		

Source:
• ESMO Minimum Clinical Recommendations for diagnosis, treatment and follow-up of chronic lymphocytic leukemia 2005.
http://annonc.oupjournals.org/cgi/reprint/16/suppl_1/i50.

Prognostic Factors in Chronic Myelogenous Leukemia

Prognostic Factors	Tumor Related	Host Related	Environment Related
Essential	Additional chromosomal abnormalities	HLA matched donor[44]	
Additional	Blast crisis Minimal residual disease Cytogenetic and molecular response Time from diagnosis to treatment	Myelosupression after imatinib Response to Imatinib Response to IFN	
New and promising	Clonal evolution Presence of point mutations in abl $-9q$ Bone marrow fibrosis		

Sources:
• National Cancer Institute: Chronic Myelogenous Leukemia (PDQ®): Treatment Guidelines 2005.
http://www.cancer.gov/cancertopics/pdq/treatment/CML/healthprofessional/.
• ESMO Minimum Clinical Recommendations for diagnosis, treatment and follow-up of chronic myelogeneous leukaemia 2005.
http://annonc.oupjournals.org/cgi/reprint/16/suppl_1/i52.
• NCCN Clinical Practice Guidelines in Oncology: Chronic Myelogenous Leukemia 2005.
http://www.nccn.org/professionals/physician_gls/PDF/cml.pdf.

REFERENCES

1. Harris NL, Jaffe ES, Diebold J, et al.: The World Health Organization classification of hematological malignancies report of the Clinical Advisory Committee Meeting, Airlie House, Virginia, November 1997. *Mod Pathol* 13:193–207, 2000.

2. Gupta V, Chun K, Yi QL, et al.: Disease biology rather than age is the most important determinant of survival of patients > or = 60 years with acute myeloid leukemia treated with uniform intensive therapy. *Cancer* 103:2082–2090, 2005.

3. Tallman MS, Andersen JW, Schiffer CA, et al.: All-trans retinoic acid in acute promyelocytic leukemia: long-term outcome and prognostic factor analysis from the North American Intergroup protocol. *Blood* 100:4298–4302, 2002.

4. Byrd JC, Mrozek K, Dodge RK, et al.: Pretreatment cytogenetic abnormalities are predictive of induction success, cumulative incidence of relapse, and overall survival in adult patients with de novo acute myeloid leukemia: results from Cancer and Leukemia Group B (CALGB 8461). *Blood* 100:4325–4336, 2002.

5. Frohling S, Scholl C, Gilliland DG, et al.: Genetics of myeloid malignancies: pathogenetic and clinical implications. *J Clin Oncol* 23:6285–6295, 2005.

6. Burnett AK: Evaluating the contribution of allogeneic and autologous transplantation to the management of acute myeloid leukemia in adults. *Cancer Chemother. Pharmacol* 48:S53–S58, 2001.

7. Slovak ML, Kopecky KJ, Cassileth PA, et al.: Karyotypic analysis predicts outcome of preremission and postremission therapy in adult acute myeloid leukemia: a southwest oncology Group/Eastern cooperative oncology group study. *Blood* 96:4075–4083, 2000.

8. Andre M, Mounier N, Leleu X, et al.: Second cancers and late toxicities after treatment of aggressive non-Hodgkin lymphoma with the ACVBP regimen: a GELA cohort study on 2837 patients. *Blood* 103:1222–1228, 2004.

9. Marie JP, Legrand O: MDR1/P-GP expression as a prognostic factor in acute leukemias. *Adv Exp Med Biol* 457:1–9, 1999.

10. Keating MJ, Kantarjian H, Smith TL, et al.: Response to salvage therapy and survival after relapse in acute myelogenous leukemia. *J Clin Oncol* 7:1071–1080, 1989.

11. Estey EH, Shen Y, Thall PF: Effect of time to complete remission on subsequent survival and disease-free survival time in AML, RAEB-t, and RAEB. *Blood* 95:72–77, 2000.

12. Valk PJ, Verhaak RG, Beijen MA, et al.: Prognostically useful gene-expression profiles in acute myeloid leukemia. *N Engl J Med* 350:1617–1628, 2004.

13. Baldus CD, Tanner SM, Ruppert AS, et al.: BAALC expression predicts clinical outcome of de novo acute myeloid leukemia patients with normal cytogenetics: a Cancer and Leukemia Group B Study. *Blood* 102:1613–1618, 2003.

14. Greiner J, Ringhoffer M, Simikopinko O, et al.: Simultaneous expression of different immunogenic antigens in acute myeloid leukemia. *Exp Hematol* 28:1413–1422, 2000.

15. Dohner K, Schlenk RF, Habdank M, et al.: Mutant nucleophosmin (NPM1) predicts favorable prognosis in younger adults with acute myeloid leukemia and normal cytogenetics – interaction with other gene mutations. *Blood* 2005.

16. Bassan R, Gatta G, Tondini C, et al.: Adult acute lymphoblastic leukaemia. *Crit Rev Oncol Hematol* 50:223–261, 2004.

17. Plasschaert SL, Kamps WA, Vellenga E, et al.: Prognosis in childhood and adult acute lymphoblastic leukaemia: a question of maturation? *Cancer Treat Rev* 30:37–51, 2004.

18. Brandwein JM, Gupta V, Wells RA, et al.: Treatment of elderly patients with acute lymphoblastic leukemia-Evidence for a benefit of imatinib in BCR-ABL positive patients. *Leuk Res* 2005.

19. Lee KH, Lee JH, Choi SJ, et al.: Clinical effect of imatinib added to intensive combination chemotherapy for newly diagnosed Philadelphia chromosome-positive acute lymphoblastic leukemia. *Leukemia* 19:1509–1516, 2005.

20. de Bont JM, Holt B, Dekker AW, et al.: Significant difference in outcome for adolescents with acute lymphoblastic leukemia treated on pediatric vs adult protocols in the Netherlands. *Leukemia* 18:2032–2035, 2004.

21. Offidani M, Corvatta L, Malerba L, et al.: Comparison of two regimens for the treatment of elderly patients with acute lymphoblastic leukaemia (ALL). Leuk. *Lymphoma* 46:233–238, 2005.

22. Ferrando AA, Neuberg DS, Staunton J, et al.: Gene expression signatures define novel oncogenic pathways in T cell acute lymphoblastic leukemia. *Cancer Cell* 1:75–87, 2002.

23. Ye Z, Song H: Glutathione s-transferase polymorphisms (GSTM1, GSTP1 and GSTT1) and the risk of acute leukaemia: a systematic review and meta-analysis. *Eur J Cancer* 41:980–989, 2005.

24. Bruggemann M, Raff T, Flohr T, et al.: Clinical significance of minimal residual disease quantification in adult patients with standard risk acute lymphoblastic leukemia. *Blood* 2005.

25. Yeoh EJ, Ross ME, Shurtleff SA, et al.: Classification, subtype discovery, and prediction of outcome in pediatric acute lymphoblastic leukemia by gene expression profiling. *Cancer Cell* 1:133–143, 2002.

26. Pui CH, Schrappe M, Ribeiro RC, et al.: Childhood and adolescent lymphoid and myeloid leukemia. *Hematology* (Am. Soc. Hematol. Educ. Program.) 118–145, 2004.

27. Anonymous: A clinical evaluation of the International Lymphoma Study Group classification of non-Hodgkin's lymphoma. The Non-Hodgkin's Lymphoma Classification Project. *Blood* 89:3909–3918, 1997.

28. Byrd JC, Stilgenbauer S, Flinn IW: Chronic lymphocytic leukemia. *Hematology* (Am. Soc. Hematol. Educ. Program.) 163–183, 2004.

29. Rassenti LZ, Huynh L, Toy TL, et al.: ZAP-70 compared with immunoglobulin heavy-chain gene mutation status as a predictor of disease progression in chronic lymphocytic leukemia. *N Engl J Med* 351:893–901, 2004.

30. Dohner H, Stilgenbauer S, Benner A, et al.: Genomic aberrations and survival in chronic lymphocytic leukemia. *N Engl J Med* 343:1910–1916, 2000.

31. Shanafelt TD, Geyer SM, Kay NE: Prognosis at diagnosis: integrating molecular biologic insights into clinical practice for patients with CLL. *Blood* 103:1202–1210, 2004.

32. Staal FJ, van der BM, Wessels LF, et al.: DNA microarrays for comparison of gene expression profiles between diagnosis and relapse in precursor-B acute lymphoblastic leukemia: choice of technique and purification influence the identification of potential diagnostic markers. *Leukemia* 17:1324–1332, 2003.

33. Falt S, Merup M, Gahrton G, et al.: Identification of progression markers in B-CLL by gene expression profiling. *Exp Hematol* 33:883–893, 2005.

34. Haslinger C, Schweifer N, Stilgenbauer S, et al.: Microarray gene expression profiling of B-cell chronic lymphocytic leukemia subgroups defined by genomic aberrations and VH mutation status. *J Clin Oncol* 22:3937–3949, 2004.

35. Moreton P, Kennedy B, Lucas G, et al.: Eradication of minimal residual disease in B-cell chronic lymphocytic leukemia after alemtuzumab therapy is associated with prolonged survival. *J Clin Oncol* 23:2971–2979, 2005.

36. Simonsson B, Kloke O, Stahel RA: ESMO Minimum Clinical Recommendations for the diagnosis, treatment and follow-up of chronic myelogenous leukemia (CML). *Ann Oncol* 16:i52–i53, 2005.

37. Hasford J, Pfirrmann M, Hehlmann R, et al.: Prognosis and prognostic factors for patients with chronic myeloid leukemia: nontransplant therapy. *Semin Hematol* 40:4–12, 2003.

38. Kantarjian HM, O'Brien S, Cortes JE, et al.: Complete cytogenetic and molecular responses to interferon-alpha-based therapy for chronic myelogenous leukemia are associated with excellent long-term prognosis. *Cancer* 97:1033–1041, 2003.

39. Hughes TP, Kaeda J, Branford S, et al.: Frequency of major molecular responses to imatinib or interferon alfa plus cytarabine in newly diagnosed chronic myeloid leukemia. *N Engl J Med* 349:1423–1432, 2003.

40. Marin D, Kaeda J, Szydlo R, et al.: Monitoring patients in complete cytogenetic remission after treatment of CML in chronic phase with imatinib: patterns of residual leukaemia and prognostic factors for cytogenetic relapse. *Leukemia* 19:507–512, 2005.

41. Kantarjian HM, O'Brien S, Cortes J, et al.: Imatinib mesylate therapy improves survival in patients with newly diagnosed Philadelphia chromosome-positive chronic myelogenous leukemia in the chronic phase: comparison with historic data. *Cancer* 98: 2636–2642, 2003.

42. Huntly BJ, Guilhot F, Reid AG, et al.: Imatinib improves but may not fully reverse the poor prognosis of patients with CML with derivative chromosome 9 deletions. *Blood* 102:2205–2212, 2003.

43. Willis SG, Lange T, Demehri S, et al.: High-sensitivity detection of BCR-ABL kinase domain mutations in imatinib-naive patients: correlation with clonal cytogenetic evolution but not response to therapy. *Blood* 106:2128–2137, 2005.

44. Goldman JM, Druker BJ: Chronic myeloid leukemia: current treatment options. *Blood* 98:2039–2042, 2001.

CHAPTER 43

Multiple Myeloma

JESÚS F. SAN MIGUEL and NORMA C. GUTIÉRREZ

The outcome of multiple myeloma patients is highly heterogeneous with a survival ranging from a few months to >10 years. This heterogeneity relates to specific characteristics of the tumor itself and of the host. The main reason for studying prognostic factors is the identification of risk groups in order to adapt patient treatment according to the expected outcome. This would be particularly important upon evaluating new therapeutic strategies.

A high proportion of myelomatous plasma cells (PC) in the bone marrow (BM), a diffuse pattern of BM infiltration and the presence of circulating PC reflect a high tumor burden, but their prognostic influence is modest. Similarly, the impact of skeletal lesions, evaluated by X-ray or bone resorption markers is not clear. By contrast, disease complications, such as anemia, thrombocytopenia, and particularly renal insufficiency, have a relevant influence. The most important factor is β_2-microglobulin (B2-M) levels that increase as a result of both tumor burden growth and renal function deterioration. The higher the value the worst the prognosis. CRP is a surrogate marker for IL-6 (a major PC growth factor), which also correlates with outcome.

Recently a new International Staging System (ISS) derived from >11,000 patients has shown that B2-M and albumin are the best combination of easily available markers to discriminate prognostic subgroups: stage I (B2-M < 3,5 and Albumin > 3,5 mg/dL), stage III (B2-M > 5.5), and stage II (the rest).[1] In the next several years, an improved staging system incorporating cytogenetics and S-phase analyses will be developed.

The favorable influence of a good performance status (ECOG 0-2) and young age (65–70 years) are well established. Moreover, it has been reported that patients under 40-years old with normal renal function and low β_2-M have a median survival of >8 years. By contrast, neither gender nor race has prognostic influence. The role in immune surveillance of T and NK cells is well established,[2] and low numbers of mature NK and CD4 cells have been reported in advanced stage MM. In addition,

Prognostic Factors in Cancer, *Third Edition*, edited by Mary K. Gospodarowicz, Brian O'Sullivan, and Leslie H. Sobin.

patients who develop expanded T-cell clones (CD8$^+$CD57$^+$CD28$^-$), which can recognize autologous idiotypic Ig structures, display improved prognosis.

An important cohort of prognostic factors is those that reflect specific characteristics of myelomatous PC and include morphology, immunophenotyping, cytogenetics, oncogenes, multidrug resistance, and the proliferative activity of PC. Immature/plasmablastic morphology is associated with poor outcome.[3] Conflicting results have been reported for immunophenotyping. A down-regulation of CD117 (C-Kit) and CD56, and expression of CD28 and CD19 are associated with poor prognosis.[4] As occurs with acute leukemia, cytogenetics is emerging as one of the most important prognostic tools for MM.[5,6] The investigation of cytogenetic changes (either by karyotyping or FISH) should be used in all newly diagnosed MM patients. Deletions of chromosome 13 are associated with shortened survival. Other chromosomal changes associated with poor survival are t(4;14)(p16;q32), t(14;16)(q32;q23), and 17p13 deletion (p53), while t(11;14) is a favorable prognostic factor or at least does not influence outcome negatively.[7–9] Moreover, the presence of complex as well as nonhyperdiploid karyotypes, which are strongly associated with del 13 and t(4;14) also bear treatment failure.[10] Similarly, patients with chromosome losses detected by comparative genomic hybridization display a very short survival.[11] Other potential adverse cytogenetic features are gains on 1q and deletion of chromosome 22.[12] By contrast, hyperdiploid tumors with multiple trisomies involving chromosomes 3, 5, 7, 9, 11, 15, 19, and 21 tend to have a favorable prognostic influence.[13] In line with this latter observation, we have shown that patients with hyperdiploid DNA cell content (defined by flow cytometry) have a favorable outcome.

The development and progression of MM implies a multistep process of oncogenic events. The p53 and K-ras mutations or c-myc overexpression are associated with progressive disease and relapse.[14] In addition, we have observed that methylation of p16 is associated with high proliferative activity of PC and poor prognosis.[15] Conflicting results have been reported regarding the independent prognostic value of MDR-1 expression, while recent data suggests that LRP may afford more important information. Finally, the proliferative activity of the malignant PC, as assessed either by the labeling index (LI) with bromodeoxyuridine or by flow cytometry with PI, is one of the most important prognostic markers for MM.[16] In our experience, the number of PC in S-phase together with cytogenetics, β_2M, PS and age, represents the best combination of disease characteristics for survival prediction.

Patients with indolent myeloma should be observed. Most patients, however, present with symptomatic MM and require treatment. High-dose chemotherapy (melphalan) with stem cell support for patients up to 70 years and conventional dose melphalan–prednisone is considered the standard therapy for myeloma. A better understanding of the biology of MM has provided the framework for development of new drugs that target not only the myeloma cells, but also the microenvironment. These new agents include immunomodulatory drugs, such as Thalidomide and lenalidomide, and proteasome inhibitors (bortezomib), which have shown high efficacy in refractory/relapse patients and are currently being explored in newly diagnosed patients. With these new treatment strategies hopefully this incurable disease (median survival: 3–5 years) may become a chronic disorder.

■■■■■■■ SUMMARY TABLE

Prognostic Factors in Multiple Myeloma

Prognostic Factors	Tumor Related	Host Related	Environment Related
Essential	β_2-Microglobulin Albumin *RB, p53* Cytogenetics/FISH: t(4;14), t(11;14)		

Additional	Plasma cell
	  proliferation
	Immunophenotyping
	  markers
		Age
		
		Performance status	

New and promising	Gene molecular
	  markers: *p27*
	CKS1B (1q21)
	Circulating
	  clonotypic PC
	COX-2
	sRANKL
		Immune status	

Sources:
• NCCN Clinical Practice Guidelines in Oncology: Multiple Myeloma.
http://www.nccn.org/professionals/physician_gls/PDF/myeloma.pdf.
• ESMO Minimum Clinical Recommendations for diagnosis, treatment and follow-up of multiple myeloma.
http://annonc.oupjournals.org/cgi/reprint/16/suppl_1/i45.

REFERENCES

1. Greipp PR, San Miguel J, Durie BG, et al.: International staging system for multiple myeloma. *J Clin Oncol* 23:3412–3420, 2005.

2. Kay NE, Leong TL, Bone N, et al.: Blood levels of immune cells predict survival in myeloma patients: results of an Eastern Cooperative Oncology Group phase 3 trial for newly diagnosed multiple myeloma patients. *Blood* 1;98:23–28, 2001.

3. San Miguel JF, García-Sanz R: Multiple myeloma: differential diagnosis and prognosis, in Gahrton G, Durie BGM, Samson D (eds.): *Multiple myeloma and related disorders*. London: Arnold, 2004, pp. 179–199.

4. Mateo G, Gutiérrez NC, López-Berges C, et al.: Immunophenotype of the malignant clone. Implications for management. *Haematologica* (Suppl) 90:3, 2005.

5. Bergsagel PL: Prognostic factors in multiple myeloma: it's in the genes. *Clin Cancer Res* 9:533–534, 2003.

6. Magrangeas F, Lode L, Wuilleme S, et al.: Genetic heterogeneity in multiple myeloma. *Leukemia* 19:191–194, 2005.

7. Chang H, Qi C, Yi QL, et al.: p53 gene deletion detected by fluorescence in situ hybridization is an adverse prognostic factor for patients with multiple myeloma following autologous stem cell transplantation. *Blood* 105:358–360, 2005.

8. Fonseca R, Blood E, Rue M, et al.: Clinical and biologic implications of recurrent genomic aberrations in myeloma. *Blood* 101:4569–4575, 2003.

9. Moreau P, Facon T, Leleu X, et al.: Recurrent 14q32 translocations determine the prognosis of multiple myeloma, especially in patients receiving intensive chemotherapy. *Blood* 100:1579–1583, 2002.

10. Fonseca R, Barlogie B, Bataille R, et al.: Genetics and cytogenetics of multiple myeloma: a workshop report. *Cancer Res* 64:1546–1558, 2004.

11. Gutiérrez NC, García JL, Hernández JM, et al.: Prognostic and biologic significance of chromosomal imbalances assessed by comparative genomic hybridization in multiple myeloma. *Blood* 104:2661–2666, 2004.

12. Zhan F, Hanamura I, Burington B, et al.: The transcriptome of multiple myeloma defines disease subgroups with distinct genetic and clinical features and also allows identification of genes highly correlated with an aggressive clinical course. *Haematologica* (Suppl) 90:33–34, 2005.

13. Hideshima T, Bergsagel PL, Kuehl WM, et al.: Advances in biology of multiple myeloma: clinical applications. *Blood* 104:607–618, 2004.

14. Rasmussen T, Kuehl M, Lodahl M, et al.: Possible roles for activating RAS mutations in the MGUS to MM transition and in the intramedullary to extramedullary transition in some plasma cell tumors. *Blood* 105:317–323, 2005.

15. Mateos MV, García-Sanz R, López-Perez R, et al.: p16/INK4a gene inactivation by hypermethylation is associated with aggressive variants of monoclonal gammopathies. *Hematol J* 2:146–149, 2001.

16. García-Sanz R, González-Fraile MI, Mateo G, et al.: Proliferative activity of plasma cells is the most relevant prognostic factor in elderly multiple myeloma patients. *Int J Cancer* 112:884–889, 2004.

BRAIN TUMORS

CHAPTER 44

Gliomas

GUISEPPE MINNITI, MICHAEL BRADA, PAUL KLEIHUES, and HIROKO OHGAKI

Brain tumors account for <2% of all cancer, with an overall incidence of 7–9/100,000 persons/year. Gliomas (generic term for neuro-epithelial tumors) are the most frequent intracranial tumors and account for >50% of all primary brain tumors. They are classified by the predominant cell type into astrocytomas, oligodendrogliomas, and mixed oligoastrocytomas. The WHO grading of central nervous system (CNS) tumors reflects their histological aggressiveness. WHO grade I and II are generally referred to as low-grade and WHO grade III and IV as high-grade or malignant gliomas.[1]

Clinical presentation includes features of raised intracranial pressure, seizures, and focal neurological deficits depending on the tumor site. Diagnosis requires imaging with contrast enhanced computerized tomography (CT) and/or magnetic resonance imaging (MRI). Pathologic confirmation is required in most patients with tissue obtained via closed/stereotactic biopsy or open craniotomy.

Pilocytic astrocytoma (WHO grade I) affects predominantly children and young adults and is preferentially located in the cerebellum and CNS midline structures. It is well delineated, lacks a tendency for malignant progression, and has a favorable clinical outcome, with 5-year survival rates of >90% of patients. In accessible locations away from critical structures, complete excision is curative treatment. Progressive, unresectable tumors, particularly those affecting the optic chiasm, are treated in young children with primary chemotherapy and in older children and adults with often curative radiotherapy.

Diffusely infiltrating astrocytomas consist of three major entities: low-grade diffuse astrocytoma (WHO grade II), anaplastic astrocytoma (WHO grade III), and glioblastoma (WHO grade IV). They have a wide range of histopathological features and biological behavior, but they diffusely infiltrate adjacent brain structures and have an inherent tendency for malignant progression.[1]

Diffuse astrocytoma (WHO grade II) is a slowly growing tumor with an inherent tendency for malignant progression to anaplastic astrocytoma (WHO grade III) and

Prognostic Factors in Cancer, Third Edition, edited by Mary K. Gospodarowicz,
Brian O'Sullivan, and Leslie H. Sobin.

secondary glioblastoma (WHO grade IV). Management options include surveillance, surgery, radiotherapy, or a combination of these. Gross total resection is recommended in fit patients with accessible localized tumors although there is no convincing data to demonstrate that this approach is associated with survival benefit.[2] Radiotherapy achieves tumor and symptom control and is usually employed in patients with progressive disease or histological evidence of transition to anaplastic astrocytoma. In cases with no evidence of progressive disease, some centers prefer a wait and see attitude. Randomized studies suggest no disadvantage for delayed rather than immediate radiotherapy.[3–5] High-dose therapy (64.8 Gy/36 fractions) is associated with shorter survival and somewhat more frequent radionecrosis than low-dose radiotherapy (50.4 Gy/28 fractions).[5] The role of chemotherapy is currently not defined and it is used at the time of recurrence/progression after failure of surgery and radiotherapy. The main prognostic factors for survival are age, tumor size, and neurological/performance status. Overexpression of VEGF, p53 mutation, higher proliferation rate (MIB-1 labeling index) and tumors with a significant fraction of gemistocytes (gemistocytic astrocytomas) have been correlated with shorter survival.[6]

Anaplastic astrocytoma (AA, WHO grade III) typically develops from diffuse astrocytomas and progresses to secondary glioblastoma within ~2 years. The overall median survival is 2–3 years.

Glioblastoma multiforme (GBM, WHO grade IV) is an aggressive tumor with a median survival in the range of 10–12 months. Most cases (>90%) are primary GBMs that develop *de novo*, that is, without a clinically or histopathologically identifiable less malignant precursor lesion. Treatment options include surgery, radiotherapy, and chemotherapy. Although gross total resection is associated with improved survival, it is not clear whether the extent of surgery rather than patient selection for resectability is the determinant of improved outcome.[7] Radical external beam radiotherapy to a dose of 60 Gy in 30 fractions improves the median survival of glioblastoma patients. Dose intensification with stereotactic radiotherapy, radiosurgery boost, brachytherapy, IMRT, or altered dose fractionation have not improved results further. A shorter course of palliative radiotherapy or supportive care alone may be appropriate in patients with poor prognosis. Recent data indicate that radiotherapy with concomitant then adjuvant chemotherapy with temozolomide compared to radiotherapy alone confers a further survival benefit of 2.5 months; the 2-year survival rate increased from 10 to 26%.[8] A small survival advantage in high-grade glioma patients (glioblastomas and anaplastic astrocytomas) from 40 to 46% at 1 year after combined radiotherapy and adjuvant PCV chemotherapy (procarbazine, CCNU/lomustine and vincristine) was demonstrated in a meta-analysis.[9]

The main prognostic factors in patients with malignant glioma are tumor grade, age, and performance status. Patients >70 years with poor performance status have the worst prognosis. Promoter methylation of the repair protein 0^6-methylguanine-DNA methyltransferase (MGMT) in conjunction with adjuvant chemotherapy has emerged as an additional independent prognostic factor.[10] Loss of heterozygosity (LOH) of 10q has been associated with worse prognosis,[11] while a negative impact of overexpression of the EGF receptor (EGFR) and mutational inactivation of the p53 and PTEN tumor-suppressor genes was not confirmed in a large, population-based study.[11]

Oligodendroglioma (WHO Grade II) is a slowly growing tumor, often with a long history of epileptic seizures. It may progress to anaplastic oligodendroglioma (WHO Grade III). The median survival is in the range of 8–10 years.[6] Management is similar to that of diffuse astrocytomas with the options of surveillance, surgery, and radiotherapy, although oligodendrogliomas are more chemoresponsive with a 60–70% rate of response to treatment with PCV[12] and temozolomide used in recurrent or primary tumors.[13] Favorable prognostic factors include gross total resection, young age and good performance status. Allelic loss at 1p and/or 19q, which is present in up to 80% of tumors,[6] has been confirmed as favorable predictor of survival and chemosensitivity.[14–16]

Anaplastic oligodendroglioma (AO, WHO Grade III) is a more aggressive variant of oligodendroglioma, with a median survival of ~3 years. Management is similar to anaplastic astrocytoma (AA) with primary surgery and radiotherapy. Although AO demonstrates high response rate to chemotherapy with PCV or temozolomide, especially in patients with deletions of the 1p and/or 19q, no survival benefit has been demonstrated with adjuvant chemotherapy.[17] As in patients with grade II oligodendroglioma, younger patients and a good performance status combined with LOH on 1p/19q are associated with better survival outcome.

Oligoastrocytoma (WHO grade II) and anaplastic oligoastrocytoma (WHO Grade III) are mixed gliomas composed of both astrocytic and oligodendroglial components and represent 4–8% of gliomas. Treatment is similar to astrocytic tumors; survival tends to be in between oligodendrogliomas and astrocytomas of corresponding grades.

Prognostic Factors in Gliomas

Glioma Type	Prognostic Factor	Tumor Related	Host Related	Treatment Related
Diffuse low-grade astrocytoma	Essential	Size	Age PS	Gross total resection
	Additional	Gemistocytes (poor) MIB-1 index VEGF expression p53 mutation		Radiotherapy Chemotherapy
Malignant gliomas (Anaplastic astrocytoma and glioblastoma)	Essential		Age PS	Radiotherapy Concomitant and adjuvant temozolomide chemotherapy (for GBM)
	Additional	Necrosis (poor) Grade LOH on 10q		Gross total resection
	New and promising	MGMT promoter methylation		
Oligodendrogliomas	Essential	LOH on 1p and/or 19q	Age PS	Gross total resection
	Additional			PCV or temozolomide chemotherapy (tumors with LOH on 1 p and/or 19q) Radiotherapy[a]

[a]An essential factor for anaplastic Oligodendrogliomas.

Sources:

• Central Nervous System Cancers. Practice Guidelines in Oncology: National Comprehensive Cancer Network. http://www.nccn.org. 2005.

• Brain Tumors Treatment Guidelines: National Cancer Institute http://cancer.gov. 2005.

REFERENCES

1. Kleihues P, Cavenee WK (eds.): *WHO Classification of tumours. Pathology and genetics of tumors of the nervous system*, Lyon, IARC Press, 2000.

2. Keles GE, Lamborn KR, Berger MS: Low-grade hemispheric gliomas in adults: a critical review of extent of resection as a factor influencing outcome. *J Neurosurg* 95:735–745, 2001.

3. Glioma Meta-analysis Trialists (GMT) Group: Chemotherapy in adult high-grade glioma: A systematic review and meta-analysis of individual patient data from 12 randomized trials. *Lancet* 359:1011–1018, 2002.

4. Karim AB, Afra D, Cornu P: Randomized trial on the efficacy of radiotherapy for cerebral low-grade glioma in the adult: European Organization for Research and Treatment of Cancer study 22845 with the Medical Research Council study BR04: An interim analysis. *Int J Radiat Oncol Biol Phys* 52:316–324, 2002.

5. Shaw E, Arusell R, Scheithauer B: Prospective randomized trial of low- versus high-dose radiation therapy in adults with supratentorial low-grade glioma: Initial report of a North Cancer Central Treatment Group/Radiation Therapy Oncology Group/Eastern Cooperative Oncology Group study. *J Clin Oncol* 20:2267–2276, 2002.

6. Okamoto Y, Di Patre PL, Burkhard C, et al.: Population-based study on incidence, survival rates, and genetic alterations of low-grade diffuse astrocytomas and oligodendrogliomas. *Acta Neuropathol (Berlin)* 108:49–56, 2004.

7. Laws ER, Parney IF, Huang W, et al.: Survival following surgery and prognostic factors for recently diagnosed malignant glioma: data from the Glioma Outcomes Project. *J Neurosurg* 99:467–473, 2003.

8. Stupp R, Mason WP, van den Bent MJ, et al.: Radiotherapy plus concomitant and adjuvant temozolomide for glioblastoma. *N Engl J Med* 352:987–996, 2005.

9. Stewart LA: Chemotherapy in adult high-grade glioma: a systematic review and meta-analysis of individual patient data from 12 randomised trials. *Lancet* 359:1011–1018, 2002.

10. Hegi ME, Diserens AC, Gorlia T, et al.: MGMT gene silencing and benefit from temozolomide in glioblastoma. *N Engl J Med* 352:997–1003, 2005.

11. Ohgaki H, Dessen P, Jourde B, et al.: Genetic pathways to glioblastoma: a population-based study. *Cancer Res* 64:6892–6899, 2004.

12. Buckner JC, Gesme D Jr, O'Fallon JR, et al.: Phase II trial of procarbazine, lomustine, and vincristine as initial therapy for patients with low-grade oligodendroglioma or oligoastrocytoma: efficacy and associations with chromosomal abnormalities. *J Clin Oncol* 21:251–255, 2003.

13. Van den Bent MJ, Taphoorn MJ, et al.: Phase II study of first-line chemotherapy with temozolomide in recurrent oligodendroglial tumors: the European Organization for Research and Treatment of Cancer Brain Tumor Group Study 26971. *J Clin Oncol* 21:2525–2528, 2003.

14. Smith JS, Perry A, Borell TJ, et al.: Alterations of chromosome arms 1p and 19q as predictors of survival in oligodendrogliomas, astrocytomas, and mixed oligoastrocytomas. *J Clin Oncol* 18:636–645, 2000.

15. Felsberg J, Erkwoh A, Sabel MC, et al.: Oligodendroglial tumors: refinement of candidate regions on chromosome arm 1p and correlation of 1p/19q status with survival. *Brain Pathol* 14:121–130, 2004 Apr.

16. Van den Bent MJ: Diagnosis and management of oligodendroglioma. *Semin Oncol* 31:645–652, 2004 Oct.

17. Cairncross G, Seiferheld W, Shaw E, et al.: An intergroup randomized controlled clinical trial (RCT) of chemotherapy plus radiation (RT) versus RT alone for pure and mixed anaplastic oligodendrogliomas: Initial report of RTOG 94-02. *J Clin Oncol* 2004. ASCO Annual Meeting Proceedings 22, 14S (Suppl), 1500, 2004.

PEDIATRIC CANCERS

CHAPTER 45

Pediatric Cancers

ERIC BOUFFET, DAVID C. HODGSON, and ENG-SIEW KOH

PEDIATRIC CENTRAL NERVOUS SYSTEM TUMORS

Brain tumors represent ~20% of all pediatric malignancies. Gliomas, medulloblastomas/primitive neuroectodermal tumors and ependymomas account for >75% of all pediatric central nervous system (CNS) tumors. These tumors are seen in all age groups, with a peak incidence between 5- and 10-years old. Some tumors are more common during infancy and early childhood, such as choroid plexus carcinomas, rhabdoid tumors, and to some extent, ependymomas.

The most common staging system in use for pediatric CNS tumors is the Chang system,[1] initially used for medulloblastoma (Table 45.1). Metastatic spread is not specific for malignant tumors, as dissemination can also be observed in low-grade "benign" tumors, such as low-grade gliomas or myxopapillary ependymomas. Three factors are paramount for the management of these tumors: the histological diagnosis, the location/extent of the tumor, and the age of the patient. Although progress has been seen over the last two decades, the outcome of children with CNS tumors is still unsatisfactory, either because of the poor survival rates (e.g., in diffuse brainstem glioma and rhabdoid tumors) or the long-term toxicities of treatment on the growing brain.

The diversity of pediatric CNS brain tumors precludes any firm statement regarding prognostic factors. Studies have suggested a link between the duration of presenting symptoms and survival in ependymoma, brainstem glioma, and spinal cord astrocytoma.[2–4] The extent of resection is the strongest prognostic factor in most nonmetastatic tumors, with some exceptions, such as CNS germ cell tumors for which the degree of resection has no influence on outcome. Recent studies have pointed out the role of molecular prognostic markers, particularly in medulloblastoma and high-grade gliomas.[1,5,6] However, this latter information is not yet been fully incorporated into a risk stratification system to guide treatment.

Prognostic Factors in Cancer, Third Edition, edited by Mary K. Gospodarowicz, Brian O'Sullivan, and Leslie H. Sobin.
Copyright © 2006 John Wiley & Sons, Inc.

TABLE 45.1   Chang Staging System for Medulloblastoma[a]

Classification		Stages	
T1	Tumor <3 cm in diameter and limited to the classic midline position in the vermis, the roof of the fourth ventricle, and less commonly to the cerebellar hemispheres	M0	No evidence of subarachnoid or hematogenous metastases
T2	Tumor ≥3 cm in diameter and invading one adjacent structure or partly filling the fourth ventricle	M1	Tumor cells found in cerebrospinal fluid on microscopic analysis
T3a	Tumor further invading two adjacent structures or completely filling the fourth ventricle, with extension into the aqueduct of Sylvius, foramen of Magendie, or foramen of Luschka, thus producing prominent internal hydrocephalus	M2[b]	Gross nodular seeding in cerebellum, cerebral subarachnoid space, or in third or fourth ventricles
T3b	Tumor arising from floor of fourth ventricle and filling the fourth ventricle	M3[b]	Gross nodular seeding in spinal subarachnoid space
T4	Tumor spread through aqueduct of Sylvius to involve third ventricle, midbrain, or down into upper cervical cord	M4	Extraneuraxial metastasis

[a]The T classification has no prognostic significance and tends to be abandoned. The M staging is used for most malignant paediatric CNS tumors (e.g., germ cell tumors, ependymomas, rhabdoid tumours).
[b]Both M2 and M3 are often pooled in a M2/3 category.

Recognition that the clinical outcome in some pediatric CNS tumors varies according to prognostic indicators has led to the development of risk stratified treatments. Patients with average risk medulloblastoma are those older than 3 years of age with no evidence of metastatic disease (M0) and totally or near totally resected tumor (<1.5 cm^2 residual on postoperative imaging). Patients who do not meet these criteria are classified as high risk. Postoperative treatment will differ according to the risk category. Similarly, the postoperative management of children with intracranial ependymoma will differ, depending on the extent of resection.

NEUROBLASTOMA

Neuroblastoma (NBL) is the fourth most common pediatric malignancy, accounting for 7–10% of all childhood cancers and the most common cancer diagnosed during

TABLE 45.2   International Neuroblastoma Staging System

Stage	Description
1	Localized tumor with complete gross excision, with or without microscopic residual disease; representative ipsilateral lymph-nodes negative for tumor microscopically (lymph-nodes adherent to and removed with primary may be positive)
2A	Localized tumor with incomplete gross excision; representative ipsilateral nonadherent lymph nodes negative for tumor microscopically
2B	Localized tumor with or without complete gross excision, with ipsilateral nonadherent lymph-nodes positive for tumor; enlarged contralateral lymph nodes must be negative microscopically
3	Unresectable unilateral tumor infiltrating across the midline, with or without regional lymph-node involvement; or localized unilateral tumor with contralateral regional lymph-node involvement; or midline tumor with bilateral extension by infiltration (unresectable) or by lymph-node involvement
4	Any primary tumor with dissemination to distant lymph nodes, bone, bone marrow, liver, skin, and/or other organs (except as defined for stage 4S)
4S	Limited to infants under 1 yr of age and localized primary tumor (as defined for stage 1, 2A, or 2B) with dissemination limited to skin, liver, and/or bone marrow (bone marrow involvement must be <10% of total nucleated cells identified as malignant on bone marrow biopsy or aspirate; more extensive bone marrow involvement is considered stage 4.

infancy with a median age at diagnosis of 18 months. Neuroblastoma originates from the autonomic nervous system, occurring most commonly in the abdomen (with an adrenal primary), or in paraspinal sympathetic ganglia, resulting in its variable presentation and extent of disease. Disseminated NBL in a subset of infants with metastatic disease involving the liver, skin, and limited infiltration of the bone marrow can undergo spontaneous differentiation and regression, whereas NBL in older children may demonstrate an aggressive course.[8,9]

NBL remains an enigmatic disease, with its marked heterogeneity serving as a model for both the clinical utility of tumor-specific biologic data for prognostication and as a guide for risk-adapted treatment strategies.[10,11]

The International Neuroblastoma Staging System (INSS) is currently recommended for NBL (Table 45.2), with stage 1–2A disease considered low stage, stage 2B–3 intermediate, and stage 4 advanced.[8]

The Children's Oncology Group (COG) has adopted a classification system based on analysis of patient age at diagnosis, INSS stage, tumor histopathology, DNA index, and *MYCN* amplification status. *MYCN* amplification, found in ~25% of primary tumors, is a marker of aggressive tumor biology in some patients and has been correlated with advanced disease, tumor progression and poor clinical outcome. Near diploid DNA content is highly associated with other adverse prognostic indicators. Patient age under 1 year is an independently favourable prognostic factor for survival.[10]

Completeness of response to dose-intensive induction chemotherapy entailing high-dose cyclophosphamide plus doxorubicin/vincristine and cisplatin/etoposide followed by complete surgical resection in high-risk disease report higher survival rates.[11] Additional survival improvement was seen with adjuvant 13-*cis*-retinoic acid in high-risk patients without progressive disease administered after myeloablative chemotherapy or transplantation.[12]

There are a multitude of postulated new molecular prognostic factors in neuroblastoma. Unbalanced gain of 1–3 additional 17q copies is associated with a more aggressive phenotype. The independent prognostic value of 1p loss of heterozygosity has been controversial.[10]

The Trk family of neurotrophin receptors (NTRK1, NTRK2, NTRK3) are important regulators of survival, growth and differentiation of normal neuronal cells. Retrospective series have demonstrated that high levels of NTRK (TrkA) expression are associated with a favourable outcome.[13] In contrast, coexpression of full-length NTRK2 (TrkB) and its ligand brain derived neurotrophic factor (BDNF) is highly associated with *MYCN* amplification. The potential future application of Trk overexpression may be as a therapeutic target utilizing small-molecule inhibitors of Trk tyrosine kinase activity.[10] Telomerase activity has been associated with advanced stage, *MYCN* amplification or 1p deletion, and adverse outcome.[14]

Other genes proposed to play a role in NBL biology include those related to multidrug resistance phenotype (MDR1 and MRP gene family), genes related to invasion and metastasis (nm23 and CD44). Allelic loss at multiple other chromosomal loci have been reported including 4p, 9p, 11q, 14q, and 19q.[10,15]

EWING'S SARCOMA

Ewing's sarcoma typically arises in bone, although commonly has a significant soft tissue component and may occur in an entirely "extra-osseous" location.[16] Stage of disease is the major predictor of outcome.[16–20] Among those with metastatic disease, those with bone marrow involvement have a worse prognosis than those with lung metastases. Histologic evidence of extensive tumor necrosis after chemotherapy is associated with favorable outcome.[19] Pelvic primary site has been found to be an adverse prognostic factor in some studies, while distal extremity sites are associated with better outcomes. This likely relates to tumor size and the ability to provide definitive local therapy (complete resection or high-dose radiation therapy), rather than anatomic site *per se*.

Young patients have better event-free survival. Other host-related adverse prognostic factors include the presence of anemia and fever, and elevated LDH.[19] Expression of certain abnormal gene fusion products are emerging as potential prognostic factors.[21]

RHABDOMYOSARCOMA

Rhabdomyosarcoma (RMS) represents 5–8% of pediatric cancers. In North America, the clinical grouping system developed by the Intergroup Rhabdomyosarcoma Study (IRS) is associated with prognosis, and is used to assign treatment on the basis of degree of primary tumor and nodal spread and extent of resection. A TNM-based (see Glossary) pretreatment staging system is also prognostic. Additional tumor factors related to prognosis include tumor site (orbit and non-bladder/prostate favorable; parameningeal and extremity sites unfavorable), bone erosion among those with parameningeal tumors, and histology.[22–25] The most common histologies of RMS are embryonal and alveolar; the latter is associated with more advanced stage at presentation, worse local control, higher relapse rate, and worse survival.[26]

Approximately 60% of alveolar RMS will have a t(2;13) translocation, and 15% will have a t(1;13) translocation. Currently, the major role of these translocations is to aid in the identification of alveolar RMS, and thereby guide appropriate treatment. Their value as an independent predictor of survival is under investigation, but expression of gene fusion products may have prognostic value for some patients with alveolar RMS.[27]

The major patient-related factor associated with prognosis is age, with patients older than 10 years faring worse than younger patients.

PROGNOSTIC FACTORS IN WILMS' TUMOR

Wilms' tumor is the most common renal tumor of childhood. The majority of known prognostic factors have been identified by analyses of large cooperative group trials. Histology is the most important prognostic factor: diffuse anaplastic histology and clear cell sarcoma of the kidney are associated with higher rates of relapse and worse survival than favorable histology Wilms' tumors.[28,29] Elements of the staging system developed by the National Wilms' Tumor Study Group (NWTS) include resection margin status, invasion of the renal sinus, penetration of the renal capsule, tumor spill, lymph node involvement, metastases, and the presence of bilateral renal tumors.[28,30]

Children under age 2 years were found to have a better prognosis than older children in NWTS-I. Several congenital syndromes (Beckwith–Wiedeman syndrome, Denys-Drash, and WAGR) are also associated with the risk of developing bilateral Wilms' tumors.[29]

TABLE 45.3   Clinical Grouping Used in IRS I-III

Clinical Group	Extent of Disease and Surgical Result
I	A. Localized tumor, confined to site of origin completely resected
	B. Localized tumor, infiltrating beyond site of origin, completely resected
II	A. Localized tumor, gross total resection, microscopic residual disease
	B. Locally extensive tumor (spread to regional lymph nodes), completely resected
	C. Extensive tumor (spread to nodes) gross total resection, microscopic residual
III	A. Localized or locally extensive tumor, gross residual after biopsy
	B. Localized or locally extensive tumor, gross residual after major resection (>50% debulking)
IV	Any size tumor with or without nodal involvement with distant metastases

TABLE 45.4   Staging System for Wilms' Tumor from National Wilms' Tumor Study Group

Stage I	Tumor limited to the kidney, completely excised. Renal capsule has an intact outer surface. Tumor not ruptured or sampled for biopsy prior to removal (fine needle aspiration excluded). Vessels of renal sinus are not involved. No evidence of tumor at or beyond the margins of resection.
Stage II	Tumor extended beyond kidney, but was completely excised. Regional extension, such as penetration of renal capsule or extensive invasion of renal sinus; blood vessels outside renal parenchyma including vessels of renal sinus, may contain tumor; biopsy performed prior to resection, excluding fine needle aspiration; spillage before or during surgery that was confined to the flank and did not involve the peritoneal surface. No evidence of tumor at or beyond the margins of resection.
Stage III	Residual nonhematogenous tumor is present, confined to the abdomen. Any of the following: a. Lymph nodes within the abdomen or pelvis involved by tumor; intrathoracic or other extra-abdominal lymph nodes are considered Stage IV. b. Tumor penetrated peritoneal surface. c. Tumor implants found on peritoneal surface. d. Gross or microscopic tumor remains postoperatively. e. Tumor not completely resectable because of local infiltration into vital structures. f. Tumor spillage not confined to the flank before or during surgery.
Stage IV	Hematogenous metastases (lung, liver, bone, brain, etc) or lymph-node metastases outside the abdominopelvic region.
Stage V	Bilateral renal involvement is present at diagnosis. Each side should be staged individually.

■■■■■■ SUMMARY TABLES

Prognostic Factors in Pediatric Central Nervous System Tumors

Prognostic Factors	Tumor Related	Host Related	Environment Related
Essential	Metastasis Tumor location		Extent of resection (medulloblastoma, ependymoma, high-grade glioma, choroid plexus tumors)
Additional	Duration of presenting symptoms (ependymoma, brainstem tumors, spinal cord astrocytoma) Histologic type (medulloblastoma, ependymoma)	Age (<3 years), which may influence the use of radiation	
New and promising	Overexpression of p53 (high-grade glioma) Trk-C and Erb-B2 expression, c-Myc expression, genomic profiling (medulloblastoma)		Quality control of radiation[7]

Sources:
• National Cancer Institute: Childhood Brain Tumors (PDQ®): Treatment Guidelines U.S. National Institutes of Health July 2005.
http://www.cancer.gov/cancertopics/pdq/pediatrictreatment.
http://www.cancer.gov/cancertopics/pdq/treatment/childmedulloblastoma/healthprofessional/.

Prognostic Factors in Neuroblastoma

Prognostic Factors	Tumor Related	Host Related	Environment Related
Essential	INSS stage MYCN amplification Shimada (histopathology) DNA ploidy (children <2 years)	Age (<1 year favorable)	Treatment by multidisciplinary team with experience in pediatric oncology
Additional			Complete response to induction dose-intensive chemotherapy followed by complete resection (high risk) Myeloablative therapy with autologous bone marrow transplant, 13 *cis*-retinoic acid (high risk)
New and promising	Gain of chromosome 17 LOH chromosome 1p TRK A expression Telomerase activity Allelic loss at multiple chromosomal loci (4p, 9p, 11q, 14q, and 19q) CD44		

Sources:
• National Cancer Institute: Cancer Information Summaries—Pediatric Treatment Childhood Neuroblastoma (PDQ®): Treatment Guidelines U.S. National Institutes of Health July 2005.
http:// www.cancer.gov/cancertopics/pdq/treatment/neuroblastoma/healthprofessional/.

Prognostic Factors in Ewing's Sarcoma

Prognostic Factors	Tumor Related	Host Related	Environment Related
Essential	Stage Size Site of primary Sites of metastases	Age	Treatment by multidisciplinary team with experience in pediatric oncology
Additional	Histologic response to chemotherapy	Elevated LDH Fever Anemia	
New and promising	Type of EWS and FLI1 gene fusion Molecular evidence of micrometastatic marrow involvement		

Sources:
• National Cancer Institute: Cancer Information Summaries—Pediatric Treatment—Ewings Family of Tumors (PDQ®): Treatment Guidelines U.S. National Institutes of Health September 2005. http://www.cancer.gov/cancertopics/pdq/treatment/ewings/healthprofessional/.

Prognostic Factors in Rhabdomyosarcoma

Prognostic Factors	Tumor Related	Host Related	Environment Related
Essential	Histologic type Stage Clinical group Tumor site	Age	Treatment by multidisciplinary team with experience in pediatric oncology
Additional	Tumor size Number of metastatic sites Sites of metastases		
New and promising	t(2;13) and t(1;13)		

Source:
• National Cancer Institute : Cancer Information Summaries—Pediatric Treatment.
• Rhabdomyosarcoma (PDQ®): Treatment Guidelines U.S. National Institutes of Health September 2005. http://www.cancer.gov/cancertopics/pdq/treatment/childrhabdomyosarcoma/healthprofessional/.

Prognostic Factors in Wilms' Tumor

Prognostic Factors	Tumor Related	Host Related	Environment Related
Essential	Stage Histology	Age (<2 favorable)	Treatment by multidisciplinary team with experience in pediatric oncology
Additional	Size Lymphatic vessel invasion	Associated clinical syndromes: Beckwith–Wiedeman Denys–Drash WAGR	
New and promising	Loss of heterozygosity in 16q or 1p DNA index Monosomy 22		

Source:
• National Cancer Institute: Cancer Information Summaries—Pediatric Treatment.
• Wilms' Tumor and Other Childhood Kidney Tumors (PDQ®): Treatment Guidelines U.S. National Institutes of Health August 2005.
http://www.cancer.gov/cancertopics/pdq/treatment/wilms/health professional/.

REFERENCES

1. Gilbertson RJ: Medulloblastoma: signalling a change in treatment. *Lancet Oncol* 5:209–218, 2004.

2. Van Veelen-Vincent ML, Pierre-Kahn A, Kalifa C, et al.: Ependymoma in childhood: prognostic factors, extent of surgery, and adjuvant therapy. *J Neurosurg* 97:827–835, 2002.

3. Desai KI, Nadkarni TD, Muzumdar DP, et al.: Prognostic factors for cerebellar astrocytomas in children: a study of 102 cases. *Pediatr Neurosurg* 35:311–317, 2001.

4. Fernandez C, Figarella-Branger D, Girard N, et al.: Pilocytic astrocytomas in children: prognostic factors—a retrospective study of 80 cases. *Neurosurgery* 53:544–553; discussion 554–545, 2003.

5. Fernandez-Teijeiro A, Betensky RA, Sturla LM, et al.: Combining gene expression profiles and clinical parameters for risk stratification in medulloblastomas. *J Clin Oncol* 15;22:994–998, 2004.

6. Pollack IF, Finkelstein SD, Woods J, et al.: Children's Cancer Group. Expression of p53 and prognosis in children with malignant gliomas. *N Engl J Med* 346:420–427, 2002.

7. Freeman CR, Taylor RE, Kortmann RD, et al.: Radiotherapy for medulloblastoma in children: a perspective on current international clinical research efforts. *Med Pediatr Oncol* 39:99–108, 2002.

8. Brodeur GM, Maris JM: Neuroblastoma in Pizzo PA, Poplack DG (eds.): *Principles and Practice of Pediatric Oncology.* 4th ed. Phildelphia, JB Lippincott, 895–938, 2002.

9. Maris JM: The biologic basis for neuroblastoma heterogeneity and risk stratification. *Curr Opin Pedi* 17:7–13, 2005.

10. Riley RD, Heney D, Jones DR, et al.: A systematic review of molecular and biological tumor markers in Neuroblastoma. *Clin Cancer Res* 10:4–12, 2004.

11. Adkins R, Sawin R, Gerbing W, et al.: Efficacy of complete resection for high-risk neuroblastoma: a children's cancer group study. *J Ped Surg* 39: 931–936 E, 2004.

12. Valteau-Couanet D, Fillipini B, Benhamou E, et al.: Results of induction chemotherapy in children older than 1 year with a stage 4 neuroblastoma treated with the NB 97 French Society of Pediatric Oncology (SFOP) protocol. *J Clin Oncol* 23:532–540, 2005.

13. Shimada H, Nakagawa A, Peters J, et al.: TrkA expression in peripheral neuroblastic tumors: prognostic significance and biological relevance. *Cancer* 101:1873–1881, 2004.

14. Nozaki C, Horibe K, Iwata H, et al.: Prognostic impact of telomerase activity in patients with neuroblastoma. *Inter J Oncol* 17:341–345, 2000.

15. Attiyeh EF, London WB, Mosse YP, Wang Q, Winter C, Khazi D, McGrady PW, Seeger RC, Look AT, Shimada H, Brodeur GM, Cohn SL, Matthay KK, Maris JM: Children's Oncology Group. Related Articles, Links Chromosome 1p and 11q deletions and outcome in neuroblastoma. *N Engl J Med* 353:2243–2253, 2005.

16. Carvajal R, Meyers P: Ewing's Sarcoma and Primitive Neuroectodermal Family of Tumors. *Hematol Oncol Clin N Am* 19:501–525, 2005.

17. Cotterill SJ, Ahrens S, et al.: Prognostic factors in Ewing's tumor of bone: analysis of 975 patients from the European Intergroup Cooperative Ewing's Sarcoma Study Group. *J Clin Oncol* 18:3108–3114, 2000.

18. Rodriguez-Galindo C, Spunt SL, et al.: Treatment of Ewing sarcoma family of tumors: current status and outlook for the future. *Med Pediatr Oncol* 40:276–287, 2003.

19. Bacci G, Ferrari S, et al.: Prognostic factors in non-metastatic Ewing's sarcoma of bone treated with adjuvant chemotherapy: analysis of 359 patients at the Istituto Ortopedico Rizzoli. *J Clin Oncol* 18:4–11, 2000.

20. Oberlin O, Deley MC, et al.: Prognostic factors in localized Ewing's tumors and peripheral neuroectodermal tumours: the third study of the French Society of Paediatric Oncology (EW88 study). *Br J Cancer* 85:1646–1654, 2001.

21. Burchill SA: Ewing's sarcoma: diagnostic, prognostic, and therapeutic implications of molecular abnormalities. *J Clin Pathol* 56:96–102, 2003.

22. Crist WM, Anderson JR, Meza JL, et al.: Intergroup rhabdomyosarcoma study-IV: results for patients with nonmetastatic disease. *J Clin Oncol* 19:3091–3102, 2001.

23. Carli M, Colombatti R, et al.: European intergroup studies (MMT4-89 and MMT4-91) on childhood metastatic rhabdomyosarcoma: final results and analysis of prognostic factors. *J Clin Oncol* 22:4787–4794, 2004.

24. Stevens MCG: Treatment for childhood rhabdomyosarcoma: the cost of cure. *Lancet Oncol* 6: 77–84, 2005.

25. Breneman JC, Lyden E, et al.: Prognostic factors and clinical outcomes in children and adolescents with metastatic rhabdomyosarcoma—a report from the Intergroup Rhabdomyosarcoma Study IV. *J Clin Oncol* 21:78–84, 2003.

26. Raney RB, Anderson JR, Barr FG, et al.: Rhabdomyosarcoma and undifferentiated sarcoma in the first two decades of life: a selective review of intergroup rhabdomyosarcoma

study group experience and rationale for Intergroup Rhabdomyosarcoma Study V. *J Pediatr Hematol Oncol* 23:215–220, 2001.

27. Sorensen PH, Lynch JC, et al.: PAX3-FKHR and PAX7-FKHR gene fusions are prognostic indicators in alveolar rhabdomyosarcoma: a report from the children's oncology group. *J Clin Oncol* 20:2672–2679, 2002.

28. Wu HY, Snyder HM 3rd, D'Angio GJ: Wilms' tumor management. *Curr Opin Urol* 15:273–276, 2005.

29. Rump P, Zeegers MP, van Essen AJ: Tumor risk in Beckwith-Wiedemann syndrome: A review and meta-analysis. *Am J Med Genet A* 136:95–104, 2005.

30. Kalapurakal JA, Dome JS, et al.: Management of Wilms' tumor: current practice and future goals. *Lancet Oncol* 5: 37, 2004.

The process of rendering prognosis is an essential part of the practice of medicine, and it is especially important in cancer, a disease associated with an overwhelming fear of death. With progress in treatment of cancer, attention has shifted away from prognosis to diagnosis and treatment. Indeed, none of the major cancer textbooks devote space to the formal consideration of the study of prognosis. This book has been written to continue to fill the gap in this area and to place some order on the field of prognosis in cancer.

The second edition of the *Prognostic Factors in Cancer*[1] presented a framework for considering prognostic factors as an activity of medical practice, within a concept of a management scenario. As previously, the third edition of *Prognostic Factors in Cancer* contains two parts. Part I considers the principles for studying prognosis, and for reflecting upon and deliberating about prognostic factors in cancer. Just as the TNM classification allows an orderly consideration and coding of the anatomic extent of disease, the prognostic factor classification provides a similar framework for prognostic factors. The management scenario, which includes the tumor, host, and environment prognostic factors at a specific point in time, is used to project outcome in the context of a planned intervention. Several concepts and classifications are empasized. The subject-based classification of prognostic factors (tumor, host, environment) allows for the inclusion of all attributes, while the relevance-based classification (essential, additional, new and promising) focuses the reader's attention on the current use of prognostic factor information. The former provides the capacity for including all the important factors, while the latter focuses on the application of prognostic factors in everyday practice.

While we do not expect the subject-based classification to change with time, it is expected that the relevance-based classification will change with the introduction of new treatments and with discovery of new factors. Progress in technology has fueled a veritable "prognostic factor industry" that is expected to fill the literature with the flurry of new attributes.[2] The literature is crowded with studies of prognostic factors in cancer that suffer from methodological weaknesses. The most common problems include failure to formulate hypotheses, failure to provide adequate sample size or adequate follow-up with a sufficient number of events, inappropriate multiple significance

Prognostic Factors in Cancer, Third Edition, edited by Mary K. Gospodarowicz, Brian O'Sullivan, and Leslie H. Sobin.
Copyright © 2006 John Wiley & Sons, Inc.

testing, overfitting the model, and failure to verify prognostic factors with an independent data set. We attempt to highlight the importance of proper methodology of studying prognostic factors. In view of the importance of prognosis in the practice of oncology, we consider it relevant to describe the issues surrounding the measurement of the accuracy of prognosis.

To write Part B of the book, Prognostic Factors in Specific Cancers, we invited an international group of experts to outline the prognostic factors for specific cancers using the classifications and format described in Part A Chapter 2. The authors comprise a diverse group of experts representing both many countries and many professional disciplines dealing with cancer patients including pathologists, surgeons, radiation and medical oncologists, epidemiologists, and biostatisticians from different countries. Moreover, $\sim$30% of the authors are new to this third edition, thereby adding new perspective to the discussion of prognostic factors. This diversity is by design and reflects the international mandate of the UICC.

In this edition, we have attempted to a certain extent to reduce the considerable heterogeneity in the approach to prognostic factors for the specific cancers contained in Part B. The remaining variability reflects the state of the art in this area. We have restructured the chapters so that they present a very concise management overview for the specified cancer, any current management controversies, as well as a discussion of relevant prognostic factors.

Most authors of disease-specific chapters have concentrated on factors that effect prognosis in the newly diagnosed cancer patient. However, the proposed framework for prognostic factors viewed in the context of a management scenario does not have to be restricted to only the initial presentation. It may equally be applied at the time of recurrence, or at any time in the course of the disease. The authors have also focused on prognostic factors for overall survival. The proposed framework is applicable to any management scenario with any endpoint, as long as both are defined. The authors gave most attention to *tumor* related factors, as they are most commonly studied and described in the literature. The *host* and *environment* related factors are much less frequently considered and only limited data are available to substantiate their importance. In spite of this, environmental factors have a profound impact on the outcome of cancer patients. Furthermore, in many instances, no new knowledge is required to influence these factors and improve the results of cancer. Progress in cancer biology, biochemistry, and genetics opened the door to the study of new targets for prognostic factor study. Although thousands of papers are published each year dealing with the immunohistochemical factors, proliferation markers, apoptosis and other factors, the clinical relevance of the newer prognostic factors still awaits confirmation. While there is now more information about the molecular prognostic factors, few of them were assigned to the essential category. In fact, the time honored and well-tested factors, such as anatomic extent of disease, and tumor type, and application of appropriate treatment intervention are consistently considered essential in today's clinical practice.

This edition of *Prognostic Factors in Cancer* further develops the framework for handling prognostic factors in the context of a management scenario. What is the future of prognostic factor study and their application in clinical practice? With the advent of the DNA microarray methodology, many new molecular prognostic factors are expected to arrive in the next few years. New and improved computational and statistical methods are required to handle the enormous amount of information and to test the clinical relevance of these putative prognostic factors. With progress in computer science, handling of large amounts of data is already possible. Besides the progress in computing and data analysis, standardization of terminology is urgently needed. The field of medical informatics deals with data recording, storage retrieval, and analysis. Further development of a medical lexicon is needed to ascertain a uniform and unambiguous use of terms being computed and represent one of the challenges faced by the discipline of medical informatics.[3] Implementation of better standards for the presentation of the results of prognostic factors research in peer-reviewed journals would assist in improving the understanding of the subject. A more difficult venture is the development of the standards for application of prognostic factors to clinical practice, cancer research, and cancer control programs.

M. K. Gospodarowicz, *Toronto, Canada*
B. O'Sullivan, *Toronto, Canada*
L. H. Sobin, *Washington, DC*

REFERENCES

1. *Prognostic Factors in Cancer* (2nd ed). New York, Wiley-Liss, 2001.
2. Hall PA, Going JJ: Predicting the future: a critical appraisal of cancer prognosis studies. *Histopathology* 35:489–494, 1999.
3. Coiera E: Medical informatics. *BMJ* 310:1381–1387, 1995.

Accuracy   The closeness of a measurement or judgment to the true value of the quantity of interest.

Additional prognostic factor   An attribute that allows refinements in predicting outcome, although they are not currently used in a decision making process (e.g., do not alter treatment).

Adjuvant therapy   Treatment given following the primary treatment to enhance the effectiveness of the primary treatment. Adjuvant therapy may be chemotherapy, radiation therapy, or hormone therapy.

Ageism   Prejudice or discrimination against a particular age-group and especially the elderly.

Biomarkers   Substances sometimes found in an increased amount in the blood, other body fluids, or tissues, and that may suggest the presence of some types of cancer. Biomarkers include CA 125 (ovarian cancer), CA 15-3 (breast cancer), CEA (ovarian, lung, breast, pancreas, and GI tract cancers), and PSA (prostate cancer); also called tumor markers.

Calibration   Determination, by measurement or comparison with a standard, of the correct value of each scale reading on a meter or other measuring instrument; or determination of the settings of a control device that correspond to particular values of voltage, current, frequency, or other output.

Clinical decision making   The process of making a selective intellectual judgment when presented with several complex alternatives consisting of several variables, and usually defining a course of action or an idea.

Clinical practice guidelines   Systematically developed statements designed to help practitioners and patients make decisions about appropriate healthcare for specific circumstances.

Clinical significance   A matter of judgment taking into account the clinical importance and applicability of the results, measured in terms of a clinical or biological outcome; unrelated to statistical significance.

Combined modality therapy Two or more types of treatments used to supplement each other. For example, surgery, radiation, chemotherapy, hormonal, or immunotherapy may be used alternatively or together for maximum effectiveness.

Confidence interval A measure of the precision of an estimated value. The interval represents the range of values, consistent with the data, that is believed to encompass the "true" value with high probability (usually 95%).

Cox regression model A multivariable regression model for describing how the time to an event of interest (e.g., death) depends on values of several predictor variables. The strength of effect for each variable is expressed as a hazard ratio.

DNA arrays Matrix of a large number of known DNA molecules (or parts of molecules) attached to an inert substrate. Such matrices can be hybridized with unknown mixtures of mRNAs or DNAs to identify which genes are being expressed or are the subject of genomic imbalance in the cells from which the mixtures were derived.

Discrimination The extent to which a test or judgment distinguishes between two states or items.

Ellipsis Omission; a figure of syntax, by which one or more words, which are obviously understood, are omitted.

Endpoint A category of data used to compare the outcome in different arms of a clinical trial. Common endpoints are severe toxicity, disease progression, or fall in such surrogate markers as PSA level, or death.

Environment The aggregate of social and cultural conditions that influence the life of an individual or community; the sum of all external conditions affecting the life, development, and survival of an organism.

Environment-related prognostic factor A factor that operates external to the patient and affect the prognosis; examples include socioeconomic status, treatment, quality of care, healthcare system, and so on.

Error The difference between the approximate result and the true result; used particularly in the rule of double position.

Error analysis The study of the observed discrepancies between the data and the values predicted by a model, often aimed at checking assumptions and diagnosing faults in the model.

Errors of measurement The part of the variation in the distribution of items that is due to faulty measurement instruments, observation errors, and other human factors.

Essential prognostic factor A factor that is fundamental to decisions about the goals and choice of treatment including details of selection of treatment modality, and specific interventions (e.g., anatomic extent of tumor; must be prescribed by published evidence or consensus-based clinical practice guidelines under conditions where access to best standard of care is available).

Event Something that happens; an occurrence.

Evidence-based practice Is the conscientious, explicit, and judicious use of current best evidence in making decisions about the care of individual patients.

Frequency   Number of occurrences in a given class (e.g., percentage of cancers that are lymphomas).

Hazard ratio   The ratio of the rates at which people in two groups have a specified event.

Health services accessibility   The degree to which individuals are inhibited or facilitated in their ability to gain entry to, and to receive care and services from, the healthcare system. Factors influencing this ability include geographic, architectural, transportational, and final considerations, amongst others.

Health services research   The integration of epidemiologic, sociological, economic, and other analytic sciences in the study of health services. Health services research is usually concerned with relationships between need, demand, supply, use, and outcome of health services. The aim of the research is evaluation, particularly in terms of structure, process, output, and outcome.

Host-related prognostic factor   Inherent characteristics, such as age, gender, and racial origin, and other factors, such as performance status, comorbid conditions, and immune status that affect the prognosis, but are not related to the presence of tumor.

Incidence   Rate, range, or amount of occurrence or influence (e.g., number of new cases of cancer occurring in 100,000 people of a defined population per year).

Independent prognostic factors   See statistical independence. Not dependent on another quantity in respect to value or rate of variation; said of quantities or functions.

Independent variable   The terms *dependent* and *independent* variable apply mostly to experimental research where some variables are manipulated, and in this sense they are "independent" from the initial reaction patterns, features, intentions, and so on of the subjects.

Management scenario   Comprises the setting for the host with a set of prognostic attributes existing at the time, in a given environment. The prognosis associated with a scenario is influenced by the history of prior events, the choice of planned intervention and the outcome of interest. A scenario is a chapter in the history of the disease. It is characterized by the date of diagnosis of the disease for the first time or the date of a recurrence for a subsequent scenario and ends with elimination of disease for an appropriate period of time for that disease or until last follow-up. A new scenario normally exists when disease recurrence manifests, but persisting disease at the same site would, in contrast, comprise continuation of the same scenario.

Meta-analysis   A quantitative method of combining the results of independent studies (usually drawn from the published literature) and synthesizing summaries and conclusions that may be used to evaluate therapeutic effectiveness or to plan new studies.

Milieu   The physical or social setting in which something occurs or develops.

Molecular prognostic factor   A substance, usually a protein, that controls tumor growth and spread, and may predict for the presence of occult metastatic spread, virulence of the cancer, or the response to specific therapies (e.g., Ki67). Molecular factors may also be themselves the targets for newer forms of therapy.

Multivariate analysis Statistical analysis (often multiple regression) in which the associations between several variables and a particular outcome are examined simultaneously (e.g., time to recurrence in relation to a tumor marker).

Natural history of disease The course and features of a disease, particularly in the absence of treatment.

New and promising prognostic factor A factor for which currently there is, at best, incomplete evidence of an independent effect on outcome or prognosis.

Oncogene Mutated and/or overexpressed version of a normal gene of animal cells (the proto-oncogene) that in a dominant fashion can release the cell from normal restraints on growth and thus alone or in concert with other changes, convert a cell into a tumor cell.

Outcome Endpoint, something assessed on each patient during or at the end of a study, such as disease recurrence.

Outcome assessment Research aimed at assessing the quality and effectiveness of healthcare as measured by the attainment of a specified end result or outcome. Measures include parameters, such as improved health, lowered morbidity or mortality, and improvement of abnormal states.

p53 A gene that encodes a protein that regulates cell growth and is able to cause potentially cancerous cells to destroy themselves.

p-value In testing, the probability of observing a value of the test as discrepant from the null hypothesis as the one actually observed. Small p-values are taken to be evidence that the null hypothesis should be rejected.

Palliative therapy Treatment given to relieve symptoms caused by advanced cancer. Palliative therapy does not alter the course of a disease, but improves the quality of life.

Pharmacogenomics The application of genomics information and technologies in drug discovery and development so as to identify, on the basis of genetic make-up, those individuals who will respond most favorably to a drug or those who are at risk of serious side-effects. Also describes the use of genetic approaches to identify drug targets linked to a critical disease pathway and to understand the genetic variation in those targets.

Physician Data Query (PDQ) A comprehensive database produced by the National Cancer Institute that provides up-to-date cancer information. The PDQ contains peer-reviewed information summaries on screening, prevention, supportive care, genetics, and treatment of cancer. These summaries are provided in two versions: one written in technical language for healthcare professionals, and a second written in nontechnical language. Editorial boards comprising cancer experts review the current medical literature to develop and update the content of PDQ each month. The PDQ also contains a registry of ∼1800 cancer clinical trials that are open to patients worldwide; and directories of physicians, genetics professionals, and organizations that provide cancer care.

Power The probability that a clinical trial will be able to detect a real difference between two treatments. The power of a study depends strongly on its sample size.

Practice guidelines Directions or principles presenting current or future rules of policy for the healthcare practitioner to assist them in patient care decisions regarding diagnosis, therapy, or related clinical circumstances. The guidelines may be developed by government agencies at any level, institutions, professional societies, governing boards, or by the convening of expert panels. The guidelines form a basis for the evaluation of all aspects of healthcare and delivery.

Precision   The extent to which a measurement is free of random error. Precision reflects the ability to reach the same value each time one measures the same object. It is the reciprocal of variability.

Prediction   Any declaration or estimate regarding the future.

Predictive factor   Any patient or tumor characteristic that is predictive of the patient's response to a specified treatment. Response is usually measured in terms of overall survival, disease free survival, and/or death.

Predictive model   A statistical combination of at least two predictive factors to predict response to a specified treatment.

Probability   The measure of the uncertainty associated with events of unknown outcome. Interpretations of probability include physical properties of phenomena, subjective states of uncertainty, and logical relations between sentences.

Prognosis   The act or art of foretelling the course of a disease. A forecast as to the probable outcome of an attack or disease, the prospect as to recovery from a disease as indicated by the nature and symptoms of the case.

Prognostic factor   A detectable feature of a cancer or patient that can be used to predict the likely outcome of treatment of the cancer. Any patient or tumor characteristic that is predictive of the patient's outcome. Outcome is usually measured in terms of overall survival, disease free survival, and/or death.

Prognostic index   Numerical score indicating risk of an adverse outcome calculated from a prognostic model.

Prognostic model   A statistical combination of at least two separate prognostic variables to predict patient outcome.

Quality assurance (healthcare)   Activities and programs intended to assure or improve the quality of care in either a defined medical setting or a program. The concept includes the assessment or evaluation of the quality of care; identification of problems or shortcomings in the delivery of care; designing activities to overcome these deficiencies; and follow-up monitoring to ensure effectiveness of corrective steps.

Quality of life   A generic concept reflecting concern with the modification and enhancement of life attributes (e.g., physical, political, moral, and social environment).

Quality of healthcare   The levels of excellence that characterize the health service or healthcare provided based on accepted standards of quality.

Random error   A random variable included in a variety of statistical models to summarize discrepancies between the data and the model that are due to unpredictable sources or to sampling variation.

Randomized clinical trial   A study in which participants are assigned by chance to separate groups that compare different treatments. Neither the researcher nor the participant can choose the group. Using chance to assign people means that the groups will be similar and the treatments they receive can be compared. At the time of the trial, there is no way for the researchers to know which of the treatments is best or who may be in control groups.

Rb Tumor suppressor gene encoding a nuclear protein that, if inactivated, enormously raises the chances of development of cancer, classically retinoblastoma, but also other sarcomas and carcinomas.

Recurrence The point when cancer cells from the primary tumor are detected following the primary treatment for the cancer.

Relative risk The ratio of the risk of an event (e.g., death) in two groups of patients.

Risk The probability that an event will occur. It encompasses a variety of measures of the probability of a generally unfavorable outcome.

Risk factor A clearly defined occurrence or characteristic that has been associated with the increased rate of a subsequently occurring disease.

Response to treatment The regression of cancer following treatment, or spontaneously. Usually categorized as complete response or partial response.

> **Complete response** The disappearance of all clinical evidence of disease, confirmed at 4 weeks (as per WHO and RECIST criteria). This does not necessarily mean cure, as microscopic metastases may remain undetected, are likely to regrow and become resistant to treatment.

> **Partial response** A decrease of at least 50% (WHO criteria) or 30% (RECIST criteria) in a study confirmed at 4 weeks.

Resection margins The edges delineating the resected and the remaining tissues following biopsy or surgical excision of a lesion. Normally these are described in relation to whether tumor extends to the resection margin or whether there is a definite layer of normal tissue separating the resection margin from the edge of the tumor within the resected specimen.

ROC curve A graphic means for assessing the ability of a screening test to discriminate between healthy and diseased persons; may also be used in other studies (e.g., distinguishing stimuli responses as to a faint stimuli or nonstimuli).

Receiver-operating-characteristics (ROC) curve A technique for assessing the efficacy of a diagnostic test based on knowledge of the true- and false-positive rates for the test in question.

Scenario See management scenario.

Sensitivity The probability that a diagnostic test will identify those patients who have a given disease or attribute.

Specificity The probability that a negative diagnostic test will correctly identify those patients who do not have a given disease or attribute.

Shared decision making Two way exchange of information with decisions shared between by the doctor and the patient, not only about risks and benefits, but also patient specific characteristics and values.

Statistical independence   The case in which the occurrence of one event does not affect, nor is affected by, the occurrence of another event.

Statistical significance   In hypothesis testing, a description of the situation when the observed p-value is less than a prespecified value, often 0.05. Formally, a statistically significant finding suggests that the null hypotheses of no effect should be rejected.

Stage   The extent to which cancer has spread from its original site. Usually denoted by a number from stage I (least severe) (e.g., small and organ confined), to stage IV (most advanced) (i.e., distant metastasis).

Staging   In cancer: The *grouping* of cases with similar features of anatomic spread and similar prognosis. The TNM system classifies the tumor by its size, site, and spread. The numbers I, II, III, and IV are used to denote the grouping of Ts, Ns, and Ms into stages, and each number refers to a possible combination of TNM factors. For example: a stage I cancer can include both: *T1, N0, M0*, where T1—tumor is small, N0— no regional lymph node metastasis, M0—no distant metastasis and *T2, N0, M0* (a larger localized primary tumor) if their prognoses are similar. It is important to separate the concepts of "staging" as an activity involving investigations and procedures to define the extent of disease versus "staging" as a process to classify and permanently record the stage using the TNM nomenclature.

Supportive care   Treatment given to prevent, control, or relieve complications and side effects and to improve the patient's comfort and quality of life.

Surrogate marker   A measurement that indirectly indicates the effect of treatment on disease state; a prognostic factor that indirectly reflects another prognostic factor, for example, mitotic activity may be a surrogate marker for proliferation as measured by the Ki-67 index.

Systematic error   A sampling error that causes the resulting measurement to be incorrect in a systematic way.

TNM   A system that classifies the anatomic extent of cancer. The letter T refers to the size or extent of spread of the primary tumor; N refers to the presence or absence of tumor in regional lymph nodes, and M to the presence or absence of distant metastases.

Treatment intervention   Planned action in the management of the disease; may involve observation, surgery, chemotherapy, radiation therapy, or a combination of any of the above.

Tumor-related prognostic factor   The characteristics of the tumor, or the effects of the tumor on the host, that affect the prognosis, for example, extent of tumor (TNM) and histologic grade.

Tumor marker   A substance detected (usually in excess) in the body, that indicates the presence of cancer. These markers may be specific for certain types of cancer and are usually detected in tumor tissue or in the blood. Tumor markers include CA 125 (ovarian cancer), CA 15-3 (breast cancer), CEA (ovarian, lung, breast, pancreas, and GI tract cancers), and PSA (prostate cancer).

Tumor registry   A site in which data on cancer patients is recorded.

Tumor suppressor gene   A gene that encodes a product that normally negatively regulates the cell cycle and that must be mutated or otherwise inactivated before a cell can proceed to rapid division.

Univariate analysis   Statistical analysis in which the association between one variable and a particular outcome is examined (e.g., time to recurrence in relation to a tumor marker).

Variable   Items that are measured, controlled, or manipulated, particularly in research.

Prognostic Factors in Cancer, Third Edition, edited by Mary K. Gospodarowicz,
Brian O'Sullivan, and Leslie H. Sobin.
Copyright © 2006 John Wiley & Sons, Inc.